Medical Statistics

Medical Statistics

A Textbook for the Health Sciences

Fifth Edition

Stephen J. Walters
Medical Statistics Group
School of Health and Related Research
University of Sheffield
Sheffield, UK

Michael J. Campbell
Medical Statistics Group
School of Health and Related Research
University of Sheffield
Sheffield, UK

David Machin
Medical Statistics Group
School of Health and Related Research
University of Sheffield
Leicester Cancer Research Centre
University of Leicester
Leicester, UK

WILEY Blackwell

Registered Office(s)
John Wiley & Sons, Inc., 111 River Street, Hoboken, NJ 07030, USA
John Wiley & Sons Ltd, The Atrium, Southern Gate, Chichester, West Sussex, PO19 8SQ, UK

Editorial Office
9600 Garsington Road, Oxford, OX4 2DQ, UK

For details of our global editorial offices, customer services, and more information about Wiley products visit us at www.wiley.com.

Wiley also publishes its books in a variety of electronic formats and by print-on-demand. Some content that appears in standard print versions of this book may not be available in other formats.

Library of Congress Cataloging-in-Publication Data
Names: Campbell, Michael J., 1950- author. | Walters, Stephen John, author.
  | Machin, David, 1939- author.
Title: Medical statistics : a textbook for the health sciences / Stephen J.
  Walters, Michael J. Campbell, David Machin.
Description: Fifth edition. | Hoboken, NJ : Wiley-Blackwell, 2021. |
  Michael J. Campbell's name appears first in earlier editions. | Includes
  bibliographical references and index.
Identifiers: LCCN 2020029691 (print) | LCCN 2020029692 (ebook) | ISBN
  9781119423645 (paperback) | ISBN 9781119423669 (adobe pdf) | ISBN
  9781119423652 (epub)
Subjects: MESH: Biometry–methods | Research Design | Statistics as Topic
Classification: LCC R853.S7 (print) | LCC R853.S7 (ebook) | NLM WA 950 |
  DDC 610.72/7–dc23
LC record available at https://lccn.loc.gov/2020029691
LC ebook record available at https://lccn.loc.gov/2020029692

Cover Design: Wiley
Cover Images: Doctor taking patients blood pressure in examination room, © Hero Images/Getty Images; Cardiogram of heart on paper, © Shevchuk Boris/ Getty Images; Crowded Istiklal street in Istanbul, © Todor Tsvetkov/Getty Images

Set in 9.5/12.5pt STIXTwoText by SPi Global, Pondicherry, India

SKY10078841_070224

Contents

The statistical tables, questions and answers, video links as well as SPSS and CSV versions of the data files from the print book are available for download from the book's web page (www.wiley.com/go/walters/medicalstatistics).

Preface

It is more than 13 years since the last edition of Medical Statistics: A Textbook for the Health Sciences was published and it has proven to be popular. This preface outlines the major changes and updates made since that edition was published.

All the chapters have been revised and updated. With simpler statistical methods it is useful to be able to carry out an analysis for oneself, to help fully understand its usefulness and its limitations. However, with the advent of public domain software for the analysis of data, ever more complex statistical methods are available to the researcher. These advanced methods have been incorporated in many elementary medical statistics syllabuses. A student today needs to understand the application and limitations of these methods to be able to fully evaluate articles in many main stream medical journals. To this end we have introduced new chapters on diagnostic tests, linear modelling, logistic modelling and a further one covering briefly more advanced topics such as random effects modelling and Poisson regression. At all times the emphasis is on understanding why such techniques should be used, their limitations, and how the results of such analyses are to be displayed.

Since the last edition, medical statistics has faced a number of challenges. One of the main ones is the problem of replication. A study is published, with a significant P-value, but another study addressing the same research question fails to replicate this result. This can often cause consternation amongst among readers of research. We discuss this issue in Chapter 18 on Meta-analysis. A related issue is the mis-use of P-values. This has been a major discussion point in the research community and we include this in our coverage of P-values in Chapter 6.

We have found that quizzes within lectures are a useful method of consolidating a student's understanding of a topic. Each chapter contains a new set of multiple-choice questions that can be used to test knowledge for the individual reader, or can be used by a lecturer, perhaps with a polling device to see how many students have understood a particular point.

Stephen J. Walters
Michael J. Campbell
David Machin
July 2020

1 Uses and Abuses of Medical Statistics

Medical Statistics: A Textbook for the Health Sciences, Fifth Edition. Stephen J. Walters, Michael J. Campbell, and David Machin.
© 2021 John Wiley & Sons Ltd. Published 2021 by John Wiley & Sons Ltd.
Companion website: www.wiley.com/go/walters/medicalstatistics

Summary

Statistical analysis features in the majority of papers published in health care journals. Most health care practitioners will need a basic understanding of statistical principles, but not necessarily full details of statistical techniques. Medical statisticians should be consulted early in the planning of a study as they can contribute in a variety of ways and not just once all the data have been collected. Thus, medical statistics can influence good research by improving the design of studies as well as suggesting the optimum analysis of the results and their reporting.

1.1 Introduction

Although some health care practitioners may not carry out medical research, they will definitely be consumers of medical research. Thus, it is incumbent on them to be able to discern good studies from bad, to be able to verify whether the conclusions of a study are valid and to understand the limitations of such studies. The current emphasis on evidence-based medicine (EBM), or more comprehensively evidence-based health care (EBHC), requires that health care practitioners consider critically all evidence about whether a specific treatment works and this requires basic statistical knowledge.

Statistics is not only a discipline in its own right but it is also a fundamental tool for investigation in all biological and medical sciences. As such, any serious investigator in these fields must have a grasp of the basic principles. With modern computer facilities there is little need for familiarity with the technical details of statistical calculations. However, a health care professional should understand when such calculations are valid, when they are not and how they should be interpreted.

The use of statistical methods pervades the medical literature. In a survey of 305 original articles published in three UK journals of general practice: *British Medical Journal* (*General Practice Section*), *British Journal of General Practice* and *Family Practice,* over a one-year period, Rigby et al. (2004) found that 66% used some form of statistical analysis. Another review by Strasak et al. (2007) of 91 original research articles published in *The New England Journal of Medicine (NEJM)* in 2004 (one of the prestigious peer-reviewed medical journals) found an even higher figure with 95% containing inferential statistics, for example, testing hypotheses and deriving estimates. It appears, therefore, that the majority of papers published in these journals require some statistical knowledge for a complete understanding.

1.2 Why Use Statistics?

To students schooled in the 'hard' sciences of physics and chemistry it may be difficult to appreciate the variability of biological data. If one repeatedly puts blue litmus paper into acid solutions it turns red 100% of the time, not most (say 95%) of the time. In contrast, if one gives aspirin to a group of people with headaches, not all of them will experience relief. Penicillin was perhaps one of the few 'miracle' cures where the results were so dramatic that little evaluation was required. Absolute certainty in medicine is rare.

Measurements on human subjects seldom give exactly the same results from one occasion to the next. For example, O'Sullivan et al. (1999), found that the systolic blood pressure (SBP) in normal healthy children has a wide range, with 95% of children having SBPs below 130 mmHg when they were resting, rising to 160 mmHg during the school day, and falling again to below 130 mmHg at night. Furthermore, Hansen et al. (2010) in a study of over 8000 subjects found that increasing variability in blood pressure over 24 hours was a significant and independent predictor of mortality and of cardiovascular and stroke events.

Diagnostic tests are not perfect. Simply because a test for a disease is positive does not mean that the patient necessarily has the disease. Similarly, a negative test does not mean the patient is necessarily disease free. The UK National Health Service invites all women aged 50–70 for breast screening every three years. According to the NHS Breast Screening Information Leaflet (2018, https://assets.publishing.service.gov.uk/government/uploads/system/uploads/attachment_data/file/840343/Breast_screening_helping_you_decide.pdf): if 100 women have breast screening; 96 will have a normal result and 4 will need more tests. Of these, 1 cancer will be confirmed whilst 3 women will have no cancer detected.

One would think that pathologists, at least, would be consistent. However, a review by Elmore et al. (2017) showed that when it came to diagnosing melanotic skin lesions, in only 83% of cases where a lone pathologist made a diagnosis would the same diagnosis be confirmed by an independent panel. In 8% of cases the lone pathologist would give a worse prognosis, and in 9% of cases they would have underestimated the severity of the disease.

This variability is also inherent in responses to biological hazards. Most people now accept that cigarette smoking causes lung cancer and heart disease, and yet nearly everyone can point to an apparently healthy 80-year-old who has smoked for many years without apparent ill effect. Although it is now known from the report of Doll et al. (2004) that about half of all persistent cigarette smokers are killed by their habit, it is usually forgotten that until the 1950s, the cause of the rise in lung cancer deaths was a mystery and commonly associated with general atmospheric pollution from, for example, exhaust fumes of cars. It was not until the carefully designed and statistically analysed case–control and cohort studies of Richard Doll and Austin Bradford Hill and others, that smoking was identified as the true cause. Enstrom et al. (2003) moved the debate on to ask whether or not passive smoking causes lung cancer. This is a more difficult question to answer since the association is weaker. However, studies by Cao et al. (2015) have now shown that it is a major health problem and scientists at the International Agency for Research on Cancer (IARC) have concluded that there is sufficient evidence that second-hand smoke causes lung cancer (IARC 2012). Restrictions on smoking in public places have been one consequence and in England and Wales since 1 October 2015 it has been illegal to smoke in a vehicle carrying anyone under the age of 18.

With such variability, it follows that in any comparison made in a medical context, such as people on different treatments, differences are almost bound to occur. These differences may be due to real effects, random variation or variation in some other factor that may affect an outcome. It is the job of the analyst to decide how much variation should be ascribed to chance or other factors, so that any remaining variation can be assumed to be due to a real effect. This is the art of statistics.

1.3 Statistics is About Common Sense and Good Design

A well-designed study, poorly analysed, can be rescued by a reanalysis but a poorly designed study is beyond the redemption of even sophisticated statistical manipulation. Many experimenters consult the medical statistician only at the end of the study when the data have been collected. They believe that the job of the statistician is simply to analyse the data and, with powerful computers available, even complex studies with many variables can be easily processed. However, analysis is only part of a statistician's job, and calculation of the final 'P-value' a minor one at that!

A far more important task for the medical statistician is to ensure that results are comparable and generalisable.

Example from the Literature – Drinking Coffee and Cancer (IARC 2018)

In 2016, a working group of 23 scientists from 10 countries met at IARC in Lyon, France, to review the research evidence of whether or not drinking coffee is carcinogenic and causes cancer. They reviewed the available data from more than 1000 observational and experimental studies. In rating the evidence, the working group gave the greatest weight to well-conducted studies that controlled satisfactorily for important potential confounders, including tobacco and alcohol consumption. For bladder cancer, they found no consistent evidence of an association with drinking coffee, or of a dose–response relationship, that is drinking more coffee increased the incidence of cancer. In several studies, the relative risks of cancer for those drinking coffee compared to non-drinkers were increased in men but women were either not affected or the risk decreased. IARC (2018) concluded from this that there was no evidence that drinking coffee caused bladder cancer and, as Loomis et al. (2016) stated 'that positive associations reported in some studies could have been due to inadequate control for tobacco smoking, which can be strongly associated with heavy coffee drinking'.

In the above example tobacco and alcohol consumption are examples of confounding variables as illustrated in Figure 1.1. In this example, the individuals exposed or drinking coffee are typified by their tobacco and alcohol consumption, and these same factors are also known to influence cancer incidence rates.

Any observational study that compares populations distinguished by a particular variable (such as a comparison of coffee drinkers and non-coffee drinkers) and ascribes the differences found in other variables (such as bladder cancer rates) to the first variable is open to the charge that the observed differences are in fact due to some other, confounding, variables. Thus, the difference in bladder cancer rates between coffee drinkers and non-drinkers has been ascribed to genetic factors; that is, some factor that makes people want to drink coffee also makes them more susceptible bladder cancer. The difficulty with observational studies is that there is an infinite source of potential confounding variables. An investigator can measure all the variables that seem reasonable to him but a critic can always think of another, unmeasured, variable that just might explain the result. It is only in prospective randomised studies that this logical difficulty is avoided. In randomised trials, where the alternative interventions (the exposure variables) are assigned purely by a chance mechanism, it can be assumed that unmeasured confounding variables are comparable, on average, in the two groups. Unfortunately, in many circumstances it is not possible to randomise

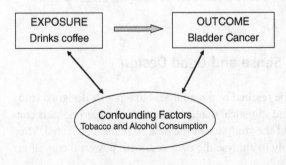

Figure 1.1 Graphical representation of how confounding variables may influence both exposure (drinking coffee) and bladder cancer incidence.

the exposure variable as part of the experimental design, as in the case of drinking coffee and bladder cancer, and so alternative interpretations are always possible. Observational studies are further discussed in Chapter 14.

1.4   How a Statistician Can Help

Statistical ideas relevant to good design and analysis are not easy and we would always advise an investigator to seek the advice of a statistician at an early stage of an investigation. Here are some ways the medical statistician might help.

Sample Size and Power Considerations

One of the commonest questions asked of a consulting statistician is: how large should my study be? If the investigator has a reasonable amount of knowledge as to the likely outcome of a study, and potentially large resources of finance and time, then the statistician has tools available to enable a scientific answer to be made to the question. However, the usual scenario is that the investigator has either a research grant of a limited size, or limited time, or a limited pool of patients. Nevertheless, given certain assumptions the medical statistician is still able to help. For a given number of patients, the probability of obtaining effects of a certain size can be calculated. If the outcome variable is simply success or failure, the statistician will need to know the anticipated percentage of successes in each group so that the difference between them can be judged of potential clinical relevance. If the outcome variable is a quantitative measurement, the statistician will need to know the size of the difference between the two groups, and the expected variability of the measurement. For example, in a survey to see if patients with diabetes have raised blood pressure the medical statistician might say 'with 100 diabetics and 100 healthy subjects in this survey and a possible difference in blood pressure of 5 mmHg, with standard deviation 10 mmHg, you have a 20% chance of obtaining a statistically significant result at the 5% level'. (The term 'statistically significant' will be explained in Chapter 6.) This statement means that one would anticipate that in only one study in five (20%) of the proposed size would a statistically significant result be obtained. The investigator would then have to decide whether it was sensible or ethical to conduct a survey with such a small probability of success. One option would be to increase the size of the survey until success (defined as a statistically significant result if a difference of 5 mmHg or more does truly exist) becomes more probable.

Questionnaires

Rigby et al. (2004), in their survey of original articles in three UK general practice journals, found that the most common design was that of a cross-sectional or questionnaire survey, with approximately one third of the articles classified as such.

For all but the smallest data sets it is desirable to use a computer for statistical analysis. The responses to a questionnaire will need to be easily coded for computer analysis and a medical statistician may be able to help with this. It is important to ask for help at an early stage so that the questionnaire can be piloted and modified before use in a study. Further details on questionnaire design and surveys are given in Chapter 14.

interested in. This is further discussed in Chapter 7. A statistician can advise on the choice of summary statistics, the type of analysis and the presentation of the results.

Medical Statistics and Data Science

Because of the availability of large amounts of data over the last few decades, the term data science has emerged to describe the substantial current intellectual effort around research with the goal of extracting information from these data. The type of data currently available in all sorts of application domains is often massive in size, very heterogeneous and far from being collected under designed or controlled experimental conditions. Nonetheless, it contains information, often substantial information, and it has been argued that data science is a new interdisciplinary approach that makes maximal use of this information. However, data alone is typically not that informative and (machine) learning from data needs conceptual frameworks. Data science would seem to encompass statistics. However, we would argue that statistics is crucial for providing conceptual frameworks that enhance the understanding of fundamental phenomena, highlight limitations and provide a formalism for properly founded data analysis, information extraction and quantification of uncertainty, as well as for the analysis and development of algorithms that carry out these key tasks.

As taught at a number of universities, data science differs from statistics in a number of ways. Statistics originated before the computer and its core concern is with statistical models. However, no serious statistician is beguiled into confusing their model with reality ('All models are wrong, but some are useful' to quote the famous statistician John Tukey). However, models are very useful in describing how the world might be, and for making generalisations beyond the data. Data science is empirical, reliant on large data sets, whereas one of the key successes of statistics is doing inference on relatively small data sets, such as those available in agriculture and laboratories. Data science is often used for prediction, and the idea is that with the vast amounts of data now available electronically (such as that provided by national health services) one can look at empirical relationships and build up accurate predictors, such as how drugs will behave in individuals. These predictions are often highly successful, but lacking models it can be difficult to know why it makes some predictions, and how generalizable the predictions might be. Data science is related to the concept of 'big data'. However, simply because a sample is large does not mean it is unbiased.

A case in point is the reported link between taking hormone replacement therapy (HRT) and *lower* heart disease rates observed in some large data sets. However, a key issue is whether women who use HRT are already more health conscious. It can be difficult to know whether this fact is adequately accounted for in conclusions drawn from the big data. Thus, it was only when the results of the randomised controlled trial of the use of HRT (Writing Group for the Women's Health Initiative Investigators 2002) became available that HRT was shown not to protect against heart disease. In fact, the trial identified an increased risk for total cardiovascular disease with hazard ratio 1.22 and 95% confidence interval 1.09 to 1.36 (the technical terms will be explained in Chapter 11). In this example, big data led to a wrong conclusion.

2   Displaying and Summarising Data

Medical Statistics: A Textbook for the Health Sciences, Fifth Edition. Stephen J. Walters, Michael J. Campbell, and David Machin.
© 2021 John Wiley & Sons Ltd. Published 2021 by John Wiley & Sons Ltd.
Companion website: www.wiley.com/go/walters/medicalstatistics

Summary

This chapter describes different types of data that the reader is likely to encounter. It illustrates methods of summarising and displaying categorical data (bar charts, pie chart). It describes the different ways of summarising continuous data by measures of location or central tendency (mean, median, mode) and measures of spread or variability (range, variance, standard deviation, inter-quartile range). It also illustrates how to display continuous data (dot-plots, histograms, box-and-whisker plots).

2.1 Types of Data

Just as a farmer gathers and processes a crop, a statistician gathers and processes data. For this reason, the logo for the UK Royal Statistical Society is a sheaf of wheat. Like any farmer who knows instinctively the difference between oats, barley, and wheat, a statistician becomes an expert at discerning different types of data. Sections of this book will refer to different data types and so we start by considering these distinctions. Figure 2.1 shows a basic summary of types, although some data do not fit neatly into these categories.

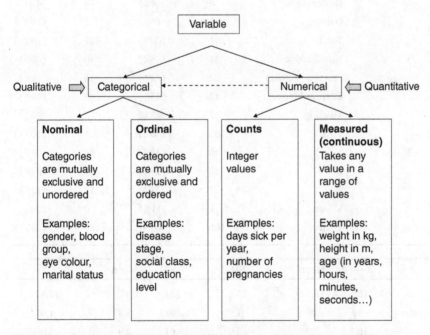

Figure 2.1 Broad classification of the different types of data with examples.

Example from the Literature – Salicylic Acid Plasters for Treatment of Foot Corns

Table 2.1 gives a typical table reporting baseline characteristics of a set of patients entered into a randomised controlled trial that investigated the effectiveness of salicylic acid plasters compared with usual scalpel debridement for treatment of foot corns (Farndon et al. 2013). Corns and calluses are areas of hard, thickened skin that develop when the skin is exposed to excessive pressure or

Table 2.1 Baseline characteristics of participants in a randomised control trial of the effectiveness of salicylic acid plasters compared with 'usual' scalpel debridement of foot corns by treatment group (*Source:* Farndon et al. 2013).

		Group			
		Corn plaster		Scalpel	
		n	%	*n*	%
Gender	Male	42	(42%)	42	(42%)
	Female	59	(58%)	59	(58%)
	Total	101	(100%)	101	(100%)
Centre	Central	58	(58%)	52	(52%)
	Manor	13	(13%)	20	(20%)
	Jordanthorpe	10	(10%)	14	(14%)
	Limbrick	3	(3%)	6	(6%)
	Firth Park	7	(7%)	4	(4%)
	Huddersfield	5	(4%)	4	(4%)
	Darnall	5	(5%)	1	(1%)
	Total	101	(100%)	101	(100%)
Smoking History	Non-Smoker	34	(35%)	40	(40%)
	Previous Smoker	22	(22%)	16	(16%)
	Current Smoker	42	(43%)	43	(43%)
	Missing	3	(3%)	2	(2%)
	Total	101	(100%)	101	(100%)
Number of corns evaluated	1	48	(48%)	66	(65%)
	2	28	(28%)	23	(23%)
	3	24	(24%)	12	(12%)
	Missing	1	(1%)	0	(0%)
	Total	101	(100%)	101	(100%)

	n	Mean	SD	*n*	Mean	SD
Age	101	58.5	15.6	101	59.7	17.5
Size of index corn (mm)	99	3.9	1.7	101	3.8	1.8
VAS pain (0–10)	100	5.7	2.9	101	4.9	3.0

	n	Median	25–75th centile	*n*	Median	25–75th centile
EQ-5D tariff	98	0.73	(0.59–0.80)	101	0.73	(0.66–0.80)
EQ 5D VAS (0–100)	100	80.0	(60.0–90.0)	99	79	(60.0–90.0)

friction. They commonly occur on the feet and can cause pain and discomfort when you walk. We will discuss the different types of data given in this paper.

Categorical or Qualitative Data

Nominal Categorical Data

Nominal or categorical data are data that one can name and put into categories. They are not measured but simply counted. They often consist of unordered 'either-or' type observations that have two categories and are often know as binary. For example: dead or alive; male or female; cured or not cured; pregnant or not pregnant. In Table 2.1 gender is a binary variable. However, categorical data often can have more than two categories, for example: blood group O, A, B, AB, country of origin, ethnic group or social class. The methods of presentation of nominal data are limited in scope. Thus Table 2.1 gives the number and percentage of people treated at each of the seven centres in each of the two randomised groups. Categorical data is sometimes referred to as 'qualitative', to distinguish it from 'quantitative' which we will discuss later. However, there is a whole area of methodology called 'qualitative research' and so to avoid confusion we will not us this term.

Ordinal Data

If there are more than two categories of classification it may be possible to order them in some way. For example, after treatment a patient may be either improved, the same or worse. In Table 2.1 smoking history is given in three categories: non-smoker, previous smoker, and current smoker. Thus, someone who is a current smoker has more recent exposure to tobacco than someone who is an ex-smoker and someone who has never smoked. However, without further knowledge (of the current and past levels of tobacco consumption) it would be wrong to ascribe a numerical quantity to the category, for example, non-smoker = 0; previous smoker = 1; current smoker = 2, as one cannot say that someone who is a current smoker has twice the levels of tobacco consumption as someone who is a previous smoker. This type of data is also known as *ordered categorical* or *ordinal data*.

Ranks

In some studies it may be appropriate to assign ranks. For example, patients with corns may be asked to order their preference for treatment, for example, hard skin (corn) removal by scalpel; special rehydration creams for thickened skin; customised soft padding or foam insoles; corn plaster containing salicylic acid. Here although numerical values from 1 to 4 may be assigned to each treatment we cannot treat them as numerical values. They are in fact only codes for best, second best, third choice, and worst.

Numerical or Quantitative Data

Count Data

Table 2.1 gives details of the number of corns each participant had at the start of the trial, since this can only be a whole number or integer value, for example, 0, 1, 2, or 3 in this trial, this is termed count data. Other examples are often counts per unit of time such as the number of deaths in a hospital per year, or the number of attacks of asthma a person has per month. In dentistry, a common measure is the number of decayed, filled or missing teeth (DFM).

Measured or Numerical Continuous

Such data are measurements that can, in theory at least, take any value within a given range. These data contain the most information, and are the ones most commonly used in statistics. Examples of continuous data in Table 2.1 are age, size of index corn, visual analogue scale (VAS), pain score and EQ-5D tariff.

However, for simplicity, it is often the case in medicine that continuous data are *dichotomised* to make binary data. Thus, diastolic blood pressure, which is continuous, is converted into hypertension (>90 mmHg) and normotension (≤90 mmHg). This clearly leads to a loss of information. There are two main reasons for dichotomising data. It is easier to describe a population by the proportion of people affected, for example, the proportion of people in the population with hypertension is 10%. Further one often has to make a decision: if a person has hypertension, then they will get treatment, and this too is easier if high blood pressure has been categorised.

One can also divide a continuous variable into more than two groups. For example, we could divide age into age bands of equal lengths of, say 10 years such as: 0–9; 10–19; 20–29, etc. When categorising continuous data authors should give an indication as to why they chose these cut-off points, and a reader has to be very wary to guard against the fact that the cuts may be chosen to make a particular point. Some statisticians have termed the habit of categorising continuous variables as 'dichotomania', which they regard as poor practice since it loses information and assumes a discontinuous relationship that is unlikely in nature.

Interval and Ratio Scales

One can distinguish between *interval* and *ratio* scales. In an *interval* scale, such as body temperature or calendar dates, a difference between two measurements has meaning, but their ratio does not. Consider measuring temperature (in degrees centigrade) then we cannot say that a temperature of 20 °C is twice as hot as a temperature of 10 °C. In a *ratio* scale, however, such as bodyweight, a 10% increase implies the same weight increase whether expressed in kilogrammes or pounds. The crucial difference is that in a ratio scale, the value of zero has real meaning, whereas in an interval scale, the position of zero is arbitrary.

One difficulty with giving ranks to ordered categorical data is that one cannot assume that the scale is interval. Thus, as we have indicated when discussing ordinal data, one cannot assume that risk of a corn healing for a current smoker, relative to a non-smoker, is the same as the risk for a previous smoker relative to a non-smoker. Were Farndon et al. (2013) simply to score the three levels of smoking as 0, 1, 2 in their subsequent analysis, then this would imply in some way the intervals between the levels or scores have equal numerical value.

2.2 Summarising Categorical Data

Binary data are the simplest type of data in which each individual has a label that takes one of two values such as: male or female; corn healed or not healed. A simple summary would be to count the different types of label. However, a raw count is rarely useful. For example, in Table 2.1 there are more non-smokers in the scalpel group (40 out of 99 or 40%) compared to corn plaster group (34 out of 98 or 35%). It is only when this number is expressed as a *proportion* that it becomes useful. Hence the first step to analysing categorical data is to count the number of observations in each category and express them as proportions of the total sample size.

Illustrative Example – Salicylic Acid Plasters for Treatment of Foot Corns

Farndon et al. (2013) reports a randomised controlled trial that investigated the effectiveness of salicylic acid plasters compared with usual scalpel debridement for treatment of foot corns. As we have already mentioned one categorical variable recorded was the centre where each trial participant was treated. Trial participants were treated at one of seven centres and the corresponding categories as displayed in Table 2.2. The first column shows category (treatment centre) names, whilst the second shows the number of individuals in each category together with its percentage contribution to the total. Since the total sample size is more than 100 we have reported the percentages to one decimal place. Table 2.2 clearly shows that the majority (54.5%) of patients were treated at the 'Central' treatment centre.

In addition to tabulating each variable separately, we might be interested in whether the distribution of patients across each centre is the same for each randomised group. Table 2.3 shows the distribution of the number of patients treated at centre by randomised group; in this case it can be said that treatment centre has been *cross-tabulated* with randomised group. Table 2.3 is an example of a *contingency* table with seven rows (representing treatment centre) and two columns

Table 2.2   Treatment centre for 202 patients with corns who were recruited to a randomised control trial of the effectiveness of salicylic acid plasters compared with 'usual' scalpel debridement for the treatment of corns (*Source:* data from Farndon et al. 2013).

Treatment centre	Frequency	Percentage
Central	110	54.5%
Manor	33	16.3%
Jordanthorpe	24	11.9%
Limbrick	9	4.5%
Firth Park	11	5.4%
Huddersfield	9	4.5%
Darnall	6	3.0%
Total	202	100.0

Table 2.3   Cross-tabulation of treatment centre by randomised group for 202 patients with corns who were recruited to a randomised control trial of the effectiveness of salicylic acid plasters compared with 'usual' scalpel debridement for the treatment of corns (*Source:* data from Farndon et al. 2013).

	Randomised group		
	Corn plaster *n* (%)	Scalpel *n* (%)	All *n* (%)
Central	58 (57)	52 (52)	110 (54.5)
Manor	13 (13)	20 (20)	33 (16.3)
Jordanthorpe	10 (10)	14 (14)	24 (11.9)
Limbrick	3 (3)	6 (6)	9 (4.5)
Firth Park	7 (7)	4 (4)	11 (5.4)
Huddersfield	5 (5)	4 (4)	9 (4.5)
Darnall	5 (5)	1 (1)	6 (3.0)
Total	101 (100)	101 (100)	202 (100)

Choice of Sample and of Control Subjects

The question of whether one has a representative sample is a typical problem faced by statisticians. For example, it used to be believed that migraine was associated with intelligence, perhaps on the grounds that people who used their brains were more likely to get headaches, but a subsequent population study failed to reveal any social class gradient and, by implication, any association with intelligence. The fallacy arose, perhaps, because intelligent people were more likely than the less intelligent to consult their physician about migraine.

In many studies an investigator will wish to compare patients suffering from a certain disease with healthy (control) subjects. The choice of the appropriate control population is crucial to a correct interpretation of the results. This is discussed further in Chapter 14.

Design of Study

It has been emphasised that design deserves as much consideration as analysis, and a statistician can provide advice on design. In a clinical trial, for example, what is known as a double-blind randomised design is nearly always preferable (see Chapter 15), but not always achievable. If the treatment is an intervention, such as a surgical procedure, it might be impossible to prevent individuals knowing which treatment they are receiving but it should be possible to shield their assessors from knowing. We also discuss methods of randomisation and other design issues in Chapter 15.

Laboratory Experiments

Medical investigators often appreciate the effect that biological variation has in patients, but overlook or underestimate its presence in the laboratory. In dose–response studies, for example, it is important to assign treatment at random, whether the experimental units are humans, animals or test tubes. A statistician can also advise on quality control of routine laboratory measurements and the measurement of within- and between-observer variation.

Displaying Data

A well-chosen figure or graph can summarise the results of a study very concisely. A statistician can help by advising on the best methods of displaying data. For example, when plotting histograms, choice of the group interval can affect the shape of the plotted distribution; with too wide an interval important features of the data will be obscured; too narrow an interval and random variation in the data may distract attention from the shape of the underlying distribution. Advice on displaying data is given in Chapter 2.

Choice of Summary Statistics and Statistical Analysis

The summary statistics used and the analysis undertaken must reflect the basic design of the study and the nature of the data. In some situations, for example, a median is a better measure of location than a mean. (These terms are defined in Chapter 2.) In a matched study, it is important to produce an estimate of the difference between matched pairs, and an estimate of the reliability of that difference. For example, in a study to examine blood pressure measured in a seated patient compared with that measured when he or she is lying down, it is insufficient simply to report statistics for seated and lying positions separately. The important statistic is the change in blood pressure as the patient changes position and it is the mean and variability of this difference that we are (randomised group). Note that we are interested in the distribution of patients across the seven centres in each randomised group (to see whether or not we have similar numbers of patients randomised to each treatment within each centre), and so the percentages add to 100 down each column, rather than across the rows. In this example since we have 101 and 101 patients in each randomised group the percentages are almost the same as the raw counts. However, for most studies you are unlikely to have exactly 100 participants in each group!

Labelling Binary Outcomes

For binary data it is common to call the outcome 'an event' or 'a non-event'. For example, having your corn healed and resolved after three months of treatment may be an 'event'. We often score an 'event' as 1 and a 'non-event' as 0. These may also be referred to as a 'positive' or 'negative' outcome or 'success' and 'failure'. It is important to realise that these terms are merely labels and the main outcome of interest might be a success in one context and a failure in another. Thus, in a study of a potentially lethal disease the outcome might be death, whereas in a disease that can be cured it might be being alive.

2.3 Displaying Categorical Data

Two methods of displaying categorical data are a *bar chart* or a *pie chart*. Figure 2.2 shows in a bar chart the recruiting centres of 202 patients with foot corns treated in the trial of Farndon et al. (2013). Along the horizontal axis are the different treatment centre categories whilst on the vertical axis is the percentage. Each bar represents the percentage of the total patient population in that

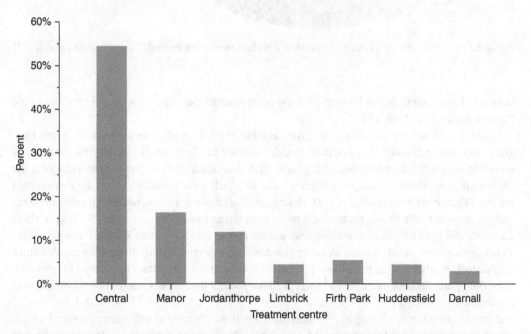

Figure 2.2 Bar chart showing where 202 patients with corns were treated (*Source:* Farndon et al. 2013).

(a)

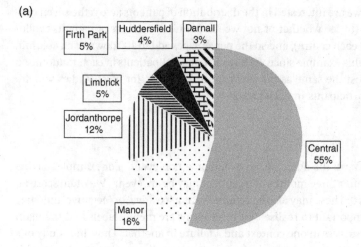

(b)

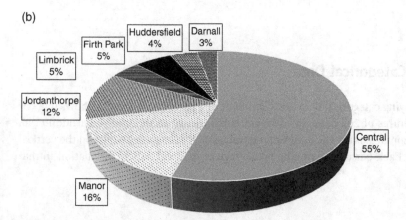

Figure 2.3 Pie chart showing where 202 patients with foot corns were treated (*Source:* Farndon et al. 2013).

category. For example, it can be seen that the percentage of participants who were treated in the Central centre was about 55%.

Figure 2.3a shows the same data displayed as a pie chart. One often sees pie charts in the literature. However, generally they are to be avoided as they can be difficult to interpret, particularly when the number of categories becomes greater than five. In addition, unless the percentages in the individual categories are displayed (as here) it can be much more difficult to estimate them from a pie chart than from a bar chart. For both chart types it is important to include the number of observations on which it is based, particularly when comparing more than one chart. Neither of these charts should be displayed in three dimensions (see Figure 2.3b for a three-dimensional pie chart). Three-dimensional charts feature in many spreadsheet packages, but are not recommended since they distort the information presented. They make it very difficult to extract the correct information from the figure, and, for example in Figure 2.3b the sectors that appear nearer the reader are over emphasised.

If the sample is further classified into whether the patient was treated with corn plasters or scalpel then it becomes impossible to present the data as a single pie or bar chart. We could present the data

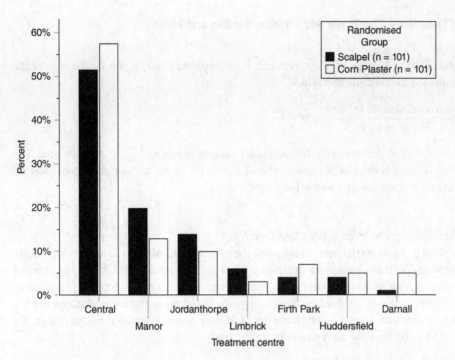

Figure 2.4 Clustered bar chart showing where 202 patients with foot corns were treated by randomised group (*Source:* Farndon et al. 2013).

as two separate pie-charts or bar charts side by side but it is preferably to present the data in one graph with the same scales and axes to make the visual comparisons easier.

In this case we could present the data as a *clustered* bar chart, as shown in Figure 2.4. This clearly shows that the distribution of the frequency of patients at each treatment centre by randomised treatment group is broadly similar. It is preferable to use the relative frequency scale on the vertical axis rather than the actual counts, particularly when the two groups are of different sizes, although in this example where the groups are of similar size this will not make much difference here.

If you do use the relative frequency scale as we have, then it is recommended good practice to report the actual total sample sizes for each group in the legend. In this way, given the total sample size and relative frequency (from the height of the bars) we can work out the actual numbers treated in each centre.

2.4 Summarising Continuous Data

A quantitative measurement contains more information than a categorical one, and so summarising these data is more complex. One chooses summary statistics to condense a large amount of information into a few intelligible numbers, the sort that could be communicated verbally. The two most important pieces of information about a quantitative measurement are 'what is the average value?' and 'what is the spread of the data?' These are categorised as measures of location (sometimes 'central tendency') and measures of spread or variability. A measure of location (average) and variability (spread) provides an informative but brief summary of a set of observations.

Measures of Location – The Three 'Ms' – Mean, Median and Mode

Mean or Average

The arithmetic mean or average of n observations $\bar{x}$ (pronounced x bar) is simply the sum of the observations divided by their number; thus

$$\bar{x} = \frac{\text{Sum of all sample values}}{\text{Size of sample}} = \frac{\sum_{i=1}^{n} x_i}{n}.$$

In the above equation, x_i represents the individual sample values and $\sum_{i=1}^{n} x_i$ their sum. The Greek letter 'Σ' (sigma) is the Greek capital 'S' and stands for 'sum' and simply means 'add up the n observations x_i from the first to the last (nth)'.

Example – Calculation of the Mean – Corn Size Data (mm)

In the randomised controlled trial that investigated the effectiveness of salicylic acid plasters compared with usual scalpel debridement for treatment of foot corns (Farndon et al. 2013), the baseline size of the index corn (at its widest diameter in mm) was measured by an independent podiatrist (foot specialist) who was not involved in the subsequent treatment of the patients. Consider the following 16 baseline corn sizes in mm, listed in ascending order, selected randomly from the 200 patients, with valid baseline corn size data, in the trial.

1, 2, 2, 2, 2, 2, 3, 3, 3, 3, 4, 4, 5, 6, 6, 10

The sum of these 16 observations is

$(1 + 2 + 2 + 2 + 2 + 2 + 3 + 3 + 3 + 3 + 4 + 4 + 5 + 6 + 6 + 10) = 58$.

Thus, the mean $\bar{x} = 58/16 = 3.625$ mm or 3.6 mm. It is usual to quote one more decimal place for the mean than the data recorded.

The major advantage of the mean is that it uses all the data values and is, in a statistical sense, therefore efficient. The mean also characterises some important statistical distributions to be discussed in Chapter 4. The main disadvantage of the mean is that it is vulnerable to what are known as outliers. Outliers are single observations that, if excluded from the calculations, have noticeable influence on the results. For example, if we had entered '100 mm' instead of '10 mm', for the 16th patient, in the calculation of the mean, we would find the mean changed from 3.6 to 9.3 mm. It does not necessarily follow, however, that outliers should be excluded from the final data summary, or that they result from an erroneous measurement.

If the data are binary, that is nominal and are coded 0 or 1, then $\bar{x}$ is the proportion of individuals with value 1, and this can also be expressed as a percentage. In the foot corn plaster trial, the corn had healed or resolved by a three-month follow-up in 52 out of 189 patients. If whether the corn was healed at a three-month post-randomisation follow-up is coded as a '1' for 'yes, healed', and a '0' for 'no, not healed', then the mean of this variable is 0.257 or 25.7%.

Median

The median is estimated by first ordering the data from smallest to largest, and then counting upwards for half the observations. The estimate of the median is either the observation at the centre of the ordering in the case of an odd number of observations, or the simple average of the middle two observations if the total number of observations is even.

Example – Calculation of the Median – Corn Size Data

Consider the following 16 corn sizes in millimetres selected randomly from the Farndon (2013) study. We order the 16 observations from smallest to largest (See Table 2.4); the median is the middle observation which splits the data set into two halves with equal number of observations in each half (eight in this example). As the number if observations are even ($n = 16$); the median is the average of the two central ordered values (the eighth and ninth). So, the median corn size is $(3 + 3)/2 = 3$ mm.

If we had observed an additional 17th subject with a corn size of 10 mm the median would be the 9th ordered observation, which is 3 mm.

The median has the advantage that it is not affected by outliers, so for example the median in the data would be unaffected by replacing largest corn size of '10 mm' with '100 mm'. However, it is not statistically efficient, as it does not make use of all the individual data values.

Mode

A third measure of location is termed the mode. This is the value that occurs most frequently, or, if the data are grouped, the grouping with the highest frequency. It is not used much in statistical analysis, since its value depends on the accuracy with which the data are measured; although it may be useful for categorical data to describe the most frequent category. However, the expression 'bimodal' distribution is used to describe a distribution with two peaks in it. This can be caused by mixing two or more populations together. For example, height might appear to have a bimodal distribution if one had men and women in the study population. Some illnesses may raise a biochemical measure, so in a population containing healthy individuals and those who are ill one might expect a bimodal distribution. However, some illnesses are *defined* by the measure of, say obesity

Table 2.4 The 16 corn sizes ordered and ranked from smallest to largest.

Rank order	Corn size (mm)
1	1
2	2
3	2
4	2
5	2
6	2
7	3
8	3
9	3
10	3
11	4
12	4
13	5
14	6
15	6
16	10

⟸ median (between rank 8 and 9)

or high blood pressure, and in these cases the distributions are usually unimodal with those above a given value regarded as *ill*.

Example – Calculation of the Mode – Corn Size Data
In the 16 patients with corns; 5 patients have a corn size of 2 mm; thus, the modal corn size is 2 mm.

Measures of Dispersion or Variability

We also need a numerical way of summarising the amount of spread or variability in a data set. The three main approaches to quantifying variability are: the range; interquartile range and the standard deviation.

Range
The simplest way to describe the spread of a data set is to quote the minimum (lowest) and maximum (highest) values. The range is given as the smallest and largest observations. For some data it is very useful, because one would want to know these numbers, for example in a sample the age of the youngest and oldest participant. However, if outliers are present it may give a distorted impression of the variability of the data, since only two of the data points are included in making the estimate. Thus, the range is affected by extreme values at each end of the data.

Example – Calculation of the Range – Corn Size Data
The range for the corn size data is 1 to 10 mm or described by a single number $10-1 = 9$ mm.

Quartiles and the Interquartile Range
The quartiles, namely the lower quartile, the median and the upper quartile, divide the data into four equal parts using three cut-points; that is there will be approximately equal numbers of observations in the four sections (and exactly equal if the sample size is divisible by four and the measures are all distinct). The quartiles are calculated in a similar way to the median; first order the data and then count the appropriate number from the bottom. The lower quartile is found by ranking the data and then taking the value below which 25% of the data sit. The upper quartile is the value above which the top 25% of the data points sit. The interquartile range is a useful measure of variability and is the range of values that includes the middle 50% of observations and is given by the difference between the lower and upper quartiles. The interquartile range is not vulnerable to outliers, and whatever the distribution of the data, we know that 50% of them lie within the interquartile range.

Percentiles
The median and quartiles are example of percentiles – points which divide the distribution of the data set into percentages above or below a certain value. A percentile (or a centile) is a measure used in statistics indicating the value below which a given percentage of observations in a group of observations fall. For example, the 20th percentile is the value (or score) below which 20% of the observations may be found. The median is the 50th percentile, the lower quartile is the 25th percentile and the upper quartile is the 75th percentile. With enough data any percentile can be calculated from continuous data.

Example – Calculation of the Range, Quartiles, and Inter-Quartile Range – Corn Size Data

Suppose, as in Table 2.5, we had the 16 corn sizes in millimetres arranged in increasing order (from smallest to largest) from the Farndon et al. (2013) study. The median is the average of the eighth and ninth ordered observations $(3 + 3)/2 = 3$ mm. The first or bottom or lower half of the data has eight observations; so the cut-point for the first or lower quartile is the observation that splits the eight lowest ranked observations into two halves again, that is, four observations in each 'half'. Thus, the lower quartile lies somewhere between the fourth and fifth ordered observations. When the quartile lies between two observations the easiest option is to take the mean of the two observations (although there are more complicated methods). So the lower quartile is $(2 + 2)/2 = 2$ mm.

Similarly, the upper quartile is calculated from the top half of the data (i.e. the observations with the largest values). The second or top or upper half of the data has eight observations; so again the cut-point for the upper quartile is the observation that splits the eight highest ranked observations (ordered observations 9–16 into two halves again, (i.e. four observations in each 'half'). Thus, the upper quartile lies somewhere between the 12th and 13th ordered observations. Since the quartile lies between two observations the easiest option is to take the mean of the two observations. Therefore, the upper quartile is $(4 + 5)/2 = 4.5$ mm. So, the interquartile range (IQR), for the corn size data, is from 2.0 to 4.5 mm; or a single number 2.5 mm.

Standard Deviation and Variance

A third measure of the amount of spread or variability in a data set is the standard deviation. It is based on the idea of averaging the distance each value is away from the sample mean, $\bar{x}$. For an individual with an observed value x_i the distance from the mean is $x_i - \bar{x}$. With n such observations we have a set of n such differences, one for each individual. The sum of these differences, $\sum(x_i - \bar{x})$ is always zero. However, if we square the distances before we sum them we get a positive quantity. This sum is then divided by $(n-1)$ and thus gives an average measure for the deviation from the mean. This quantity is called the *variance* and is defined as:

$$\text{Variance} = \frac{\sum_{i=1}^{n} (x_i - \bar{x})^2}{n - 1}.$$

Table 2.5 Calculating the median, quartiles, and interquartile range for the corn size data.

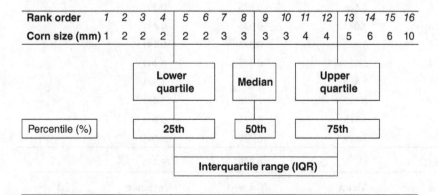

Rank order	1	2	3	4	5	6	7	8	9	10	11	12	13	14	15	16
Corn size (mm)	1	2	2	2	2	2	3	3	3	3	4	4	5	6	6	10

	Lower quartile	Median	Upper quartile
Percentile (%)	25th	50th	75th

Interquartile range (IQR)

The variance is expressed in square units and so is not a suitable measure for describing variability because it is not in the same units as the raw data. The solution is to take the square root of the variance to return to the original units. This gives us the *standard deviation* (usually abbreviated to SD or *s*) defined as:

$$SD = s = \sqrt{\frac{\sum_{i=1}^{n}(x_i - \bar{x})^2}{n-1}}.$$

Examining this expression it can be seen that if all the *x*'s were the same, then they would all equal $\bar{x}$ and so *s* would be zero. If the *x*'s were widely scattered about $\bar{x}$, then *s* would be large. In this way *s* reflects the variability in the data.

Illustrative Example – Calculation of the Standard Deviation – Foot Corn Size
The calculations to work out the standard deviation for the 16 corn sizes are given in Table 2.6.

A convenient method of removing the negative signs is by squaring the deviations, which is given in the next column, which is then summed to get 75.756 mm². Note that the majority of this sum

Table 2.6 Calculation of the variance and standard deviation for 16 subjects from the corn size data.

Subject	Corn size (*mm*)	Mean	Differences from mean	Square of differences from mean
(*i*)	(*x_i*)	($\bar{x}$)	($x_i - \bar{x}$)	($x_i - \bar{x}$)²
1	1	3.625	−2.625	6.891
2	2	3.625	−1.625	2.641
3	2	3.625	−1.625	2.641
4	2	3.625	−1.625	2.641
5	2	3.625	−1.625	2.641
6	2	3.625	−1.625	2.641
7	3	3.625	−0.625	0.391
8	3	3.625	−0.625	0.391
9	3	3.625	−0.625	0.391
10	3	3.625	−0.625	0.391
11	4	3.625	0.375	0.141
12	4	3.625	0.375	0.141
13	5	3.625	1.375	1.891
14	6	3.625	2.375	5.641
15	6	3.625	2.375	5.641
16	10	3.625	6.375	40.641
Total	**58**		**0.000**	**75.756**
	n	Mean	*df = n−1*	Variance	SD
	16	3.625 mm	15	5.050 mm²	2.247 mm

(54%) is contributed by one observation, the value of 10 mm from subject 16, which is the observation furthest from the mean. This illustrates that much of the value of an SD is derived from the outlying observations. (The standard deviation is vulnerable to outliers, so if the 10 was replaced by 100 we would get a very different result.) We now need to find the average squared deviation. Common sense would suggest dividing by n, but it turns out that this actually gives an estimate of the population variance, which is too small. This is because we use the estimated mean $\bar{x}$ in the calculation in place of the true population mean. In fact, we seldom know the population mean so there is little choice but for us to use its estimated value, $\bar{x}$, in the calculation. The consequence is that it is then better to divide by what are known as the *degrees of freedom,* which in this case is $n-1$, to obtain the SD.

Why is the Standard Deviation Useful?

From the corn plaster trial data, the mean and standard deviation of the baseline corn size of the 200 trial patients are 3.8 and 1.8 mm respectively (two baseline sizes were missing). It turns out in many situations that about 95% of observations will be within two standard deviations of the mean. This is known as a *reference interval* or *reference range* and it is this characteristic of the standard deviation which makes it so useful. It holds for a large number of measurements commonly made in medicine. In particular it holds for data that follow a Normal distribution (see Chapter 4).

For example, the Association for Clinical Biochemistry and Laboratory Medicine gives a number of reference ranges in biochemistry such as for serum potassium of 3.5–5.3 mmol l^{-1} (labtestsonline 2019, https://labtestsonline.org.uk/articles/laboratory-test-reference-ranges). This means in a normal, health population we would expect 19 out of 20 people to have serum potassium levels within these limits. For the corn plaster example, we would expect the majority of corns will be sized between $3.8-1.96 \times 1.8$ to $3.8 + 1.96 \times 1.8$ or 0.2 and 7.4 mm. Table 2.7 shows that there are 10 patients out of 200 (or 5%) who have a corn size above 7.4 mm and none below 1 mm; thus 95% of the observations in the data lie with two standard deviations of the mean.

Table 2.7 Frequency distribution the size of the corn, in mm, at baseline for 200 patients with corns who were recruited to a randomised control trial of the effectiveness of salicylic acid plasters compared with 'usual' scalpel debridement for the treatment of corns (*Source:* data from Farndon et al. 2013).

Size of corn at baseline (mm)	Frequency	Percentage	Cumulative percentage
1 to <2	6	3.0	3.0
2 to <3	39	19.5	22.5
3 to <4	52	26.0	48.5
4 to <5	42	21.0	69.5
5 to <6	38	19.0	88.5
6 to <7	10	5.0	93.5
7 to <8	3	1.5	95.0
8 to <9	5	2.5	97.5
9 to <10	1	0.5	98.0
10 to <11	4	2.0	100
Total	**200**	**100**	

As we have noted, standard deviation is often abbreviated to SD in the medical literature. Sometimes for emphasis we will denote it by $SD(x)$, where the bracketed term x is included for a reason to be introduced later.

Means or Medians?

Means and medians convey different impressions of the location of data, and one cannot give a prescription as to which is preferable; often both give useful information. If the distribution is symmetric, then in general the mean is the better summary statistic, and if it is skewed then the median is less influenced by the tails. If the data are skewed, then the median will reflect a 'typical' individual better. For example, if in a country median income is £20 000 and mean income is £24 000, most people will relate better to the former number.

It is sometimes stated, incorrectly, that the mean cannot be used with binary, or ordered categorical data but, as we have noted before, if binary data are scored 0/1 then the mean is simply the proportion of 1s. If the data are ordered categorical, then again the data can be scored, say 1, 2, 3, etc. and a mean calculated. This can often give more useful information than a median for such data, but should be used with care, because of the implicit assumption that the change from score 1 to 2, say, has the same meaning (value) as the change from score 2 to 3, and so on.

2.5 Displaying Continuous Data

A picture is worth a thousand words, or numbers, and there is no better way of getting a 'feel' for the data than to display them in a figure or graph. The general principle should be to convey as much information as possible in the figure, with the constraint that the reader is not overwhelmed by too much detail.

Dot Plots

The simplest method of conveying as much information as possible is to show all of the data and this can be conveniently carried out using a dot plot. It is also useful for showing the distributions in two or more groups side by side.

Example – Dot Plot – Baseline Corn Size

The data on corn size and treatment group (corn plaster or scalpel) are shown in Figure 2.5 as a dot plot. This method of presentation retains the individual subject values and clearly demonstrates any similarities or differences between the groups in a readily appreciated manner. An additional advantage is that any outliers will be detected by such a plot. However, such presentation is not usually practical with large numbers of subjects in each group because the dots will obscure the details of the distribution. Figure 2.5 shows that the two randomised groups had similar distributions of corn sizes at baseline.

Histograms

The patterns may be revealed in large data set of a numerically continuous variable by forming a histogram with them. This is constructed by first dividing up the range of variable into several non-overlapping and equal intervals, classes, or bins, then counting the number of observations in each. A histogram for all the baseline corn sizes in the Farndon et al. (2013) trial data is shown in Figure 2.6. In this histogram the intervals corresponded to a width of 1 mm. The area of each

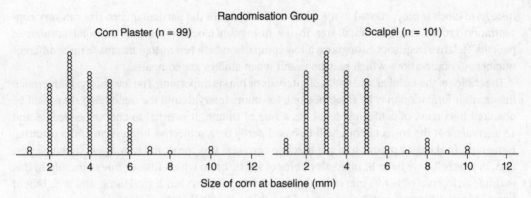

Figure 2.5 Dot plot showing corn size (in mm) by randomised treatment group for 200 patients with corns. (*Source:* data from Farndon et al. 2013).

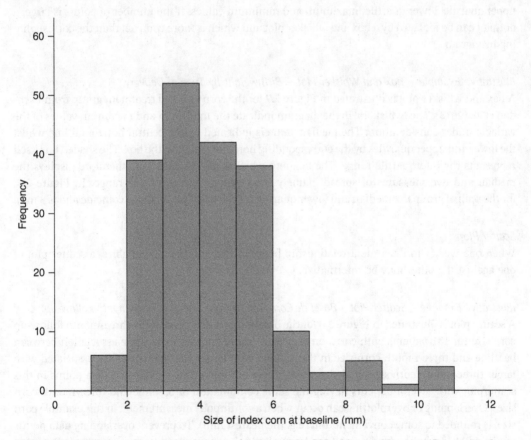

Figure 2.6 Histogram of baseline index corn size (in mm) for 200 patients with corns. (*Source:* data from Farndon et al. 2013).

histogram block is proportional to the number of subjects in the particular corn size category concentration group. Thus, the total area in the histogram blocks represents the total number of patients. Relative frequency histograms allow comparison between histograms made up of different numbers of observations which may be useful when studies are compared.

The choice of the number and width of intervals or bins is important. Too few intervals and much important information may be smoothed out; too many intervals and the underlying shape will be obscured by a mass of confusing detail. As a rule of thumb, it is usual to choose between 5 and 15 intervals, but the correct choice will be based partly on a subjective impression of the resulting histogram. In the corn plaster trial the baseline corn size was measured in integers to the nearest mm. In Figure 2.6 we have 10 intervals or bins of width 1 mm which fits our rule of thumb. In this example an interval of 1–1.99 mm covers bin 1, 2–2.99 mm covers bin 2, etc. Histograms with bins of unequal interval length can be constructed but they are usually best avoided.

Box and Whisker Plot

A box and whisker plot contains five pieces of summary information about the data: the median; upper quartile; lower quartile; maximum and minimum values. If the number of points is large, a dot-plot can be replaced by a box and whisker plot and which is more compact than the corresponding histogram.

Illustrative Example – Box and Whisker Plot – Birthweight by Type of Delivery

A box and whisker plot is illustrated in Figure 2.7 for the corn size and treatment group from Farndon et al. (2013). The 'whiskers' in the diagram indicate the minimum and maximum values of the variable under consideration. The median value is indicated by the central horizontal line whilst the lower and upper quartiles by the corresponding horizontal ends of the box. The shaded box itself represents the interquartile range. The box and whisker plot as used here therefore displays the median and two measures of spread, namely the range and interquartile range. In Figure 2.7, for the scalpel group the median and lower quartile for the baseline corn size coincide and is 3 mm.

Scatter Plots

When one wishes to illustrate a relationship between two continuous variables, a scatter plot of one against the other may be informative.

Illustrative Example – Scatter Plot – Baseline Corn Size by Corn Size at a Three month Follow-up

A scatter plot is illustrated in Figure 2.8 for the baseline corn size against the three-month follow-up corn size for 181 patients with corns on their feet. There appears to be some association between baseline and three-month corn size in this sample with larger baseline corn sizes associated with larger three-month corn sizes and vice versa. There are numerous overlapping data points in this scatterplot with several patients having the same combination of baseline and three-month corn sizes. Overlapping or overplotting can occur when a continuous measurement, in this example corn size, is rounded to some convenient unit (e.g. the nearest mm). To prevent overlapping data points in Figure 2.8, we have added a small random noise to the data called jittering. Jittering is the act of adding random noise to data in order to prevent overplotting in statistical graphs.

It is likely that baseline corn size will have an influence on corn size at three months, but vice versa cannot be the case. In this case, if one variable, x, (baseline corn size) could cause the other, y, (three-month corn size) then it is usual to plot the x variable on the horizontal axis and the y variable on the vertical axis.

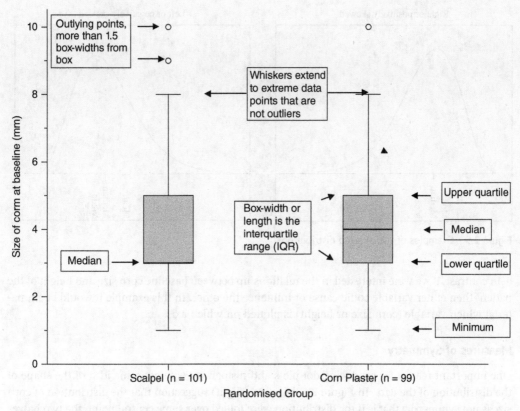

Figure 2.7 Box and whisker plot of size of corn at baseline (in mm) by randomised group for 200 patients with corns. (*Source:* data from Farndon et al. 2013).

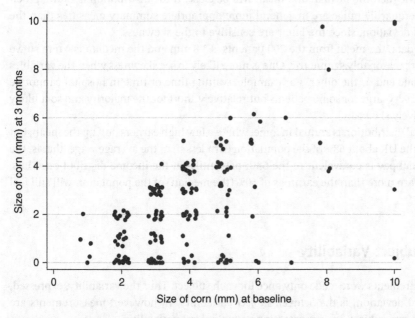

Figure 2.8 Scatter plot of baseline corn size by corn size at a three month follow-up for 181 patients with corns. (*Source:* data from Farndon et al. 2013).

Right or positively skewed

Left or negatively skewed

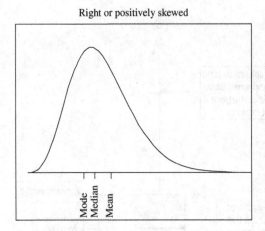 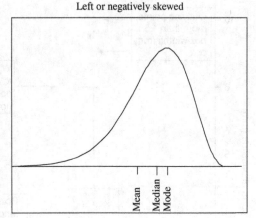

Figure 2.9 Examples of two skewed distributions.

In contrast, if we were interested in the relationship between baseline corn size and height of the patient then either variable could cause or influence the other. In this example it would be immaterial which variable (corn size or height) is plotted on which axis.

Measures of Symmetry

One important reason for producing dot plots and histograms is to get some idea of the shape of the distribution of the data. In Figure 2.6 there is a (slight) suggestion that the distribution of corn size is not symmetric; that is if the distribution were folded over some central point, the two halves of the distribution would not coincide. When this is the case, the distribution is termed *skewed*. A distribution is right (left) skewed if the longer tail is to the right (left), see Figure 2.9. If the distribution is symmetric then the median and mean will be close. If the distribution is skewed then the median and interquartile range are in general more appropriate summary measures than the mean and standard deviation, since the latter are sensitive to the skewness.

For the corn size data, the mean from the 200 patients is 3.8 mm and the median is 4 mm so we conclude the data are reasonably symmetric. One is more likely to see skewness when the variables are constrained at one end or the other. For example, waiting time or time in hospital cannot be negative, but can be very large for some patients but relatively short for the majority and so it likely to be right or positively skewed.

A common skewed distribution is annual income, where a few high earners pull up the mean, but not the median. In the UK about 68% of the population earn less than the average wage, that is, the mean value of annual pay is equivalent to the 68th percentile on the income distribution. Thus, many people who earn more than the earnings of 50% (the median) of the population will still feel under paid!

2.6   Within-Subject Variability

In Figure 2.1, measurements were made only once for each subject. Thus the variability, expressed, say, by the standard deviation, is the *between-subject* variability. If, however, measurements are made repeatedly on one subject, we are assessing *within-subject* variability.

Illustrative Example – Within-Subject Variability – Total Steps per Day

Figure 2.10 shows an example in which the total steps-per-day walked by one subject, assessed by a pedometer worn on the hip, was recorded every day for 100 days. The observed daily total step count is subject to day-to-day fluctuations. There is considerable day-to-day variation in steps but little evidence of any trend over time. Such variation is termed *within-subject variation*. The *within-subject* standard deviation in this case, is SD = 4959 steps with a mean daily step count of 14 107 steps over the 100 days.

If another subject had also completed this experiment, we could calculate their within-subject variation as well, and perhaps compare the variabilities for the two subjects using these summary measures. Thus a second subject had a mean step count of 12 745 with standard deviation of 4861 steps, and so has a smaller mean but similar variability.

Successive within-subject values are unlikely to be independent, that is, consecutive values will be dependent on values preceding them. For example, if a sedentary or inactive person records their step count on one day, then if the step count is low on one day it is likely to be low on the next day. This does not imply that the step count will be low, only that it is a good bet that it will be. In contrast, examples can be found in which high step counts are usually followed by lower values and vice versa. With independent observations, the step count on one day gives no indication or clue as to the step count on the next.

It is clear from Figure 2.10 that the daily step counts are not constant over the observation period. This is nearly always the case when medical observations or measurements are taken over time. Such variation occurs for a variety of reasons. For example, the step count may depend critically on the day of the week, whether the subject was on holiday or at work, whether the subject was on medication or unwell. There may be observer-to-observer variation if the successive step counts were recorded by different personnel rather than always by the same person. There may be measuring device-to-measuring-device variation if the successive step counts were recorded by different pedometers rather than always the same pedometer. The possibility of recording errors in the laboratory, transcription errors when conveying the results to the clinic or for statistical

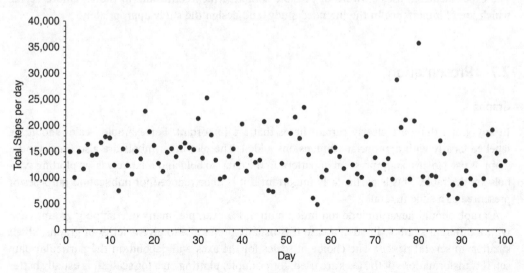

Figure 2.10 Total steps per day for 100 days for one participant in a global corporate challenge designed to increase physical activity.

analysis, should not be overlooked in appropriate circumstances. When only a single observation is made on one patient at one time only, then the influences of the above sources of variation are not assessable, but may nevertheless all be reflected to some extent in the final entry in the patient's record.

Suppose successive observations on a patient with heart disease taken over time fluctuate around some more or less constant daily step count, then the particular level may be influenced by factors within the patient. For example, step counts (and physical activity levels) may be affected by the presence of a viral infection whose presence is unrelated to the cause of the heart disease itself. Levels may also be influenced by the severity of the underlying condition and whether concomitant treatment is necessary for the patient. Levels could also be influenced by other factors, for example, alcohol, tobacco consumption and diet. The cause of some of the variation in step counts may be identified and its effect on the variability estimated. Other variation may have no obvious explanation and is usually termed *random* variation. This does not necessarily imply there is no cause of this component of the variation but rather that its cause has not been identified or is being ignored.

Different patients with heart disease observed in the same way may have differing average levels of step counts (physical activity levels) from each other but with similar patterns of variation about these levels. The variation in mean step count levels from patient to patient is termed *between-subject variation*.

Observations on different subjects are usually regarded as independent. That is, the data values on one subject are not influenced by those obtained from another. This, however, may not always be the case, particularly with subjective measures such as pain or quality of life which may be influenced by the subject's personal judgement, and different patients may assist each other when recording their quality of life.

In the investigation of total variability it is very important to distinguish within-subject from between-subject variability. In a study there may be measures made on different individuals and also repeatedly on the same individual. Between- and within- subject variation will always be present in any biological material, whether animals, healthy subjects, patients, or histological sections. The experimenter must be aware of possible sources which contribute to the variation, decide which are of importance in the intended study, and design the study appropriately.

2.7 Presentation

Graphs

In any graph there are clearly certain items that are important. For example, scales should be labelled clearly with appropriate dimensions added. The plotting symbols are also important; a graph is used to give an impression of pattern in the data, so bold and relatively large plotting symbols are desirable. This is particularly important if it is to be reduced for publication purposes or presented as a slide in a talk.

A graph should never include too much clutter; for example, many overlapping groups each with a different symbol. In such a case it is usually preferable to give a series of graphs, albeit smaller, in several panels. The choice of scales for the axes will depend on the particular data set. If transformations of the axes are used, for example, plotting on a log scale, it is usually better to mark the axes using the original units as this will be more readily understood by the reader.

Breaks in scales should be avoided. If breaks are unavoidable under no circumstances must points on either side of a break be joined. If both axes have the same units, then use the same scale for each. If this cannot be done easily, it is sensible to indicate the line of equality, perhaps faintly in the figure. False impressions of trend, or lack of it, in a time plot can sometimes be introduced by omitting the zero point of the vertical axis. This may falsely make a mild trend, for example a change from 101 to 105, into an apparently strong trend (seemingly as though from 1 to 5). There must always be a compromise between clarity of reproduction that is filling the space available with data points and clarity of message. Appropriate measures of variability should also be included. One such is to indicate the range of values covered by two standard deviations each side of a plotted mean.

It is important to distinguish between a bar chart and a histogram. Bar charts display counts in mutually exclusive categories, and so the bars should have spaces between them. Histograms show the distribution of a continuous variable and so should not have spaces between the bars. It is not acceptable to use a bar-chart to display a mean with standard error bars (see Chapter 6). These should be indicated with a data point surrounded with errors bars, or better still a 95% confidence interval.

With currently available graphics software one can now perform extensive exploration of the data, not only to determine more carefully their structure, but also to find the best means of summary and presentation. This is usually worth considerable effort.

Tables

Although graphical presentation is very desirable it should not be overlooked that tabular methods are very important (see Table 2.3). In particular, tables can give more precise numerical information than a graph, such as the number of observations, the mean and some measure of variability of each tabular entry. They often take less space than a graph containing the same information. Standard statistical computer software can be programmed to provide basic summary statistics in tabular form on many variables.

2.8 Points When Reading the Literature

1) Is the number of subjects involved clearly stated?
2) Are appropriate measures of location and variation used in the paper? For example, if the distribution of the data is skewed, then has the median rather the mean been quoted? Is it sensible to quote a standard deviation, or would a range or interquartile range, be better? In general do *not* use SD for data which have skewed distributions.
3) On graphs, are appropriate axes clearly labelled and scales indicated?
4) Do the titles adequately describe the contents of the tables and graphs?
5) Do the graphs indicate the relevant variability? For example, if the main object of the study is a within-subject comparison, has the within-subject variability been illustrated?
6) Does the method of display convey all the relevant information in a study? Can one assess the distribution of the data from the information given?

2.9 Technical Details

Calculating the Sample Median

If the n observations in a sample are arranged in increasing or decreasing order, the median is the middle value. If there are n observations the median is the $\frac{1}{2}(n + 1)$th ordered value. If the number of observations, n, is *odd* there will be a unique median – the $\frac{1}{2}(n + 1)$th ordered value. If n is *even*, there is strictly no middle observation, but the median is defined by convention as the mean of the two middle observations – the $\frac{1}{2}n$th and $(\frac{1}{2}n + 1)$th.

Calculating the median for the foot corn size data, as the number of observations is even ($n = 16$), the median is the average of the two middle observations – the $\frac{1}{2}(16)$th and $([\frac{1}{2} \times 16] + 1)$th, i.e. the eighth and ninth ordered values. So the median corn size is $(3 + 3)/2 = 3$ mm.

Calculating the Quartiles and Inter Quartile Range

Arrange the n observations in increasing or decreasing order. Split the data set into four equal parts –or *quartiles* using three cut-points:

1) Lower quartile (25th centile) or the $\frac{1}{4}(n + 1)$th ordered value;
2) Median(50th centile) or the $\frac{1}{2}(n + 1)$th ordered value;
3) Upper quartile(75th centile) or the $\frac{3}{4}(n + 1)$th ordered value.

The interquartile range (IQR) is the upper quartile minus the lower quartile.

It should be noted there is not a single standard convention for calculating the quartiles. When the quartile lies between two observations the simplest option is to take the mean of the two observations. A second option is for the lower and upper quartiles to be the $\frac{1}{4}(n + 1)$th and $\frac{3}{4}(n + 1)$th ordered values respectively. A third option is for the lower and upper quartiles to be the $\frac{1}{4}n + \frac{1}{2}$ and $\frac{3}{4}n + \frac{1}{2}$ ordered values respectively. It is also common to round the $\frac{1}{4}$ and $\frac{3}{4}$ to the nearest integer and only use interpolation when this involves calculation of the midpoint of two values. Differences between the results using the different conventions are usually small and unimportant in practice.

To calculate the quartiles for the foot corn size data in Tables 2.4 and 2.5, as the number of observations is even ($n = 16$), the upper quartile is the $\frac{3}{4}(n + 1)$th ordered value or $\frac{3}{4}(17)$th $= 12\frac{3}{4}$ ordered value. When the quartile lies between two observations the easiest option is to take the mean (there are more complicated methods). The upper quartile (*simple method*) is the mean of the 12th and 13th ordered values or $(4 + 5)/2 = 4.5$ mm. *Rounding* the $12\frac{3}{4}$ ordered value to the nearest integer (the 13th ordered value) gives an upper quartile of 5 mm.

A more complicated method for estimating the upper quartile is by *interpolation* between the 12th and 13th ordered values. The interpolation involves moving $\frac{3}{4}$ of the way from the 12th ordered value towards the 13th value, i.e. $4 + \frac{3}{4} (4 \text{ to } 5) = 4.75$ mm (or 4.8 mm when rounding to one decimal place).

The lower quartile is the $\frac{1}{4}(n + 1)$th ordered value or $\frac{1}{4}(17)$th $= 4\frac{1}{4}$ ordered value. The lower quartile (simple method) is the mean of the 4th and 5th ordered values or $(2 + 2)/2 = 2.0$ mm. *Rounding* the $4\frac{1}{4}$ ordered value to the nearest integer (the 4th ordered value) gives a lower quartile of 2 mm. A more complicated method for estimating the lower quartile is by interpolation between the fourth and fifth ordered values. The interpolation involves moving $\frac{1}{4}$ of the way from the fourth ordered value towards the fifth value, i.e. $2 + \frac{1}{4} (2 \text{ to } 2) = 2$ mm (or 2.0 mm when rounding to 1 decimal place). The IQR estimated by the simple method is 2.0 to 4.5 mm vs 2.0 to 5.0 mm (using the rounding to the nearest integer method) vs 2.0 to 4.8 mm using the more complex interpolation method. As we already mentioned the differences between the results using the different conventions for calculating the quartiles are usually small and unimportant in practice.

2.10 Exercises

Figure 2.11 shows the anatomical site of the foot corn by randomised group for 201 patients (Farndon et al. 2013) who were taking part in a randomised controlled trial to investigate the effectiveness of salicylic acid plasters compared with usual scalpel debridement for treatment.

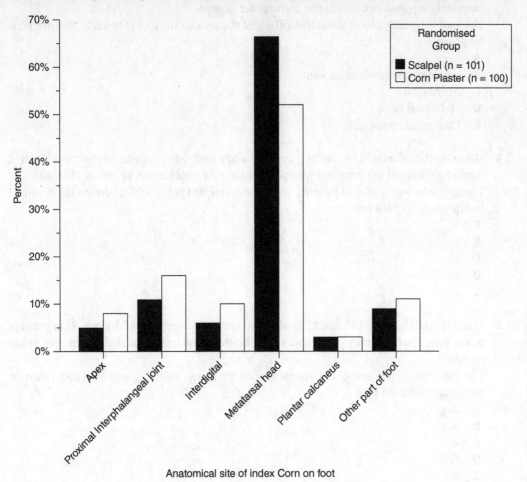

Figure 2.11 Anatomical site of corn on the foot by randomised group for 201 patients with corns (*Source:* Farndon et al. 2013).

2.1 What type of graph is Figure 2.11?
  A Bar chart
  B Pie chart
  C Histogram
  D Scatterplot
  E Dot plot

2.2 What type of data in Figure 2.11 is anatomical site of foot corn?
  A Discrete
  B Nominal

C Binary
D Ordinal
E Continuous

2.3 Using the data shown in Figure 2.11 which anatomical site of the corn on the foot was the *least* frequently reported patients in the corn plaster group?
The least frequently reported anatomical site of the corn on the foot patients in the corn plaster group was:
A Apex
B Proximal interphalangeal joint
C Interdigital
D Metatarsal head
E Plantar calcaneus

2.4 Using the data shown in Figure 2.11, approximately how many patients in the scalpel treated group had corn on the proximal interphalangeal joint (middle part of toe on the top)?
The approximate number of patients in the scalpel treated group with a corn on the proximal interphalangeal joint was:
A 5
B 8
C 11
D 50
E 100

2.5 Using the data shown in Figure 2.11, what approximate percentage of the sample of patients in the corn plaster treated group had a corn on the metatarsal head (ball of the foot at the bottom)?
The approximate percentage of patients in the corn plaster treated group who had a corn on the metatarsal head was:
A 20%
B 30%
C 40%
D 50%
E 60%

The baseline corn size, in mm, of 10 randomly selected patients from the corn plaster randomised controlled trial (RCT) (Farndon et al. 2013) are given below

| 2 | 2 | 2 | 3 | 4 | 4 | 5 | 5 | 7 | 10 |

2.6 The *mean* corn size (in mm) for this sample of 10 patients is:
A 1.0
B 2.0
C 3.0
D 4.0
E 4.4

2.7 The *median* corn size (in mm) for this sample of 10 patients is:

   A   1.0

   B   2.0

   C   3.0

   D   4.0

   E   4.4

2.8 The *modal* corn size (in mm) for this sample of 10 patients is:

   A   1.0

   B   2.0

   C   3.0

   D   4.0

   E   4.4

2.9 The *range* of corn sizes (in mm) for this sample of 10 patients is:

   A   1 to 10

   B   2 to 5

   C   2 to 10

   D   3 to 11

   E   3 to 12

2.10 The *interquartile range* (IQR) corn size (in mm) for this sample of 10 patients is:

   A   2 to 10

   B   2 to 7

   C   2 to 5

   D   3 to 7

   E   3 to 10

2.11 The *variance* in corn size (in mm^2) for this sample of 10 patients is:

   A   0.8

   B   2.5

   C   3.5

   D   4.4

   E   6.5

2.12 The *standard deviation* corn size (in mm) for this sample of 10 patients is:

   A   0.8

   B   2.5

   C   3.5

   D   4.4

   E   6.5

3 Summary Measures for Binary Data

Medical Statistics: A Textbook for the Health Sciences, Fifth Edition. Stephen J. Walters, Michael J. Campbell, and David Machin.
© 2021 John Wiley & Sons Ltd. Published 2021 by John Wiley & Sons Ltd.
Companion website: www.wiley.com/go/walters/medicalstatistics

Summary

This chapter illustrates methods of summarising binary and categorical data. It covers proportions, risk, rates, relative risk, and odds ratios. The importance of considering the absolute risk difference (ARD) as well as the relative risk is emphasised.

3.1   Summarising Binary and Categorical Data

Categorical data are simply data which can be put into categories. Binary data are the simplest type of categorical data. Each individual has a label which takes one of two types. A simple summary would be to count the different types of label. However, a raw count is rarely useful. For example, there were 45 656 new cases of breast cancer registered in England in 2016. On its own this sounds like a large number, but there were 303 135 new cases of all cancers registered in 2016. Thus breast cancer accounts for 15.2% (45 656/303 135) of all new cancer registrations in England. Proportions are a special example of a *ratio*. When time is also involved (as in counts per year) then it is known as a *rate*. The mid-year population of England in 2016 was estimated as 55 268 067. Thus, the breast cancer registration rate was 0.008 (45 656/55 268 067).

Ratios, Proportions, Percentages, Risk and Rates

A *ratio* is simply one number divided by another. If we measure how far a car travels in a given time then the ratio of the distance travelled to the time taken to cover this distance is the *speed*.

Proportions are ratios of counts where the numerator (the top number) is a subset of the denominator (the bottom number). Thus in a study of 50 patients, 30 are depressed, so the proportion is 30/50 or 0.6. It is usually easier to express this as a percentage (%), so we multiply the proportion by 100, and state that 60% of the patients are depressed. Clearly proportions must lie between 0 and 1 and percentages between 0 and 100%.

A proportion is known as a *risk* if the numerator counts events which happen prospectively. Hence if 100 students start an introductory statistics course and 15 drop out before the final course examination, the *risk* of dropping out is 15/100 = 0.15 or 15%.

Rates always have a time period attached. In the UK, 597 206 deaths were recorded in 2016 out of a population of 65 648 100; a death *rate* of 597 206/65 648 or 0.009 deaths per person per year. This is known as the *crude death rate* (crude because it makes no allowance for important factors such as age). Crude death rates are often expressed as deaths per thousand per year, so the crude death rate is nine deaths per thousand per year, since it is much easier to imagine 1000 people, of whom 9 die, than it is 0.009 deaths per person!

Illustrative Example – RCT of Salicylic Acid Plasters for Treatment of Foot Corns

Farndon et al. (2013) reports a randomised controlled trial which investigated the effectiveness of salicylic acid plasters compared with usual scalpel debridement for treatment of foot corns. One categorical variable recorded was the location or anatomical site of the corn on the foot in six categories as displayed in Table 3.1. The first column shows category names, whilst the second shows the number of individuals in each category together with its percentage contribution to the total. We can see that corns are most likely on the metatarsal head.

Table 3.1 Anatomical site of foot corn of 201 patients with corns (*Source:* data from Farndon et al. 2013).

Anatomical site of index corn on foot	Frequency	(%)
Apex (end of toe)	13	7
Proximal interphalangeal joint (middle part of toe – on the top)	27	13
Interdigital (between the toes)	16	8
Metatarsal head (ball of the foot – on the bottom)	119	59
Plantar calcaneus (heel)	6	3
Other part of foot	20	10
Total	201	100

Table 3.2 Cross-tabulation of anatomical site of corn by gender for 201 patients with corns on feet (*Source:* data from Farndon et al. 2013).

	Gender			
	Male		Female	
Anatomical site of index corn on foot	n	(%)	n	(%)
Apex (end of toe)	4	(5)	9	(8)
Proximal interphalangeal joint (middle part of toe – on the top)	8	(10)	19	(16)
Interdigital (between the toes)	5	(6)	11	(9)
Metatarsal head (ball of the foot – on the bottom)	54	(64)	65	(56)
Plantar calcaneus (heel)	3	(4)	3	(3)
Other part of foot	10	(12)	10	(9)
Total	84	(100)	117	(100)

We might be interested in whether the corn site is related to the gender of the patient. Table 3.2 shows the distribution of corn site by gender; in this case it can be said that corn site type has been *cross-tabulated* with gender. We can see that the distribution of sites for corns is similar for males and females. Table 3.2 is an example of a *contingency* table with six rows (representing corn site) and two columns (gender). Note that we are interested in the distribution of the site where the corn is located on the foot within gender, and so the percentages add up to 100 down each column, rather than across the rows.

As an example of the importance of considering relative proportions Furness et al. (2003) reported in Auckland, New Zealand over a one-year period that 25.6% of road accidents were to white cars. As a consequence, a New Zealander may think twice about buying a white car! White cars were the most prevalent colour on the roads with a proportion of 25.9%. So about a quarter of cars on the road are white and this is the same as the proportion of road accidents that were in white cars; thus white cars are not more dangerous than other colours.

Labelling Binary Outcomes

For binary data it is common to call the outcomes 'an event' or 'a non-event'. So having a car accident in Auckland, New Zealand may be an 'event'. We often score an 'event' as 1 and a 'non-event' as 0. These may also be referred to as a 'positive' or 'negative' outcome, or 'success' and 'failure'. It is important to realise that these terms are merely labels and the main outcome of interest might be a success in one context and a failure in another. Thus in a study of a potentially lethal disease the outcome might be death, whereas in a disease that can be cured it might be being alive.

Comparing Outcomes for Binary Data

Many studies involve a comparison of two groups. We may wish to combine simple summary measures to give a summary measure that in some way shows how the groups differ. Given two proportions one can either subtract one from the other, or divide one by the other.

Suppose the results of a clinical trial, with a binary categorical outcome (positive or negative), to compare two treatments (a new test treatment versus a control) are summarised in a two by two contingency table as in Table 3.3. The results of this trial can be summarised in a number of way sas in Table 3.3 below.

Summarising Comparative Binary Data – Differences in Proportions

From Table 3.3, the proportion of subjects with a positive outcome under the test treatment is $p_{Test} = \dfrac{a}{a+c}$ and under the control treatment is $p_{Control} = \dfrac{b}{b+d}$.

The difference in proportions is given by

$$d_{prop} = p_{Test} - p_{Control}.$$

In prospective studies the proportion is also known as the risk and the difference in proportions as the risk difference (RD)

$$RD = p_{Test} - p_{Control}.$$

When one ignores the sign, the above quantity is also known as the absolute risk difference (ARD), that is.

$$ARD = |p_{Test} - p_{Control}|,$$

where the symbols || mean to take the absolute value.

Table 3.3 Example of two by two contingency table with a binary outcome and two groups of subjects.

	Treatment group	
Outcome	Test	Control
Positive	a	b
Negative	c	d
Total	a + c	b + d

If we anticipate that the treatment to reduce some bad outcome (such as deaths) then it may be known as the *absolute risk reduction* (ARR). If we anticipate that the exposure/treatment will increase some bad outcome (such as deaths) then it may be known as the *absolute risk excess* (ARE).

Example – Summarising Results from a Clinical Trial – Corn Plasters RCT: Differences in Proportions

Table 3.4 shows the results of a randomised controlled trial conducted by Farndon et al. (2013) to investigate the effectiveness of salicylic acid plasters compared with usual scalpel debridement for treatment of foot corns. There are two study groups, the control group (randomised to receive usual care of scalpel treatment) and the experimental or intervention group (randomised to receive corn plasters). The main outcome measure was whether or not the index corn had improved or resolved (healed) at a three-month post-randomisation as assessed by an independent podiatrist 'blind' to the treatment group.

The 'risk' or proportion of patients whose corn was healed or resolved by a three-month post-randomisation is 32/95 = 0.337 or 34% in the plaster group and 20/94 = 0.213 or 21% in the scalpel group. The difference in proportions or RD is 0.337–0.213 = 0.124 or 12%. If we started with 100 patients in each arm we would expect 12 more patients' corns to have healed in the plaster arm compared to the scalpel arm by the three-month follow-up.

Summarising Comparative Binary Data – Relative Risk

The risk ratio, or relative risk (RR), is

$$RR = \frac{p_{Test}}{p_{Control}}.$$

Example – Summarising Results from a Clinical Trial – Corn Plasters RCT: Relative Risk

The relative risk for a corn healing, at three months, in the plaster group compared to the scalpel group is 0.337/0.213 = 1.582 or RR = 1.58. This is the risk of the corn healing (a good thing) with the intervention compared to the control group. Thus, patients treated with corn plasters are 1.58 times more likely to see their corn resolve compared to patients with scalpel treatment.

Table 3.4 Corn healing rates at three-months post-randomisation in patients with corns by randomised treatment group (*Source:* data from Farndon et al. 2013).

Index corn resolved/healed at a three-month post-randomisation	Corn plaster (intervention) group		Scalpel (control) group	
	n	(%)	*n*	(%)
Yes	32 (*a*)	(34%)	20 (*b*)	(21%)
No	63 (*c*)	(66%)	74 (*d*)	(79%)
Total	95 (*a* + *c*)	(100%)	94 (*b* + *d*)	(100%)

Summarising Comparative Binary Data – Number Need to Treat

A further summary measure, sometimes used in clinical trials is the *number needed to treat*. This is defined as the inverse of the ARD.

$$\text{Number needed to treat (NNT)} = \frac{1}{|p_{\text{Test}} - p_{\text{Control}}|} = \frac{1}{\text{ARD}}.$$

This is the additional number of people you would need to give a new treatment to in order to cure one extra person compared to the old treatment. Alternatively, for a harmful exposure, the number needed to treat becomes the number needed to harm and it is the additional number of individuals who need to be exposed to the risk in order to have one extra person develop the disease, compared to the unexposed group. The NNT is a number between 1 and ∞; a lower number indicates a more effective treatment. When there is no difference in outcome between the test and control groups, that is, ARD = 0, then the NNT is 1/0 which is infinity ∞.

Example – Summarising Results from a Clinical Trial – Corn Plasters RCT: NNT

The 'risk' or proportion of patients whose corn was healed or resolved by a three-month post-randomisation is 32/95 = 0.337 or 34% with the corn plaster and 20/94 = 0.213 or 21% in the scalpel control group. The difference in proportions or RD is 0.337–0.213 = 0.124 or 12%.

$$\text{NNT} = \frac{1}{|0.337 - 0.213|} = \frac{1}{0.124} = 8.065.$$

The NNT is 8.065 or 9 (rounded up to the nearest person). Thus, on average one would have to treat nine patients with corn plasters in order to expect one extra patient (compared to scalpel treatment) to have their corn resolved at a three-month follow-up.

Each of the above measures summarises the study outcomes, and the one chosen may depend on how the test treatment behaves relative to the control. Commonly one may chose an absolute RD for a clinical trial and a relative risk for a prospective study. In general the relative risk is independent of how common the risk factor is. Smoking increases ones risk of lung cancer by a factor of 10, and this is true in countries with a high smoking prevalence and countries with a low smoking prevalence. However, in a clinical trial, we may be interested in what reduction in the proportion of people with poor outcome a new treatment will make.

Issues with NNT – Always Consider all the Risks

Consider a test and a control treatment with success rates (proportion of patients on the treatment with a positive outcome) of P_{Test} and P_{Control} respectively. Table 3.5 shows several scenarios that have the same RD, $P_{\text{Test}} - P_{\text{Control}}$, of 0.1 and NNT of 10 but different risks (of a positive outcome) and relative risks ($RR_{\text{Test/Control}}$) and odds ratios ($OR_{\text{Test/Control}}$). When interpreting a NNT it is important to consider the baseline risk or event rate in the control group. For example, in scenario 1, the new test treatment still only has a success rate of 10% (compared to an admittedly poor success rate of 0.1% in the control group). That is, only one out of 10 treated patients are likely to benefit on the new treatment but this gives the same NNT as scenario 7 where the success rate on the control treatment is a much higher 80% (that is, 8 out of 10 treated patients are likely to benefit on the control treatment compared to 9 out of 10 on the new treatment).

Without stating the direction of the effect, the alternative treatment, the treatment period, and the follow-up period, information in terms of NNTs is uninterpretable. Thus when quoting an NNT one should always give the basic information about which treatments are compared, the treatment period, the follow-up period, and the direction of the effect.

Table 3.5 Seven scenarios with the same NNT but different risks.

Scenario	P_{Test}	$P_{Control}$	$P_{Test} - P_{Control}$	NNT	$RR_{Test/Control}$	$OR_{Test/Control}$
1	0.1001	0.0001	0.1	10	1001	1112
2	0.101	0.001	0.1	10	101	112
3	0.11	0.01	0.1	10	11	12
4	0.15	0.05	0.1	10	3	3
5	0.2	0.1	0.1	10	2	2
6	0.6	0.5	0.1	10	1.2	2
7	0.9	0.8	0.1	10	1.1	2

Example – Importance of Considering both Absolute Risk and Relative Risk

Women of reproductive age not using the combined oral contraceptive pill have a risk of deep vein thrombosis (DVT) of about 2 per 10 000 women per year (Stegeman et al. 2013). Use of combined oral contraceptives increases the risk of DVT compared with non-use by a relative risk of 4 to 8 per 10 000 women per year, which would seem a large extra risk. However, the absolute increase in risk is 8/10 000 – 2/10 000 = 6/10 000 = 0.0006, or an additional 6 women with DVTs in 10 000 years of exposure. This increased risk is very small and hence may be considered worth taking, when balanced against other factors such as cost or convenience. Also, it is worth mentioning that a pregnant woman has a risk of a DVT of about 11 per 10 000 per year (Kourlaba et al. 2016); so the risk of DVT if you are pregnant is greater than the risk of a DVT when using the contraceptive pill, of 8 per 10 000 per year. Thus when one reads in the newspapers about a new risk to health that has been discovered, often only the relative risk is quoted, but one should ask about the baseline risk or incidence of the outcome (given you are not exposed to the risk factor) and the ARD, which may be negligible. If you are at very low risk, then you will remain at very low risk even when exposed to a hazard, unless the relative risk for the hazard is enormous!

Summarising Binary Data – Odds and Odds Ratios

A further method of summarising the results is to use the odds of an event rather than the probability. The odds of an event are defined as the ratio of the probability of occurrence of the event to the probability of non-occurrence, that is, $p/(1-p)$.

Using the notation of Table 3.3 we can see that the odds of a positive outcome for the test group relative to the odds of a positive outcome for control group, the odds ratio (OR), is:

$$\frac{p_{Test}/(1-p_{Test})}{p_{Control}/(1-p_{Control})}.$$

The odds ratio (OR) from Table 3.3 is

$$OR_{Test/Control} = \frac{a}{c} / \frac{b}{d} = \frac{ad}{bc}.$$

What does an odds ratio of less than 1 mean? There is a negative association between exposure and outcome (people in the exposed group less likely to experience outcome of interest). What does an odds ratio of more than 1 mean? There is a positive association between the exposure and outcome (people in the exposed group more likely to experience the outcome of interest).

Example – Summarising Results from a Clinical Trial– Corn Plasters: Odds Ratio

From Table 3.4, the odds of the corn resolving by three-months in the plaster group is $0.337/(1 - 0.337) = 0.508$; whilst the odds of resolution in the scalpel group is $0.213/(1 - 0.213) = 0.270$. Thus, the odds ratio for the corn resolving by three months in the plaster compared to the scalpel treated group is $0.508/0.270 = 1.88$. You can also calculate the odds ratio by using the four cell counts in the 2×2 contingency table of Table 3.3. The odds ratio for the corn resolving in the plaster group compared to the scalpel group is OR $= (32 \times 74)/(20 \times 63) = 1.88$.

The OR $= 1.88$ and RR $= 1.58$ with these trial data are clearly different. However, when the probability of an event happening is rare, the odds and probabilities are close, because when a is much smaller than c then the risk $a/(a + c)$ is approximately a/c. Further if b is much smaller than d then $b/(b + d)$ is approximately b/d, then RR $= (a/c)/(b/d)$. Thus, the OR approximates the RR when the successes are rare, say with a maximum incidence less than 10% of either p_{Test} or $p_{Control}$ Sometimes the odds ratio is referred to as 'the approximate relative risk'. The approximation is demonstrated in Table 3.6.

Why Should One Use the Odds Ratio?

The calculation for an OR may seem rather perverse, given that we can calculate the relative risk directly from the 2×2 table and the odds ratio is only an approximation of this. However, the OR appears quite often in the literature, so it is important to be aware of it. It has certain mathematical properties which render it attractive as an alternative to the RR as a summary measure. The OR features in logistic regression (see Chapter 10) and as a summary measure for case-control studies (see Section 14.8). An example where the authors quote an odds ratio is given below.

One point about the OR that can be seen immediately from the formula is that the odds ratio for failure as opposed to the odds ratio for success in Table 3.3 is given by OR $= bc/ad$. Thus, the OR for failure is just the inverse of the OR for success.

Thus in the corn plaster trial, the odds ratio for the corn *not healing* or resolving at three months in the plaster group compared to the scalpel group is $(20 \times 63)/(32 \times 74) = 0.532$; which is the same as the reciprocal or inverse of the odds ratio for the corn resolving at three months in the plaster group compared to the scalpel group or $1/1.879 = 0.53$. In contrast the relative risk ratio for the corn *not healing* or resolving at three months in the plaster group compared to the scalpel group $(1 - 0.337)/(1 - 213) = 0.842$, which is not the same as the inverse of the relative risk for the corn resolving at three months in the plaster compared to the scalpel group, which is $1/1.583 = 0.632$. This symmetry of interpretation of the OR is one of the reasons for its continued use.

Table 3.6 Comparison of RR and OR for different baseline rates.

p_{Test}	$p_{Control}$	RR	OR	RR and OR
0.05	0.1	0.5	0.47	Close
0.1	0.2	0.5	0.44	Close
0.2	0.4	0.5	0.38	Not close
0.4	0.2	2	2.66	Not close
0.2	0.1	2	2.25	Close
0.1	0.05	2	2.11	Close

Table 3.7 Example of a two by two contingency table with a binary outcome (alive or dead) and two groups of subjects (exposed or not exposed).

Outcome	Test treatment exposed	Control treatment not exposed
Alive	0.96	0.99
Dead	0.04	0.01
Total	1.00	1.00

The Odd Ratios are Symmetrical but the Relative Risk Is Not

Consider the data in the 2×2 contingency table of Table 3.7 where the relative risk of being alive in the exposed compared to the not exposed group is relative risk (alive) = 0.96 /0 99 = 0.97; the reciprocal is 1/relative risk (alive) = 1/ 0.97 = 1.03. The relative risk (dead) = 0.04/0.01 = 4. Thus, note that the relative risk (dead) is not equal to 1 / relative risk (alive).

The odds ratio (alive) = (0.96/0.04) / (0.99/0.01) = 0.24; the reciprocal is: 1/odds ratio (alive) = 1/ 0.24 = 4.13. The odds ratio (dead) = (0.04/0.96)/(0.01/0.99) = 4.13; and hence the odds ratio (dead) is equal to 1/odds ratio (alive).

How Are Risks Compared?

To understand risks that are smaller than 1% (or 1 in 100) you may find it helpful to compare these risks to other risks in life. Some people use words like 'high' or 'low' to talk about risk. So Calman (1996), an expert in risk communication, has produced a 'risk classification' scale that looks at particular risks and suggests words that the public and health care professionals can use to describe them. An outline of the scale is given in Table 3.8.

Table 3.8 Risk of an individual dying (D) in one year or developing an adverse response (A) (*Source:* Calman 1996).

Term used	Risk range	Example	Risk estimate
High	>1:100	(A) Transmission to susceptible household contacts of measles and chickenpox (A) Transmission of HIV from mother to child (Europe)	1:1–1:2 1:6
Moderate	1:100–1:1000	(D) Smoking 10 cigarettes per day (D) All natural causes, age 40	1:200 1:850
Low	1:1000–1:10 000	(D) All kinds of violence (D) Influenza (D) Accident on road	1: 300 1:5000 1:8000
Very low	1:10 000–1:100 000	(D) Leukaemia (D) Playing soccer (D) Accident at work	1:12 000 1:25 000 1:43 000
Minimal	1:100 000–1:1 000 000	(D) Accident on railway	1:500 000
Negligible	<1:1 000 000	(D) Hit by lightning (D) Release of radiation by nuclear power station	1:10 000 000 1:10 000 000

3.2 Points When Reading the Literature

1) Is the number of subjects involved clearly stated in the table?
2) Are the row and columns in the table clearly labelled?
3) Do the titles adequately describe the contents of the table?
   In tables:
4) If percentages are shown, is it clear whether they add across rows or down columns? For example in Table 3.4 it is clear the percentages total down the columns, not across the rows.
5) Percentages should not have decimal places if the number of subjects in total is less than 100.
   Summary statistics:
6) If a relative risk is quoted, what is the ARD? Is this a very small number? Beware of reports that only quote relative risks and give no hint of the absolute risk!
7) If an odds ratio is quoted, is it a reasonable approximation to the relative risk? (Ask what the size of the risk in the two groups are).

3.3 Exercises

Table 3.9 shows the results of randomised controlled trial in primary care in patients with venous leg ulcers to compare a new specially impregnated bandage, called 'Band aid', with usual care. Usual care will be treatment by district nurses with standard bandages and wound dressings. The primary outcome for the study will be whether or not the index or reference leg ulcer has completely healed at a 12-month post-randomisation.

Table 3.9 Results of randomised controlled trial in primary care in patients with venous leg ulcers to compare a new specially impregnated bandage, called 'Band aid', with usual care.

	Group	
Leg ulcer completely healed	Band-aid intervention	Usual care control
Yes, healed	147	123
No, not healed	63	82
Total	210	205

From the data in Table 3.9:

3.1 What proportion of patients in the Band-aid group had a completely healed leg ulcer at 12 months?

  A 0.30
  B 0.40
  C 0.60
  D 0.65
  E 0.70

3.2 What proportion of patients had a completely healed leg ulcer at 12 months in the control group?

A 0.30
B 0.40
C 0.60
D 0.65
E 0.70

3.3 What is the difference in response (leg ulcer healing rates at 12 months) between the Band-aid and control groups?

A −0.10
B −0.05
C 0.00
D 0.05
E 0.10

3.4 Calculate the number of people needed to be treated with Band-aid dressing in order for an additional person to have a completely healed leg ulcer at 12 months compared to people usual care?

A 6
B 7
C 8
D 8
E 10

3.5 What is the *relative risk* for the leg ulcer healing at 12 months in the Band-aid group compared to the control group?

A 0.64
B 0.86
C 1.17
D 1.56
E 2.33

3.6 What is the *relative risk* for the leg ulcer healing at 12 months in the control group compared to the Band-aid group?

A 0.64
B 0.86
C 1.17
D 1.56
E 2.33

3.7 What are the *odds* for the leg ulcer healing at 12 months in the Band-aid group?

A 0.64
B 0.86
C 1.50
D 1.56
E 2.33

3.8 What are the *odds* for the leg ulcer healing at 12 months in the control group?

    A   0.64

    B   0.86

    C   1.50

    D   1.56

    E   2.33

3.9 Calculate the *odds ratio* for the leg ulcer healing at 12 months in the Band-aid group compared to the control group?

    A   0.64

    B   0.86

    C   1.17

    D   1.56

    E   2.33

3.10 Calculate the *odds ratio* for the leg ulcer healing at 12 months in the control group compared to the band-aid group?

    A   0.64

    B   0.86

    C   1.17

    D   1.56

    E   2.33

4 Probability and Distributions

Medical Statistics: A Textbook for the Health Sciences, Fifth Edition. Stephen J. Walters, Michael J. Campbell, and David Machin.
© 2021 John Wiley & Sons Ltd. Published 2021 by John Wiley & Sons Ltd.
Companion website: www.wiley.com/go/walters/medicalstatistics

Summary

Probability is defined in terms of either the long-term frequency of events, as model based or as a subjective measure of the certainty of an event happening. Examples of each type are given. The concepts of independent events and mutually exclusive events are discussed. Several theoretical statistical distributions, such as the Binomial, Poisson and Normal are described. The properties of the Normal distribution and its importance are stressed and its use in calculating reference intervals is also discussed.

4.1 Types of Probability

There are a number of ways of looking at probability and we describe three as the 'frequency', 'model-based' and 'subjective' approaches as shown in Figure 4.1.

We all have an intuitive feel for probability but it is important to distinguish between probabilities applied to single individuals and probabilities applied to groups of individuals. In recent years about 600 000 people die annually from about 65 million people in the United Kingdom. Hence, for a single individual, with no information about their age or state of health, the chance or probability of dying in any particular year is 600 000/65 000 000 = 0.009 or just under 1 in 100. This is termed the crude mortality rate as it ignores differences in individuals due, for example, to their gender or age, which are both known to influence mortality. From year-to-year this probability of dying is fairly stable (see Figure 4.2), although there has been a long-term decline over the years in the probability of dying. This illustrates that the number of deaths in a group can be accurately predicted but, despite this, it is not possible to predict exactly which particular individuals are going to die.

The basis of the idea of probability is a sequence of what are known as independent trials. To calculate the probability of an individual dying in one year we give each one of a group of individuals a trial over a year and the event occurs if the individual dies. As already indicated, the estimate of the (crude) probability of dying is the number of deaths divided by the number in the original group. The idea of independence is difficult, but is based on the fact that whether or not one individual survives or dies does not affect the chance of another individual's survival.

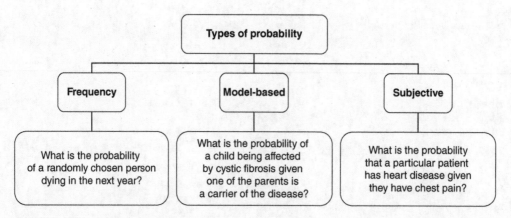

Figure 4.1 Three types of probability.

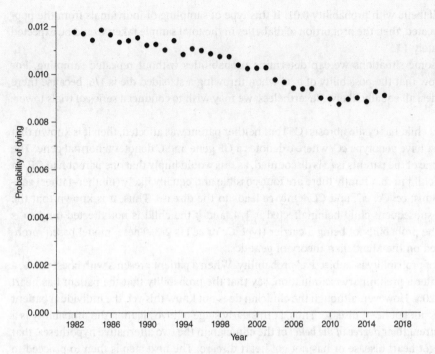

Figure 4.2 Crude mortality rates in the United Kingdom from 1982 to 2016. (*Source:* data from ONS 2017, https://www.ons.gov.uk/peoplepopulationandcommunity/birthsdeathsandmarriages/deaths/datasets/deathregistrationssummarytablesenglandandwalesdeathsbysingleyearofagetables).

On a very simple level and where the probability of an event is known in advance, consider tossing one coin repeatedly a large number of times. Each toss of the coin is an 'experiment' or 'trial' and the results of this experiment or trial will be an outcome (head or tail). If the coin is unbiased, that is one which has no preference for 'heads' or 'tails', we would expect heads half of the time and thus say the probability of a head is 0.5. This leads to *the long-term relative frequency definition* of probability, which is that the probability of a specific outcome is the proportion of times that the specific outcome would happen if we repeated the experiment a large number of times.

For example, the proportion of male births out of total births in England and Wales in 2016 was 357 046/696 271 = 0.51. Since all births in England and Wales must be registered within 42 days of the child being born and this a large sample, we can use this an estimate of the probability that a baby born in England and Wales will be male.

Similarly, when it is stated that patients with a certain disease have a 50% chance of surviving five years, this is based on past experience of other patients with the same disease. In some cases a 'trial' may be generated by randomly selecting an individual from the general population, as discussed in Chapters 5 and 14, and examining him or her for the particular attribute in question. For example, suppose the prevalence of diabetes in the population is 1%. The prevalence of a disease is the number of people in a population with the disease at a certain time divided by the number of people in the population (see Chapter 14 for further details). If a trial was then conducted by randomly selecting one person from the population and testing him or her for diabetes, the individual would be expected to be diabetic with probability 0.01. If this type of sampling of individuals from the population were repeated, then the proportion of diabetics in the total sample taken would be expected to be approximately 1%.

However, in some situations we can determine probabilities without repeated sampling. For example, we know that the possibility of a '6' when throwing a six-sided die is 1/6, because there are six possibilities, all equally likely. Nevertheless, we may wish to conduct a series of trials to verify this fact.

In genetics, if a child has cystic fibrosis (CF) but neither parent was affected, then it is known that each parent must have genotype cC, where c denotes a CF gene and C denotes a normal gene. The possibility that one of the parents is cc is discounted, as this would imply that one parent had CF. In any subsequent child in that family there are four possible and equally likely (mother–father) genotype combinations: cc, Cc, cC, and CC. Only cc leads to the disease. Thus, it is known that the probability of a subsequent child being affected is 1/4, and *if* the child is not affected (and so is Cc, cC or CC), the probability of being a carrier (type Cc or cC) is 2/3. These 'model based' probabilities are based on the Mendelian theory of genetics.

Another type of probability is 'subjective' probability. When a patient presents with chest pains, a clinician may, after a preliminary examination, say that the probability that the patient has heart disease is about 20%. However, although the clinician does not know this yet, the individual patient either has or has not got heart disease. Thus, at this early stage of investigation the probability is a measure of the strength or *degree of the belief* of the clinician in the two alternative hypotheses, that the patient has got heart disease or has not got heart disease. The next step is then to proceed to further examinations of the patient in order to modify the strength of this initial *subjective* belief so that the clinician becomes more certain of which is the true situation – the patient has heart disease or the patient does not. We commonly come across subjective probability in the gaming industry. The odds of a horse winning a race, for example, are a measure of how likely a bookmaker thinks it will win. It is based not just on how often the horse has won before, but also on other factors such as the jockey and the course conditions.

In some circumstances we will have some prior knowledge or belief about the chance or likelihood of an event and as long as it can be quantified, it is possible to combine this prior belief with the observed frequency data to give an updated and better estimate of the probability of the event. An example of this is when we apply Bayes' Theorem (see Chapter 13) to diagnostic data and use the prevalence and sensitivity to give us the positive predictive value. Further application using statistical distributions of degrees of belief to modify data gives raise to the body of statistical methods known as *Bayesian statistics*.

The three types of probability all have the following basic properties.

1) All probabilities lie between 0 and 1.
2) If two outcomes or events are mutually exclusive so that they both cannot occur at the same time, the probability of either happening is the sum of the two individual probabilities (this is known as the 'addition rule').
3) If two outcomes are independent (i.e. knowing the outcome of one experiment tells us nothing about the other experiment), then the probability of both occurring is the product of the individual probabilities (this is known as the 'multiplication rule').

When the outcome can never happen the probability is 0. When the outcome will definitely happen the probability is 1. If two events are mutually exclusive then only one can happen. For example, the outcome of a trial might be death (probability 5%) and severe disability (probability 20%). Thus, by the addition rule the probability of either death or severe disability is 25%.

If two events are independent then the fact that one has happened does not affect the chance of the other event happening. For example, the probability that a pregnant woman gives birth to a boy (event A) and the probability of white Christmas (event B). These two events are unconnected since the probability of giving birth to a boy is not related to the weather at Christmas.

Examples of Addition and Multiplication Rules – Using Dice Rolling

If we throw a six-sided die the probability of throwing a 6 is 1/6 and the probability of a 5 is also 1/6. We cannot throw a 5 and 6 at the same time (these events are mutually exclusive) using 1 die so the probability of throwing either 5 or a 6 is (by the addition rule):

$$P(5 \text{ or } 6) = P(5) + P(6) = 1/6 + 1/6 = 2/6 \text{ or } 0.333.$$

Suppose we throw two six-sided dice together. The probability of throwing a 6 is 1/6 for each die. The outcome of each die is independent of the other. Therefore, the probability of throwing two 6s together (by the multiplication rule) is:

$$P(6 \text{ and } 6) = P(6) \times P(6) = 1/6 \times 1/6 = 1/36 \text{ or } 0.028.$$

Probability Distributions for Discrete Outcomes

If we toss a two-sided coin it comes down either heads or tails. In a single toss of the coin you are uncertain whether you will get a head or a tail. However, if we carry on tossing our coin, we should get several heads and several tails. If we go on doing this for long enough, then we would expect to get as many heads as we do tails. So, the probability of a head being thrown is a half, because in the long run a head should occur on half the throws. The number of heads which might arise in several tosses of the coin is called a *random variable*, that is a variable which can take more than one value, each with a given probability attached to them.

If we toss a coin the two possibilities; head (H) – scored 1, or tail (T) – scored 0, are mutually exclusive and these are the only events which can happen. If we let X be a random variable that is the number of heads shown on a single toss and is therefore either 1 or 0, then the probability distribution, for X is: probability (H) = ½; probability (T) = ½ and is shown graphically in Figure 4.3a.

What happens if we toss two coins at once? We now have four possible events: HH, HT, TH, and TT. There are all equally likely and each has probability ¼. If we let Y be the number of heads then Y has three possible values 0, 1, and 2. $Y = 0$ only when we get TT and has probability ¼. Similarly, $Y = 2$ only when we get HH, so has probability ¼. However, $Y = 1$ either when we get HT or TH and so has probability ¼ + ¼ = ½. The probability distribution for Y is shown in Figure 4.3b. The distribution for the number of heads becomes more symmetrical as the number of coin tosses increases (Figures 4.3c and d).

In general, we can think of the tosses of the coin as trials, each of which can have an outcome of success (H) or failure (T). These distributions are all examples of what is known as the Binomial distribution. In addition, we will discuss two more distributions that are the backbone of medical statistics: the Poisson and the Normal. Each of the distributions is known as the *probability distribution function,* which gives the probability of observing an event. The corresponding formulas are given in Section 4.7. These formulas contain certain constants, known as *parameters,* which identify the particular distribution, and from which various characteristics of the distribution, such as its mean and standard deviation, can be calculated.

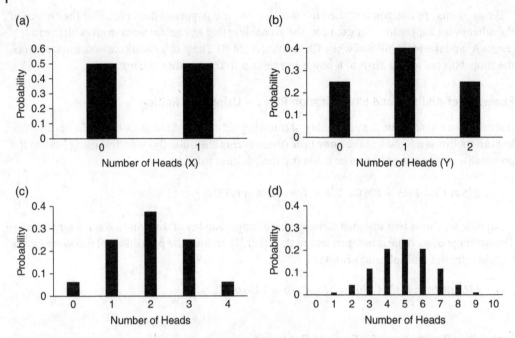

Figure 4.3 Examples of probability distributions. (a) Probability distribution for the number of heads (X) shown in one toss of a coin. (b) Probability distribution for the number of heads (Y) shown in two tosses of a coin. (c) Probability distribution for the number of heads in four tosses of a coin. (d) Probability distribution for the number of heads in ten tosses of a coin.

4.2 The Binomial Distribution

If a group of patients is given a new treatment such as acupuncture for the relief of a particular condition, such as tension type headache, then the proportion p being successfully treated can be regarded as estimating the population treatment success rate π (here, π denotes a population value and has no connection at all with the mathematical constant 3.14159). The sample proportion p is analogous to the sample mean $\bar{x}$, in that if we score zero for those s patients who fail on treatment, and unity for those r who succeed, then $p = r/n$, where $n = r + s$ is the total number of patients treated. The Binomial distribution is characterised by the parameters n (the number of individuals in the sample, or repetitions of the trial) and π (the true probability of success for each individual, or in each trial). The formula is given as Eq. (4.1) in Section 4.9.

For a fixed sample size n the shape of the Binomial distribution depends only on π. Suppose $n = 5$ patients are to be treated, and it is known that on average 0.25 will respond to this particular treatment. The number of responses actually observed can only take integer values between 0 (no responses) and 5 (all respond). The Binomial distribution for this case is illustrated in Figure 4.4a. The distribution is not symmetric; it has a maximum at one response and the height of the blocks corresponds to the probability of obtaining the particular number of responses from the five patients yet to be treated.

Figure 4.4 illustrates the shape of the Binomial distribution for various n and $\pi = 0.25$. When n is small (here 5 and 10), as in Figure 4.4a and b, the distribution is skewed to the right. The distribution becomes more symmetrical as the sample size increases (here 20 and 50) as in Figure 4.4c and d.

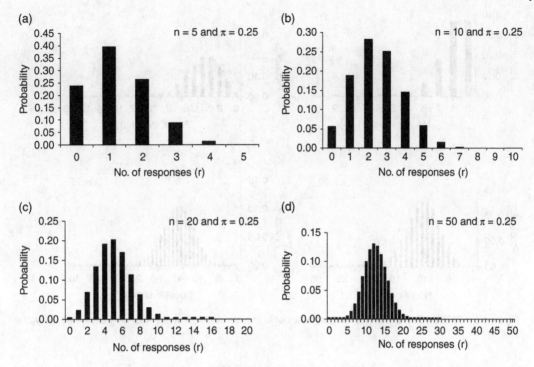

Figure 4.4 Binomial distribution for $\pi = 0.25$ and various values of n. The horizontal scale in each diagram shows the value of r the number of successes.

We also note that the width of the bars decreases as n increases since the total probability of unity is divided amongst more and more possibilities.

If π were set equal to 0.5, then all the distributions corresponding to those of Figure 4.4 would be symmetrical whatever the size of n. On the other hand, if $\pi = 0.75$ then the distributions would be skewed to the left.

We can use the properties of the Binomial distribution when making inferences about proportions, as we shall see in subsequent chapters.

Example – Probability of Corn Resolving

Farndon et al. (2013) give the successful response rate to scalpel treatment in 94 patients with foot corns as 21%. From their data we have $p = 20/94 = 0.21$. Suppose a podiatrist treated four patients with corns with scalpel debridement. What is the probability that at most one patient responds to treatment? This implies that either 0 or 1 respond. We can use formula 4.1, with $r = 0$ to give $1 \times 0.21^0 \times (1-0.21)^4 = 0.3895$ and with $r = 1$ to give $4 \times 0.21^1 \times (1-0.21)^3 = 0.4142$. Summing these two probabilities gives $P = 0.3895 + 0.4142 = 0.8037$.

4.3 The Poisson Distribution

The Poisson distribution is used to describe discrete quantitative data such as counts that occur independently and randomly in time or space at some average rate. For example, the number of

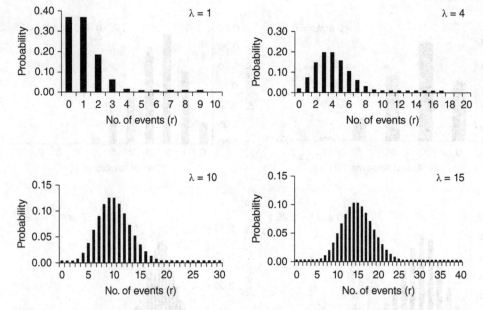

Figure 4.5 Poisson distribution for various values of λ. The horizontal scale in each diagram shows the value of *r*.

deaths in a town from a particular disease per day, or the number of admissions to a particular hospital in a day typically follows a Poisson distribution.

The Poisson random variable is the count of the number of events that occur independently and randomly in time at some rate, λ. The formula for a Poisson distribution is given as Eq. (4.2) in Section 4.9.

We can use our knowledge of the Poisson distribution to calculate the anticipated number of hospital admissions on any particular day or the number of deaths from lung cancer in a year in a town. We can use this information to compare observed and expected values, to decide if, for example, the number of deaths from cancer in an area is unusually high.

Figure 4.5 shows the Poisson distribution for four different rates λ = 1, 4, 10 and 15. For λ = 1 the distribution is very right skewed, for λ = 4 the skewness is much less and as the rate increases to λ = 10 or 15 it is more symmetrical, and looks more like the Binomial distribution in Figure 4.4.

Example from the Literature – IV Treated Exacerbations in Patients with Cystic Fibrosis

CF is a genetic disorder that affects mostly the lungs. Long-term issues include difficulty breathing and coughing up mucus as a result of frequent lung infections. There is no known cure for CF. Lung infections are treated with antibiotics which may be given intravenously (IV), inhaled, or by mouth. The build-up of mucus in the lungs causes chronic infections, meaning that people with CF struggle with reduced lung function and have to spend hours doing physiotherapy and taking nebulised treatments each day. Exacerbations (a sudden worsening of health, often owing to infection) can lead to frequent hospitalisation for weeks at a time, interfering with work and home life.

Hind et al. (2019) looked at the incidence of IV treated exacerbations in patients with CF as part of a pilot randomised controlled trial (RCT). They observed 60 IV treated exacerbations in 60 patients with CF in six months of follow-up (27 patients had no exacerbations; 14 had one; 13 had two, 4 had

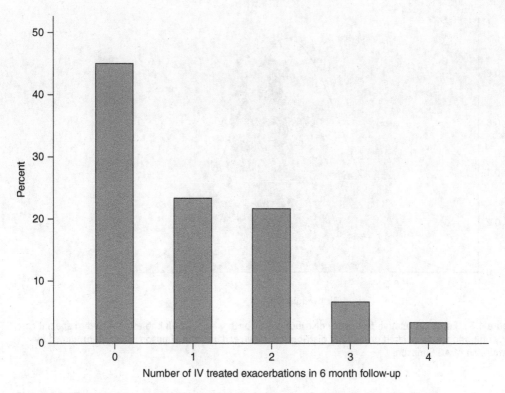

Figure 4.6 Relative frequency of IV treated exacerbations in 60 patients with cystic fibrosis over six months.

three and 2 patients had four). This gave a mean of one exacerbation per six months (see Figure 4.6). What is the probability of a patient having no exacerbations in a year assuming the data follow a Poisson distribution?

With this pilot RCT data would anticipate an average of $\lambda = 1 \times 2 = 2$ exacerbations per year. Using this value in Eq. (4.2), for $r = 0$, $P(0) = \dfrac{e^{-2}2^0}{0!} = \dfrac{0.14 \times 1}{1} = 0.14$ (since $0! = 1$ and $2^0 = 1$). Thus there is about a 1 in 7 chance of a patient with CF not getting any exacerbations in any one year.

4.4 Probability for Continuous Outcomes

So far, we have looked at what is the probability of a particular value, for example, a success or failure on treatment. The Binomial and Poisson distributions are discrete distributions that describe discrete variables that can only take a limited set of values. As the number of possible values increases the probability of any particular value decreases. Continuous probability distributions are distributions that can take any value between given limits. For continuous variables, such as birth weight and blood pressure, the set of possible values is infinite (only limited by the precision of how were take the measurements). So, we are more interested in the probability of having values between certain limits rather than one particular value. For example, what is the probability of having a systolic blood pressure of 140 mmHg or higher?

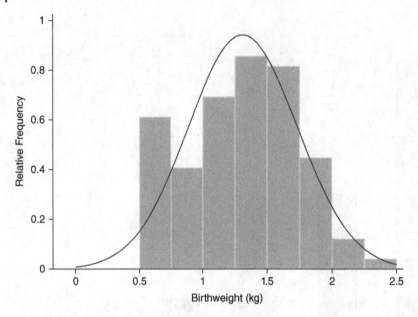

Figure 4.7 Empirical relative frequency distributions of birth weight of 98 babies admitted to special care baby unit and the associated probability distribution. (*Source:* data from Simpson 2004). Reproduced by permission of AG Simpson.

The vertical scale of histograms, such as Figure 2.6, shown so far, have been frequencies and depend on the total number of observations. As an alternative we can use the relative frequency (or %) on the vertical scale. The advantage of using the relative frequency is that the scale of different histograms, with the same outcome but different sample sizes, will be the same. Such a histogram, as in Figure 4.7 can be given the rather formal name of an empirical relative frequency distribution but it is simply the observed distribution of the data in a sample.

If we imagine for the birthweight data in Figure 4.7 that we have a very large sample (many more than 98 babies) and by taking smaller and smaller intervals to classify the birth weights (much smaller than 0.25 kg) then the histogram will start to look like a smooth curve (see Figure 4.8). In these circumstances the distribution of observations may be approximated by a smooth underlying curve, which is also shown in Figure 4.7. This curve is called a *probability distribution* and is the theoretical equivalent of an empirical relative frequency distribution. Probability distributions are used to calculate the probability that different values will occur, for example: what is the probability of having a birthweight of 2.0 kg or less? It is often the case with medical data that the histogram of a continuous variable obtained from a single measurement on different subjects will have a symmetric 'bell-shaped' distribution.

4.5 The Normal Distribution

This symmetric 'bell-shaped' distribution mentioned above is known as the Normal distribution and is one of the most important distributions in statistics. One such example is the histogram of the birthweight (in kilogrammes) of the 3226 new-born babies shown in Figure 4.9.

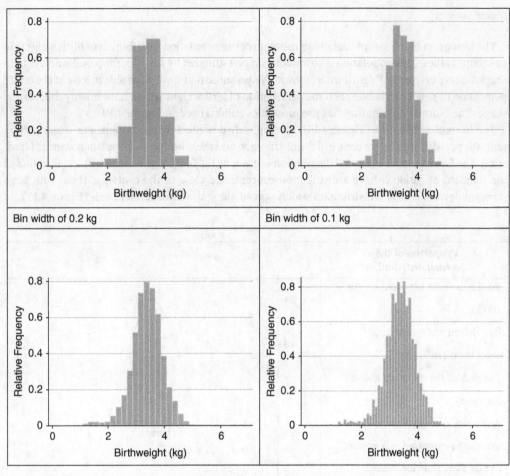

Figure 4.8 Empirical relative frequency distributions of birthweight with interval (bin) widths of 0.5, 0.25, 0.2, and 0.1 kg

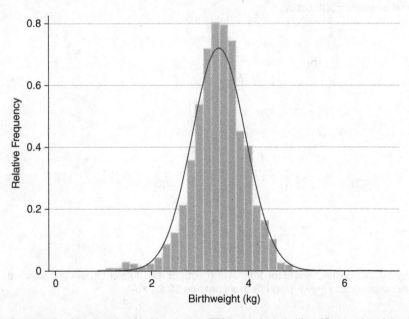

Figure 4.9 Distribution of birthweight in 3226 new-born babies. (*Source:* data from O'Cathain et al. 2002).

The histogram of the sample data is an estimate of the population distribution of birth weights in new-born babies. This population distribution can be estimated by the superimposed smooth 'bell-shaped' curve or 'Normal' distribution shown. We presume that if we were able to look at the entire population of new-born babies then the distribution of birthweight would have exactly the Normal shape. The Normal distribution has the properties summarised in Figure 4.10.

The Normal distribution (Figure 4.10), is completely described by two parameters: one, μ, represents the population mean or centre of the distribution and the other, σ, the population standard deviation. The formula for the Normal distribution is given as Eq. (4.3). Populations with small values of the standard deviation σ have a distribution concentrated close to the centre, μ; those with large standard deviation have a distribution widely spread along the measurement axis (Figure 4.11).

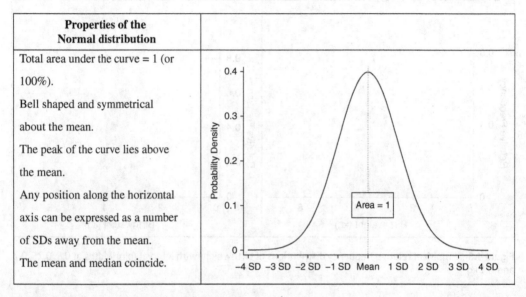

Properties of the Normal distribution	
Total area under the curve = 1 (or 100%). Bell shaped and symmetrical about the mean. The peak of the curve lies above the mean. Any position along the horizontal axis can be expressed as a number of SDs away from the mean. The mean and median coincide.	

Figure 4.10 The Normal probability distribution.

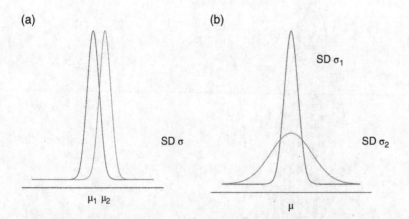

Figure 4.11 Probability distribution functions of the Normal distributions with different means and standard deviations. (a) Effect of changing mean ($\mu_2 > \mu_1$). (b) Effect of changing SD ($\sigma_2 > \sigma_1$).

Table 4.1 Selected probabilities associated with the Normal distribution.

Standardised deviate	Probability of greater deviation	
$Z = (X - \mu)/\sigma$	(i) Area in one direction	(ii) Area both directions
0	0.5000	1.0000
1.000	0.1590	0.3170
1.645	0.0500	0.0100
1.960	0.0250	0.0500
2.000	0.0230	0.0460
2.576	0.0050	0.0100
3.000	0.0013	0.0027

There are infinitely many Normal distributions depending on the values of μ and σ. The Standard Normal distribution has a mean of zero and a variance (and standard deviation) of one and a shape as shown in Figure 4.10. The formula is given as Eq. (4.4) in Section 4.9. If the random variable X has a Normal distribution with mean, μ and standard deviation, σ, then the standardised Normal deviate $Z = \dfrac{X - \mu}{\sigma}$ is a random variable that has a Standard Normal distribution.

The areas under the Standard Normal distribution curve have been tabulated in Table T1 in the appendix and some examples in Table 4.1. In column (i), the table gives for a positive value of Z, (that is the number of standard deviations above the mean of zero), the area under the Normal curve to the right of this value. The same value is obtained for the area below the same numerical, but negative, value $-Z$. Column (ii) gives the combination of these two equal areas. Using Figure 4.12 or Table 4.1, we can note that much of the area (68%) of the probability is between -1 and $+1$ SD, the large majority (95%) between -2 and $+2$ SD, and almost all (99%) between -3 and $+3$.

As can be seen from Table 4.1, using Z values of 1.96 (that is, 1.96 SD away from the mean) then exactly 95% of the Normal distribution lies between

$$\mu - 1.96 \times \sigma \quad \text{and} \quad \mu + 1.96 \times \sigma.$$

Changing the multiplier 1.96 to 2.58, exactly 99% of the Normal distribution lies in the corresponding interval.

How Do We Use the Normal Distribution?

The Normal probability distribution can be used to calculate the probability of different values occurring. We could be interested in the probability of being within 1 SD of the mean (or outside it). We can use a Normal distribution table, which tells us the probability of being outside this value.

Illustrative Example – Normal Distribution – Birthweights

Using the birthweight data from the O'Cathain et al. (2002) study let us assume that the birthweight for new born babies has a Normal distribution with a mean of 3.4 kg and a standard deviation of 0.6 kg. So, what is the probability of giving birth to baby with a birthweight of 4.5 kg or higher?

Since birthweight is assumed to follow a Normal distribution, with mean of 3.4 kg and SD of 0.6 kg, we therefore know that approximately 68% of birthweights will lie between 2.8 and

(a)

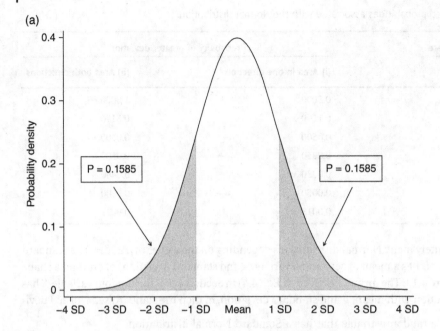

(b)

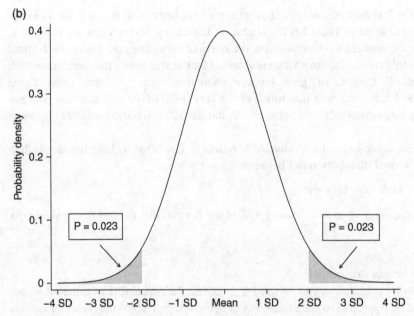

Figure 4.12 Areas (percentages of total probability) under the standard Normal curve. (a) 31.7% of observations lie outside the mean ± 1 SD. (b) 4.6% of observations lie outside the mean ± 2SD.

4.0 kg and about 95% of birthweights will lie between 2.2 and 4.6 kg. Using Figure 4.13 we can see that a birthweight of 4.5 kg is between one and two standard deviations away from the mean.

First calculate, Z, the number of standard deviations 4.5 kg is away from the mean of 3.4 kg, that is, $Z = \dfrac{4.5 - 3.4}{0.6} = 1.83$. Then look for $z = 1.83$ in Table T1 of the Normal distribution table, which

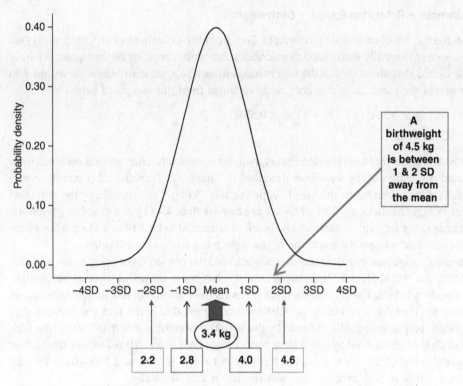

Figure 4.13 Normal distribution curve for birthweight with a mean of 3.4 kg and SD of 0.6 kg.

gives the probability of being outside the values of the mean −1.83SD to mean +1.83SD as 0.0672. Therefore the probability of having a birthweight of 4.5 kg or higher is 0.0672/2 = 0.0336 or 3.4%.

The Normal distribution also has other uses in statistics and is often used as an approximation to the Binomial and Poisson distributions. Figure 4.4 shows that the Binomial distribution for any particular value of the parameter π approaches the shape of a Normal distribution as the other parameter n increases. The approach to Normality is more rapid for values of π near 0.5 than for values near to 0 or 1. Thus, provided n is large enough, a count may be regarded as approximately Normally distributed with mean $n\pi$ and $\sqrt{[n\pi(1-\pi)]}$. The Poisson distribution with mean λ approaches Normality as λ increases (see Figure 4.5). When λ is large a Poisson variable may be regarded as approximately Normally distributed with mean λ and SD $= \sqrt{\lambda}$.

4.6 Reference Ranges

Diagnostics tests use patient data to classify individuals as either normal or abnormal. A related statistical problem is the description of the variability in normal individuals, to provide a basis for assessing the test results of other individuals. The most common form of presenting such data is as a range of values or interval that contains the values obtained from the majority of a sample of normal subjects. The reference interval is often referred to as a normal range or reference range. To distinguish the use of the same word for the Normal distribution we have used a lower case, for the normal range, and upper case convention throughout this book.

Worked Example – Reference Range – Birthweight

We can use the fact that our sample birthweight data, from the O'Cathain et al. (2002) study (see Figure 4.9); appear Normally distributed to calculate a reference range for birthweights. We have already mentioned that about 95% of the observations from a Normal distribution lie within 1.96 SDs either side of the mean. So a reference range obtained from this sample of babies is:

3.391 − (1.96 × 0.554) to 3.391 + (1.96 × 0.554)

or 2.31 to 4.47 kg.

If the baby data were *not* Normally distributed then the normal reference range is obtained from the calculated percentiles of the sample as described in Chapter 2. Thus the 2.5 percentile corresponds to 2.5% of the babies below this weight which equals 2.91 kg. Correspondingly the estimated 97.5 percentile suggests that only 2.5% of babies are heavier than 4.43 kg at birth. The percentile-based reference range for baby birthweight is therefore estimated to be 2.19 to 4.43 kg. This is very close to that obtained when we assume the birthweight has a Normal distribution.

Most reference ranges are based on samples larger than 3500 people. Over many years, and millions of births, the World Health Organization (WHO) has come up with a normal birthweight range for new-born babies. These ranges represent results than are acceptable in new-born babies and actually cover the middle 80% of the population distribution, that is, the 10th and 90th centiles. Low birthweight babies are usually defined (by the WHO) as weighing less than 2500 g (the 10th centile) regardless of gestational age, and large birth weight babies are defined as weighing above 4000 g (the 90th centile). Hence the normal birth weight range is around 2.5 to 4.0 kg. For our sample data, the 10th to 90th centile range was similar, at 2.75 to 4.03 kg.

4.7 Other Distributions

There are many other probability distributions used in statistics. In this section we briefly list and describe those that are more commonly used.

t-distribution

Student's *t*-distribution is any member of a family of continuous probability distributions that arises when estimating the mean of a Normally distributed variable (in the population) in situations where the sample size is small and the population standard deviation is unknown. It was developed by William Sealy Gosset under the pseudonym Student.

The *t*-distribution plays an important role in a number of widely used statistical analyses, including Student's *t*-test for assessing the statistical significance of the difference between two sample means, the construction of confidence intervals for the difference between two population means, and in linear regression analysis.

The *t*-distribution is symmetric and bell-shaped, like the Normal distribution, but has heavier tails, meaning that it is more prone than a Standard Normal distribution to producing values that fall far from its mean (Figure 4.14a). The exact shape of the *t*-distribution is determined by the mean and variance plus what are known as the degrees of freedom, *df*. These are derived from the sample size. As the *df* increases, the shape of the *t*-distribution becomes closer to the Normal distribution; and when the sample size (and degrees of freedom) are greater than 30, the *t*-distribution is very similar to the Standard Normal distribution.

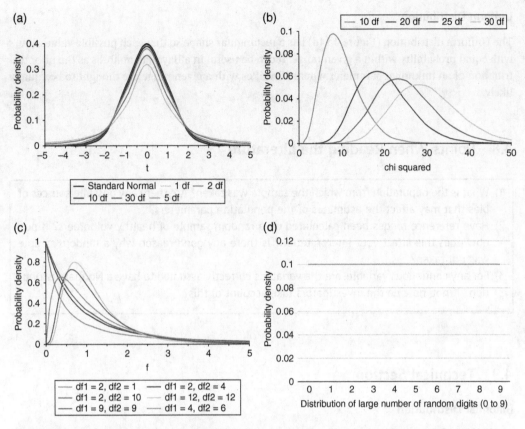

Figure 4.14 Examples of probability density/distribution functions for the *t*-, chi-squared, *F*- and Uniform distributions. (a) *t*-distribution. (b) chi-squared distribution. (c) *F*-distribution. (d) Uniform distribution.

Chi-squared Distribution

The chi-squared distribution (or χ^2-distribution) with n degrees of freedom (Figure 4.14b) is the distribution of a sum of the squares of n independent standard Normal random variables. The chi-squared distribution is always positive and its shape is uniquely determined by the degrees of freedom. The distribution becomes more symmetrical as the degrees of freedom increase and when the degrees of freedom are greater than 50, the chi-squared distribution is very similar to the Normal distribution. The chi-squared distribution is used in the common chi-squared tests for goodness of fit of an observed distribution to a theoretical one, the independence of two criteria of classification of qualitative data, and in confidence interval estimation for a population standard deviation of a Normal distribution from a sample standard deviation.

F-distribution

The *F*-distribution (Figure 4.14c) is the distribution of the ratio of two chi-squared distributions and is used in hypothesis testing when we want to compare variances, such as in one-way analysis of variance (see Section 7.3). It is always positive, but the exact shape depends on the degrees of freedom for the two chi-squared distributions that determine it.

Uniform Distribution

The Uniform distribution (Figure 4.14d) has a rectangular shape so that each possible value occurs with equal probability within a given range. It can be useful in a Bayesian analysis as the prior distribution of an unknown parameter where all values with a given range are thought to be equally likely.

4.8 Points When Reading the Literature

1) What is the population from which the sample was taken? Are there any possible sources of bias that may affect the estimates of the population parameters?
2) Have reference ranges been calculated on a random sample of healthy volunteers? If not, how does this affect your interpretation? Is there any good reason why a random sample was not taken?
3) For any continuous variable, are the variables correctly assumed to have a Normal distribution? If not, how do the investigators take account of this?

4.9 Technical Section

Binomial Distribution

Data that can take only a 0 or 1 response, such as treatment failure or treatment success, follow the *Binomial distribution* provided the underlying population response rate π does not change. The Binomial probabilities are calculated from

$$\text{Prob}(r \text{ responses out of } n) = \frac{n!}{r!(n-r)!}\pi^r(1-\pi)^{n-r} \tag{4.1}$$

for successive values of r from 0 through to n. In the above $n!$ is read as n factorial and $r!$ as r factorial. For $r = 4$, $r! = 4 \times 3 \times 2 \times 1 = 24$. Both 0! and 1! are taken as equal to unity. It should be noted that the expected value for r, the number of successes yet to be observed if we treated n patients, is $n\pi$. The potential variation about this expectation is expressed by the corresponding standard deviation $SD(r) = \sqrt{[n\pi(1-\pi)]}$.

Poisson Distribution

Suppose events happen randomly and independently in time at a constant rate. If the events happen with a rate of λ events per unit time, the probability of r events happening in unit time is

$$\text{Prob}(r \text{ events}) = \frac{exp(-\lambda)\lambda^r}{r!} \tag{4.2}$$

where $exp(-\lambda)$ is a convenient way of writing the exponential constant e raised to the power $-\lambda$. The constant e being the base of natural logarithms which is 2.718281...

The mean of the Poisson distribution for the number of events per unit time is simply the rate, λ. The variance of the Poisson distribution is also equal to λ, and so the SD $= \sqrt{\lambda}$.

Normal Distribution

The probability density, $f(x)$, or the height of the curve above the x axis (see Figures 4.7 and 4.9) of a Normally distributed random variable x, is given by the expression,

$$f(x) = \frac{1}{\sigma\sqrt{2\pi}} \exp\left[-\frac{(x-\mu)^2}{2\sigma^2}\right],$$ (4.3)

where μ is the mean value of x and σ is the standard deviation of x. Note that for the Normal distribution π, is the mathematical constant 3.14159... and not the parameter of a Binomial distribution.

The probability density simplifies for the Standard Normal distribution, since $\mu = 0$ and $\sigma = 1$, then the probability density, $f(x)$, of a Normally distributed random variable x, is

$$f(x) = \frac{1}{\sqrt{2\pi}} \exp\left[-\frac{x^2}{2}\right].$$ (4.4)

4.10 Exercises

4.1 Which ONE of the following statements about probability is INCORRECT?
  A If two binary outcomes (X and Y) are mutually exclusive the probability that either X or Y occurs is the sum of the probability that X occurs and the probability that Y occurs.
  B If two binary outcomes (X and Y) are independent, then the probability that both outcomes X and Y occur is the probability that X occurs multiplied by the probability that Y occurs.
  C When the outcome will definitely happen the probability of it happening is 1.
  D When an outcome can never happen, the probability of it happening is 1.
  E All probabilities range between 0 to 1.

4.2 Suppose we toss a single unbiased two-sided coin three times in a row and record the number of heads. What is the probability of observing a head on three successive tosses?
  A 0.500
  B 0.250
  C 0.750
  D 0.125
  E 0.050

4.3 Suppose we roll a 10-sided die (numbered 1 to 10) once.
  What is the probability of observing a score of 6 or more on this roll?
  A 0.4
  B 0.5
  C 0.6
  D 0.7
  E 0.08

4.4 Which ONE of the following statements about the Normal distribution is INCORRECT?
   A The Normal distribution is symmetrical.
   B The peak of the curve lies above the mean.
   C The total area under the Normal distribution curve is 1.
   D The mean and median will coincide.
   E The bigger the variance the taller the peak.

4.5 Which (if any) of the following statements about the Normal distribution is CORRECT?
   A Approximately 1% of the observations from a Normal distribution lie outside the mean ± 2SD.
   B Approximately 2% of the observations from a Normal distribution lie outside the mean ± 2SD.
   C Approximately 3% of the observations from a Normal distribution lie outside the mean ± 2SD.
   D Approximately 5% of the observations from a Normal distribution lie outside the mean ± 2SD.
   E Approximately 10% of the observations from a Normal distribution lie outside the mean ± 2SD

4.6 Which (if any) of the following statements about the Normal distribution is CORRECT?
   A Approximately 1% of the observations from a Normal distribution lie outside the mean ± 1SD.
   B Approximately 5% of the observations from a Normal distribution lie outside the mean ± 1SD.
   C Approximately 10% of the observations from a Normal distribution lie outside the mean ± 1SD.
   D Approximately 32% of the observations from a Normal distribution lie outside the mean ± 1SD.
   E Approximately 95% of the observations from a Normal distribution lie outside the mean ± 1SD

4.7 The systolic blood pressure in the population of middle-aged people is Normally distributed with a mean of 140 mmHg and a standard deviation of 10.

i) What is the approximate probability of having a systolic blood pressure of 120 mmHg or less?
   A 0.025
   B 0.05
   C 0.16
   D 0.32
   E 0.95

ii) What proportion of the population of middle-aged people have a systolic blood pressure between 130 and 150 mmHg?
   A 0.95
   B 0.68
   C 0.32
   D 0.16
   E 0.90

4.8 The birthweight of babies in the population is Normally distributed with a mean of 3.5 kg and a standard deviation of 0.5 kg.

i) What is the probability of giving birth to a baby weighing more than 3.5 kg?
- **A** 0.025
- **B** 0.05
- **C** 0.5
- **D** 0.75
- **E** 0.95

ii) What is the approximate probability of giving birth to a baby weighing more than 4.0 kg?
- **A** 0.025
- **B** 0.05
- **C** 0.16
- **D** 0.32
- **E** 0.95

iii) What is the approximate probability of giving birth to a baby weighing more than 4.5 kg?
- **A** 0.025
- **B** 0.05
- **C** 0.16
- **D** 0.32
- **E** 0.95

5   Populations, Samples, Standard Errors and Confidence Intervals

Medical Statistics: A Textbook for the Health Sciences, Fifth Edition. Stephen J. Walters, Michael J. Campbell, and David Machin.
© 2021 John Wiley & Sons Ltd. Published 2021 by John Wiley & Sons Ltd.
Companion website: www.wiley.com/go/walters/medicalstatistics

Summary

In this chapter the concepts of a population and a population parameter are described. The sample from a population is used to provide the estimates of the population parameters. The standard error is introduced and methods for calculating confidence intervals for population means for continuous data having a Normal distribution and for discrete data which follow Binomial or Poisson distributions are given.

5.1 Populations

In the statistical sense a *population* is a theoretical concept used to describe an entire group of individuals in whom we are interested. Examples are the population of all patients with diabetes mellitus, or the population of all middle-aged men. Parameters are quantities used to describe characteristics of such populations. Thus, the proportion of diabetic patients with nephropathy, or the mean serum potassium of middle-aged men, are characteristics describing the two populations. Generally, it is costly and labour intensive to study the entire population. Therefore, we collect data on a *sample* of individuals from the population who we believe are *representative* of that population, that is, they have similar characteristics to the individuals in the population. We then use them to draw conclusions, technically make inferences, about the population as a whole. The process is represented schematically in Figure 5.1. So, samples are taken from populations

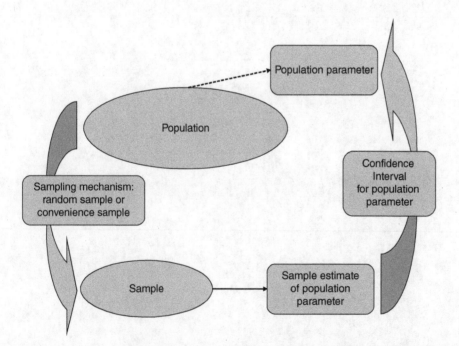

Figure 5.1 Taking a sample from the population and using the sample to estimate a population parameter.

Table 5.1 Population parameters and sample statistics.

	Population parameter	Sample statistic
Mean	μ	$\bar{x}$
Standard deviation	σ	s
Proportion	π	p
Rate	λ	r

to provide estimates of population parameters. Some common population parameters and their corresponding sample statistics or estimates are described in Table 5.1.

It is important to note that although populations are unique, samples are not, as more than one sample from the target population could be taken. Thus, for middle-aged men, there is only one (true) reference range for serum potassium. However, one investigator taking a random sample from a population of healthy middle-aged men and measuring their serum potassium may obtain a different reference range from another investigator who takes a different random sample from the same population of such men. By studying a sample of only some of the population we have introduced a sampling error. In this chapter we show how to use the theoretical probability distributions, outlined in Chapter 4, to quantify this error.

5.2   Samples

In some circumstances the sample may consist of all the members of a specifically defined population. For practical reasons, this is only likely to be the case if the population of interest is relatively small. If all members of the population can be assessed, then the *estimate* of the parameter concerned is derived from information obtained on all members and so its value will be the population parameter itself. In this idealised situation we know all about the population as we have examined all its members and the parameter is estimated with no bias. The dotted arrow in Figure 5.1 connecting the population ellipse to population parameter box illustrates this. However, this situation will rarely be the case so, in practice, we take a sample which is often much smaller in size than the population under study.

Ideally, we should aim for a *random sample*. A list of all individuals from the population is drawn up (the *sampling frame*), and individuals are selected randomly from this list, that is, every possible sample of a given size in the population has an equal chance of being chosen. Sometimes, there may be difficulty in constructing this list or we may have to 'make-do' with those subjects who happen to be available or what is termed a *convenience sample*. Essentially, if we take a random sample then we obtain an unbiased estimate of the corresponding population parameter, whereas a convenience sample may provide a biased estimate but by how much we will not know. The different types of sampling are described more fully in Chapter 14.

5.3 The Standard Error

Standard Error of the Mean

So how good is the sample mean as an estimate of the true population mean? To answer this question we need to assess the uncertainty of our single sample mean. How can we do this? We shall use the birthweight data from the O'Cathain et al. (2002) study. In Figure 4.9 of Chapter 4 we showed that the birthweights of 3226 new-born babies are approximately Normally distributed with a mean of 3.39 kg and a standard deviation of 0.55 kg. Let us assume for expository purposes that this distribution of birthweights is the whole population. Obviously, the real population would be far larger than this and consist of the birthweights of millions of babies.

Suppose we take a random sample from this population and calculate the sample mean. This information then provides us with *our* estimate of the population mean. However, a different sample *may* give us a different estimate of the population mean. So, if we take (say) 100 samples all of the same size, $n = 4$, we would get a spread of sample means which we can display visually in a dot plot or histogram like that in the top panel of Figure 5.2. These sample means range from as low as 2.6 to as high as 4.1 kg, whereas if we had taken samples of size $n = 16$ the range is less from 2.9 to 3.7 kg. This is because the mean from the larger sample absorbs or dilutes the effect of very small or very large observations in the sample more than does a sample of a smaller size which contains such observations.

The variability of these sample means gives us an indication of the uncertainty attached to the estimate of the population mean when taking only a single sample – very uncertain when the sample size is small to much less uncertainty when the sample size is large. Figure 5.2 clearly

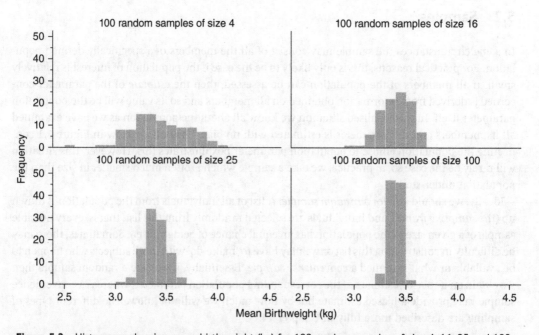

Figure 5.2 Histograms showing mean birthweight (kg) for 100 random samples of size 4, 16, 25 and 100.

shows that the spread or variability of the sample means reduces as the sample size increases. In fact, in turns out that sample means have the following properties.

Properties of the Distribution of Sample Means

The mean of all the sample means will be the same as the population mean.

The standard deviation of all possible sample means is known as the standard error (SE) of the mean or SEM.

Given a large enough sample size, the distribution of sample means, will be roughly Normal regardless of the distribution of the variable.

The standard error or variability of the sampling distribution of the mean is measured by the standard deviation of the estimates. If we know the population standard deviation, σ, then the standard error of the mean is given by SEM $= \sigma/\sqrt{n}$. In reality, an investigator will only complete a study once (although it may be repeated for confirmatory purposes by others) so this single study provides a single sample mean, $\bar{x}$, and this is our best (and only) estimate of μ. The same sample also provides s, the standard deviation of the observations, as an estimate of σ. So, with a *single* study, the investigator can then estimate the standard deviation of the distribution of the means by SEM $= s/\sqrt{n}$ without having to repeat the study at all.

Properties of Standard Errors

The standard error is a measure of the precision of a sample estimate. It provides a measure of how far from the true value in the population the sample estimate is likely to be. All standard errors have the following interpretation:

- A large standard error indicates that the estimate is imprecise.
- A small standard error indicates that the estimate is precise.
- The standard error is reduced, that is, we obtain a more precise estimate, if the size of the sample is increased.

Worked Example – Standard Error of a Mean – Birthweight of Preterm Infants
Simpson (2004) reported the birthweights of 98 infants who were born prematurely, for which $n = 98, \bar{x} = 1.31$ kg, $s = 0.42$ kg and the SEM often written SE$(\bar{x}) = 0.42/\sqrt{98} = 0.04$ kg. The standard error provides a measure of the precision of our sample estimate of the population mean birthweight. We would expect that means of repeated samples will have a Normal distribution with mean $= 1.31$ kg and a standard deviation of 0.042 kg.

5.4 The Central Limit Theorem

It is important to note that the distribution of the sample means will be nearly Normally distributed, whatever the distribution of the measurement amongst the individuals, and will get closer to a

Normal distribution as the sample size increases. Technically the fact that we can estimate the standard error from a single sample derives from what is known as the *Central Limit Theorem* and this important property enables us to apply the techniques we describe to a wide variety of situations.

To illustrate this, we will use the random number table Table T5 in the appendix. In this table each digit (0–9) is equally likely to appear and cannot be predicted from any combination of other digits. The first 15 digits (in sets of 5) read 94 071, 63 090, 23 901. Assume that our population consists of all the 10 digits (0–9) in a random numbers table. Figure 5.3 shows the population distribution of these random digits, which is clearly not Normal, (in fact it is the Uniform distribution of Section 4.7). Each digit has a frequency of 10%. The population mean value is 4.5.

Suppose we take a random sample of five digits from this distribution and calculate their mean and repeat this 500 times. So, for example, reading across the first row of Table T5, the means would be 4.2, 3.6, 3.0, etc. Each of these is an estimate of the population value. How would these sample means (of size five) be distributed? One can imagine that mean values close to 0 or 9 are very unlikely, since one would need a run of five 0s or five 9s. However, values close to 4.5 are quite likely. Figure 5.4 shows the distribution of the means of these random numbers for different sized samples. The distribution for samples of size five is reasonably symmetric but well spread out. As we take means of size 50, the distributions become more symmetric and Normally distributed.

The important point is that *whatever* the parent distribution of a variable, the distribution of the sample means will be nearly Normal, as long as the samples are large enough. Furthermore, as *n* gets larger the distribution of the sample means will become closer and closer to Normal. In practice the sample size restriction is not an issue when the parent distribution is unimodal and not particularly asymmetric (as in our example), as even for a sample size as small as 10, the distribution is close to Normal.

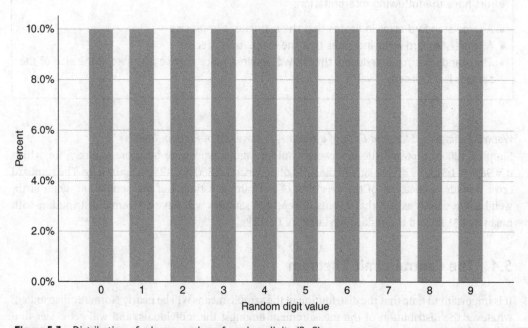

Figure 5.3 Distribution of a large number of random digits (0–9).

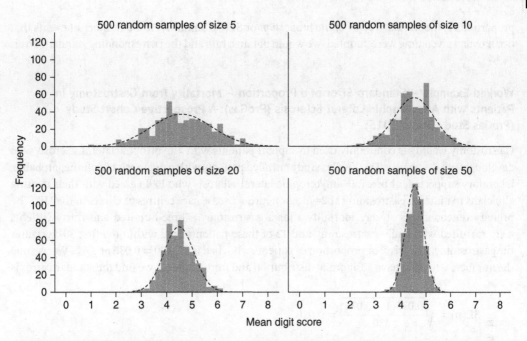

Figure 5.4 Observed distributions of the means of 500 random samples of size 5, 10, 20 and 50 taken from the distribution of random digits 0–9.

5.5 Standard Errors for Proportions and Rates

Any estimate of a parameter obtained from data has a standard error and Table 5.2 gives formulae for means, proportions and rates. For example we may be interested in the proportion of individuals in a population who possess some characteristic, such as having a disease. Having taken a sample of size n from the population, suppose r individuals have a particular characteristic. Our best estimate, p, of the population proportion, π, is given by $p = r/n$. If we were to take repeated samples of size n from our population and plot the estimates of the proportion as a histogram, then, provided $0.1 < \pi < 0.9$ and $n > 10$ the resulting sampling distribution of the proportion would approximate a Normal distribution with mean value, π. The standard deviation of this distribution of estimated

Table 5.2 Population parameters of the Normal, Binomial and Poisson distributions, their estimates and the associated standard errors (SE) for a single group.

Distribution	Parameters	Population values	Sample estimate	Standard error (SE)
Normal	Mean	μ	$\bar{x}$	$\dfrac{s}{\sqrt{n}}$
Binomial	Proportion	π	p	$\sqrt{\dfrac{p(1-p)}{n}}$
Poisson	Rate	λ	r	$\sqrt{\dfrac{r}{n}}$

proportions is the *standard error of the proportion* or SE(*p*). Similarly, if the number of events that occur over a given time were counted, we would obtain a rate and the corresponding standard error.

Worked Example – Standard Error of a Proportion – Mortality from Gastrostomy in Patients with Amyotrophic Lateral Sclerosis (ProGas): A Prospective Cohort Study (ProGas Study Group 2015)

Gastrostomy feeding is commonly used to support patients with amyotrophic lateral sclerosis who develop severe dysphagia. The ProGas study enrolled patients with a diagnosis of definite, probable, laboratory supported, or possible amyotrophic lateral sclerosis who had agreed with their treating clinicians to undergo gastrostomy at 24 motor neuron disease care centres or clinics in the UK. The primary outcome was 30 day mortality after a gastrostomy. Three-hundred and thirty patients were recruited who had a gastrostomy and 12 of these patients died within the first 30 days after the gastrostomy. The 'risk' or proportion of patients who died is 12/330 = 0.036 or 3.6%. We assume the numbers who died have a Binomial distribution and from Table 5.2 we find the standard error is

$$SE(p) = \sqrt{\frac{0.036(1 - 0.036)}{330}} = 0.010.$$

Worked Example – Standard Error of a Rate – Exacerbations in Patients with Cystic Fibrosis

Hind et al. (2019) looked at the incidence of IV treated exacerbations in patients with cystic fibrosis. As we noted in Chapter 4 they observed 60 IV treated exacerbations in 60 patients in six months of follow-up, a mean of 1.0 exacerbation per six months. With these data would anticipate an average of $r = 1.0 \times 2 = 2.0$ exacerbations per year. We assume the number of exacerbations follows a Poisson distribution and from Table 5.2 we find the standard error is

$$SE(r) = \sqrt{\left(\frac{2.0}{60}\right)} = 0.18.$$

Standard Deviation or Standard Error?

There is often confusion about the distinction between the standard error and the standard deviation. The standard error always refers to an estimate of a parameter. As such the estimate gets more precise as the number of observations gets larger, which is reflected by the standard error becoming smaller. If the term standard deviation is used in the same way, then it is synonymous with the standard error. However, if it refers to the observations then it is an estimate of the population standard deviation and does not get smaller as the sample size increases. The statistic, *s*, the calculation of which is described in Chapter 2, is an estimator of the population parameter σ, that is, the population standard deviation.

In summary, the standard deviation, *s*, is a measure of the variability between individuals with respect to the measurement under consideration, whereas the standard error, SE, is a measure of the uncertainty in the sample statistic, for example the mean, derived from the individual measurements.

5.6 Standard Error of Differences

When two groups are to be compared, then it is the standard error of the *difference* between groups that is important. The standard errors for the difference in means, proportions and rates are given in Table 5.3 in Section 5.10.

Worked Example – Standard Error of Difference in Means – Corn Size

Farndon et al. (2013) report the results of a randomised controlled trial that investigated the effectiveness of salicylic acid plasters compared with usual scalpel debridement for treatment of foot corns. One of the secondary outcomes for the trial was the size of the index corn (in mm) three months post-randomisation. Further suppose such measurements can be assumed to follow a Normal distribution. The results from the 189 patients are expressed using the group means and standard deviations (SDs) as follows:

$$n_{\text{Plaster}} = 95, \bar{x}_{\text{Plaster}} = 1.7, SD(x_{\text{Plaster}}) = s_{\text{Plaster}} = 1.6;$$

$$n_{\text{Scalpel}} = 94, \bar{x}_{\text{Scalpel}} = 2.7, SD(x_{\text{Scalpel}}) = s_{\text{Scalpel}} = 2.3.$$

From these data $d = \bar{x}_{\text{Plaster}} - \bar{x}_{\text{Scalpel}} = 1.7-2.7 = -1.0$ mm (i.e. a reduction of 1.0 mm in the size of the index corn in the plaster group compared to the scalpel treated control group and the corresponding standard error from Table 5.3 is, $SE(d) = \sqrt{\dfrac{1.6^2}{95} + \dfrac{2.3^2}{94}} = 0.29$.

Worked Example – Difference in Proportions –Haemorrhoid Recurrence at One Year (HubBLe Trial)

The results of a randomised controlled trial conducted by Brown et al. (2016) to assess the effect of haemorrhoidal artery ligation (HAL) surgery (intervention) compared with rubber band ligation (RBL) surgery (control) in patients with grade II–III haemorrhoids are summarised in Table 5.4. The primary outcome was recurrence of haemorrhoids at one year.

The corresponding proportions of patients who had a haemorrhoid recurrence with 12 months of the surgical treatment is $p_{\text{HAL}} = 48/161 = 0.298$ and $p_{\text{RBL}} = 87/176 = 0.494$. The difference in the

Table 5.3 Population parameters of the Normal, Binomial and Poisson distributions, their estimates and the associated standard errors (SE) for comparing two groups.

Distribution	Parameter	Population value	Estimated difference	SE (difference)
Normal	Mean	$\mu_1 - \mu_2$	$\bar{x}_1 - \bar{x}_2$	$\sqrt{\dfrac{s_1^2}{n_1} + \dfrac{s_2^2}{n_2}}$
Binomial	Proportion	$\pi_1 - \pi_2$	$p_1 - p_2$	$\sqrt{\dfrac{p_1(1-p_1)}{n_1} + \dfrac{p_2(1-p_2)}{n_2}}$
Poisson	Rate	$\lambda_1 - \lambda_2$	$r_1 - r_2$	$\sqrt{\dfrac{r_1}{n_1} + \dfrac{r_2}{n_2}}$

Source: data from Brown et al. 2016.

Table 5.4 Haemorrhoid recurrence rates, in HAL and RBL groups, at 12 months after the surgical procedure in patients with grade II–III haemorrhoids (Brown et al. 2016).

Haemorrhoid	HAL intervention		RBL control	
Recurrence	*n*		*n*	
Yes	48	(29.8%)	87	(49.4%)
No	113	(70.2%)	89	(50.6%)
Total	161		176	

HAL: haemorrhoidal artery ligation; RBL: rubber band ligation.

proportion of patients with a recurrence on the HAL intervention treatment compared to the RBL control treatment is $p_{HAL} - p_{RBL} = 0.298 - 0.494 = -0.196$ (i.e. a reduction in the proportion with recurrence in the HAL treated intervention group compared to the RBL treated control group). Finally, from Table 5.3 the standard error of this difference is:

$$\text{SE}(p_{HAL} - p_{RBL}) = \sqrt{\frac{0.298(1-0.298)}{161} + \frac{0.494(1-0.494)}{176}} = 0.052.$$

5.7 Confidence Intervals for an Estimate

Confidence Interval for a Mean

The sample mean, proportion or rate is the best estimate we have of the true population mean, proportion or rate. We know that the distribution of these parameter estimates from many samples of the same size will roughly be Normal. As a consequence, we can construct a confidence interval – a range of values in which we are confident the true population value of the parameter will lie. A confidence interval defines a range of values within which our population parameter is likely to lie. Such an interval for the population mean μ is defined by

$$\bar{x} - 1.96 \times \text{SE}(\bar{x}) \text{ to } \bar{x} + 1.96 \times \text{SE}(\bar{x})$$

and, in this case, is termed a 95% confidence interval as it includes the multiplier 1.96. Figure 5.5 illustrates that 95% of the distribution of sample means lies within ±1.96 standard errors (the *standard deviation* of *this* distribution) of the population mean.

A confidence interval gives the values most compatible with the data, given the assumptions. However, it does not mean that values outside the confidence interval are incompatible with the data; they are just less compatible. In fact, as Figure 5.5 shows values just outside the interval do not differ substantively from those just inside the interval. It is thus wrong to claim that an interval shows all possible values. Not all values inside the confidence interval are equally compatible with the data, given the assumptions. In Figure 5.5, the point estimate is the most compatible value, and values near it are more compatible than those near the lower and upper limits.

In strict terms the confidence interval is a range of values that is likely to cover the true but unknown population mean value, μ. The confidence interval is based on the concept of repetition of the study under consideration. Thus, if the study were to be repeated 100 times, of the 100

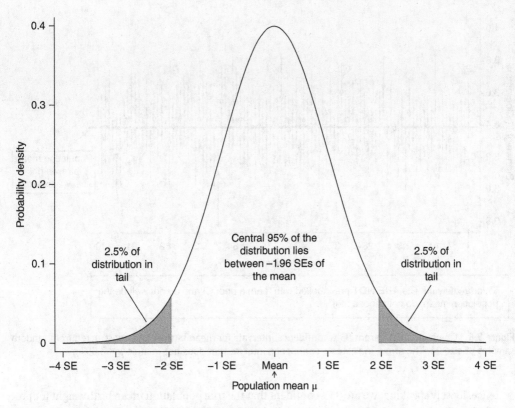

Figure 5.5 Sampling distribution of the sample mean.

resulting 95% confidence intervals, we would expect 95 of these to include the population parameter. Consequently, a reported confidence interval from a particular study *may* or *may not* include
the actual population parameter value of concern.

Figure 5.6 illustrates some of the possible 95% confidence intervals that could be obtained
from different random samples of 25 babies from the 3226 babies whose birthweight data
was recorded by O'Cathain et al. (2002). Ninety-four (94%) of these 100 confidence intervals
contain the population mean birthweight of 3.39 kg but 6 (6%) do not. This is close to what
we would expect – that the 95% confidence interval will *not* include the true population mean
5% of the time.

In an actual study, only *one* 95% confidence interval is obtained, and we would never know
without detailed further study whether, within it, it included the true population mean value.

Worked Example – Confidence Interval for a Mean – Birthweights of Pre-term Infants
Simpson (2004) reported the mean birthweight of 98 infants who were born prematurely as $\bar{x} =$
1.31 kg with $(\bar{x}) = 0.42/\sqrt{98} = 0.04$ kg. From these the 95% confidence interval for the population
mean is

$$1.31 - (1.96 \times 0.04) \text{ to } 1.31 + (1.96 \times 0.04)$$

or 1.23 to 1.39 kg.

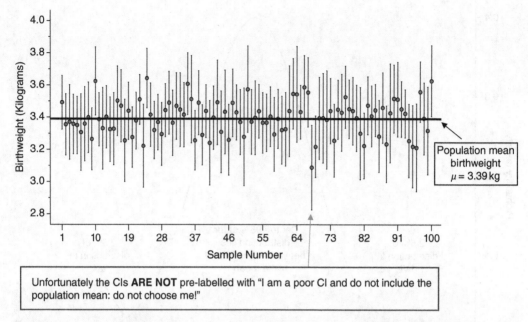

Figure 5.6 One hundred different 95% confidence intervals for mean birthweight constructed from random samples of size 25. The arrow indicates a confidence interval that does not include μ = 3.39 kg.

Hence, loosely speaking, we are 95% confident that the true population mean birthweight for pre-term infants lies between 1.23 and 1.39 kg. Our best estimate is provided by the sample mean of 1.31 kg. We could say our results suggest a mean birthweight of 1.31 kg for pre-term infants (the observed or point-estimate), is most compatible with the data. However, mean birthweights ranging from 1.23 to 1.39 kg are also reasonably compatible with our data, given the assumptions used in calculating the confidence interval.

Strictly speaking, it is incorrect to say that there is a probability of 0.95 that the population mean birthweight lies between 1.23 and 1.39 kg as the population mean is a fixed number and not a random variable and therefore has no probability attached to it. However, most statisticians, including us, often describe confidence intervals in that way. The value of 0.95 is really the probability that the limits calculated from a random sample, of size 98 from a population of premature babies, will include the population value. For 95% of the calculated confidence intervals it will be true to say that the population mean, μ, lies within this interval. The problem is, as Figure 5.6 shows, with a single study we just do not know which one of these 100 intervals in Figure 5.6 we will obtain and hence we will not know if it includes μ. So, we usually interpret a confidence interval as the range of values within which we are 95% confident that the true population mean lies.

Confidence Interval for a Proportion

Since a proportion, p, is a mean of a series of 0s and 1s, we can use a similar expression for a confidence interval for π as we did for μ with corresponding changes to the estimated parameter and the associated standard error. The Central Limit Theorem will assure Normality. The standard error is given in Table 5.2 and so the confidence interval is just the estimate $\pm 1.96 \times SE$ once more.

Example from the Literature – Confidence Interval for a Proportion –Gastrostomy in Patients with Amyotrophic Lateral Sclerosis (ProGas)

The ProGas study reported that 12 patients out of 330 died within the first 30 days after a gastrostomy giving the death rate as $p = 12/330 = 0.036$, $SE(p) = 0.016$ and a 95% confidence interval for π as $0.036 - (1.96 \times 0.01)$ to $0.036 + (1.96 \times 0.01)$ or 0.016–0.057, that is, from 1.6 to 5.7%, or 2 to 6% after rounding.

We are 95% confident that the true population proportion of amyotrophic lateral sclerosis patients with a gastrostomy who die within the first 30 days of gastrostomy surgery lies between 2 and 6% and our best estimate is a death rate of 4%.

For technical reasons, this expression given for a confidence interval for π is an approximation and is referred to as the *traditional* approach. It is also only in situations in which reasonable agreement exists between the shape of the Binomial distribution and the Normal distribution (see Chapter 4) that we would use the confidence interval expression just given. The approximation will usually be quite good provided π is not too close to 0 or 1, situations in which either almost none or nearly all of the patients respond. The approximation improves with increasing sample size n.

If n is small, however, or π close to 0 or 1, the disparity between the Normal and Binomial distributions with the same mean and standard deviation, similar to those illustrated in Figure 4.2, increases and the Normal distribution can no longer be used to approximate the Binomial distribution.

The preferred or *recommended* method described by Altman et al. (2000), and given in the Section 5.10, for calculating a confidence interval for a single proportion has better statistical properties than the traditional method just given. For the ProGas study the 95% confidence interval, from the recommended method, is from 0.021 to 0.062, that is, from 2.1 to 6.2%; and after rounding is from 2 to 6%. This is little different from the traditional approach.

Confidence Interval for a Rate

Provided the sample size is reasonably large we can use the general formula, estimate $\pm 1.96 \times SE$, for the confidence interval of a rate.

Worked Example – Confidence Interval for a Rate – Exacerbations in Patients with Cystic Fibrosis

In the example from Hind et al. (2019) the estimated exacerbation rate per year was $r = 2.00$ with $SE(r) = 0.18$. Therefore, the 95% confidence interval for the population rate λ is $2.00 - (1.96 \times 0.18)$ to $2.00 + (1.96 \times 0.18)$ or 1.65 to 2.35 exacerbations per year.

5.8 Confidence Intervals for Differences

To calculate a confidence interval for a difference in means, for example $\delta = \mu_1 - \mu_2$, the same structure for the confidence interval of a single mean is used but with $\bar{x}$ replaced by $\bar{x}_1 - \bar{x}_2$ and $SE(\bar{x})$ replaced by $SE(\bar{x}_1 - \bar{x}_2)$. Algebraic expressions for these standard errors are given in Table 5.3. Thus the 95% confidence interval is given by

$$(\bar{x}_1 - \bar{x}_2) - 1.96 \times SE(\bar{x}_1 - \bar{x}_2) \text{ to } (\bar{x}_1 - \bar{x}_2) + 1.96 \times SE(\bar{x}_1 - \bar{x}_2).$$

Example from the Literature – Confidence Interval for the Difference Between Two Means – Corn Size at Three Months

In the study by Farndon et al. (2013) described earlier there was a reduction in corn size at three months between the corn plaster intervention treated and usual care scalpel control group of 1.0 mm, with standard error 0.29 mm. Thus a 95% confidence interval is

$$1.0 - (1.96 \times 0.29) \text{ to } 1.0 + (1.96 \times 0.29)$$

which is 0.4 to 1.6 mm.

Therefore, we are 95% confident that true population mean difference in corn size between the corn plaster and scalpel treated groups lies somewhere between 0 4 and 1.6 mm, but our best estimate is 1.0. It is therefore plausible that the corn plaster intervention could reduce the corns size, at a three month follow-up, by as little as 0.4 or by as much as 1.6 mm more than scalpel.

Similar changes are needed when calculating a confidence interval for the difference between two proportions, $\pi_1 - \pi_2$, and between two rates, $\lambda_1 - \lambda_2$. Provided the sample sizes in the two groups are large, this method of calculating a confidence interval can be adapted for the comparison of two proportions with appropriate changes.

Worked Example – Confidence Interval for Difference Between Two Proportions – Haemorrhoid Recurrence at One Year (HubBLe Trial)

In the study by Brown et al. (2016) described in Table 5.4 the difference in recurrence proportions was 0.196, with SE = 0.052. Thus the 95% confidence interval for the true difference in proportions is given by 0.196 – (1.96 × 0.052) to 0.196 + (1.96 × 0.052) or 0.094 to 0.298.

Therefore, we are 95% confident that the true population estimate of the effect of this intervention lies somewhere between 0.094 (9.4%) and 0.298 (29.8%) but our best estimate is 0.196 (19.6%). These data are therefore consistent with the HAL intervention reducing (improving) the haemorrhoid recurrence rate over control by between 9 and 30%, with a best estimate of a 20% reduction.

5.9 Points When Reading the Literature

Some authors (and with more than 800 signatories) have suggested that we rename confidence intervals as 'compatibility intervals' and 'interpret them in a way that avoids over-confidence' (Amrhein et al. 2019). In particular, they recommend that 'Authors describe the practical implications of all values inside the confidence interval, especially the observed effect (or point estimate) and the lower and upper limits. In doing so, they should remember that all the values between the interval's limits are reasonably compatible with the data, given the statistical assumptions used to compute the interval. Therefore, singling out one particular value (such as the null value) in the interval as "shown" makes no sense'.

When interpreting a confidence interval we are interested in three main issues.

1) How wide is the confidence interval?
   A wide interval shows that the estimate is imprecise; a narrow interval shows a more precise estimate. The width of the confidence interval is determined by the size of the standard error, which in turn depends on the sample size and, when considering a quantitative numerical variable, the variability of the data. Therefore, small studies on data with a wide range of values will give wider confidence intervals than larger studies on less variable data.

2) What clinical implications can be drawn from the interval?
   The upper and lower limits of the interval provide a means of judging whether the results are clinically or practically important.
3) Does the interval include any values of particular interest?
   We can check whether a hypothesised value for the population parameter falls with the estimated confidence interval. If so, then our results are consistent with this hypothesised value. If the confidence interval excludes our hypothesised value, then we have little evidence for the hypothesised value being the true population parameter.

---

1) When authors give the background information to a study they often quote figures of the form $a \pm b$. Although it is usual that a represents the value of the sample mean, it is not always clear what b is. When the intent is to describe the variability found in the sample then b should be the SD. When the intent is to describe the precision of the mean then b should be the SE. This $\pm$ method of presentation tends to cause confusion and should be avoided.
2) A useful mnemonic to decide which measure of variability to use is: 'If the purpose is *descrip*tive use standard *d*eviation, if the purpose is *e*stimation, use the standard *e*rror'.
3) What is the population from which the sample was taken? Are there any possible sources of bias that may affect the estimates of the population parameters?
4) Have reference ranges been calculated on a random sample of healthy volunteers? If not, how does this affect your interpretation? Is there any good reason why a random sample was not taken?
5) Have confidence intervals been presented? Has the confidence level been specified?
6) Has a Normal approximation been used to calculate confidence intervals for a Binomial proportion or Poisson rate? If so, is this justified?

5.10 Technical Details

Standard Errors

More Accurate Confidence Intervals for a Proportion

To use this method we first need to calculate three quantities:

$$A = 2r + z^2; B = z\sqrt{z^2 + 4r(1 - p)}; \text{ and, } C = 2(n + z^2)$$

where z is as before the appropriate value, $z_{1-\alpha/2}$, from the Standard Normal distribution of Table T1. Then the recommended confidence interval for the population proportion is given by:

$$\frac{(A - B)}{C} \text{ to } \frac{(A + B)}{C}.$$

When there are no observed events, $r = 0$ and hence $p = 0/n = 0$ (0%), the recommended confidence interval simplifies to 0 to $\dfrac{z^2}{(n + z^2)}$, whilst when $r = n$ so that $p = 1$ (100%), the interval becomes $\dfrac{n}{(n + z^2)}$ to 1.

Another approximation, for a rate, when there are no events is that the upper limit of the rate is $3/n$ (known unsurprisingly as the '$3/n$ rule') (Eypasch et al. 1995). This can be very useful for a quick approximation and can be used to help determine a sample size. For example, if an investigator was comparing two devices and found no difference in a binary outcome 100 patients, then the upper 95% limit of any difference will be 3/100, i.e. 3%. If, on the other hand the investigator wanted to know how many patients to investigate so that, if there were no differences found, they could be 95% sure the difference was no greater than 10% then they would require $3/0.1 = 30$ subjects, each tested on both devices.

Worked Example – Confidence Interval for a Proportion – Gastrostomy in Patients with Amyotrophic Lateral Sclerosis (ProGas)

The ProGas study reported that 12 patients out of 330 died with the first 30 days after gastrostomy. Here $p = 12/330 = 0.036$, $r = 12$ and $n = 330$. To calculate the recommended 95% confidence interval:

$$A = 2 \times 12 + 1.96^2 = 27.84;$$

$$B = 1.96 \times \sqrt{\left(1.96^2 + 4 \times 12 \times (1 - 0.036)\right)} = 13.87;$$

$$C = 2 \times \left(330 + 1.96^2\right) = 667.68.$$

Then the 95% confidence interval for the 30 day mortality or death rate in the population of patients in amyotrophic lateral sclerosis who have undergone a gastrostomy is

$$\frac{(27.84 - 13.87)}{667.68} = 0.021 \text{ to } \frac{(27.84 + 13.87)}{667.68} = 0.062$$

that is, from 2.1 to 6.2%.

5.11 Exercises

5.1 Which (if any) of the following statements about the standard error is CORRECT?
  A The standard error (of the mean) is a measure of the precision of the sample estimate of the mean.
  B If we take repeated samples (of the same size) from a population, calculate the sample mean, then the standard deviation of these sample means is known as the standard error.
  C A large standard error indicates the estimate is imprecise.
  D The standard error is reduced, if the size of the sample is increased.
  E The standard error (of the mean) is the square root of the sample standard deviation.

5.2 The mean birthweight of a sample of 100 babies is 3500 g with a standard deviation of 500 g. The standard error of the mean birthweight is:
  A 25 g
  B 50 g
  C 100 g
  D 500 g
  E 3500 g

5.3   The mean birthweight of a sample of 25 babies is 3500 g with a standard deviation of 500 g. The standard error of the mean birthweight is:

A   25 g
B   50 g
C   100 g
D   500 g
E   3500 g

5.4   Which (if any) of the following statements about a 95% confidence interval for a mean is CORRECT?

A   The 95% confidence interval will include the true population mean.
B   The 95% confidence interval will include the observed mean.
C   If the study were repeated 100 times, of the 100 resulting 95% confidence intervals for the mean, we would expect 95 of these to include the true population mean.
D   There is a probability of 0.95 that the true population mean lies between the lower and upper limits of the confidence interval.
E   A 95% confidence interval is a range of values which will include the true population mean for 90% of possible samples.

5.5   The mean birthweight of sample of 100 babies is 3500 g with a standard deviation of 500 g. Thus an approximate 95% confidence interval for the mean birthweight is:

A   3000 to 4000 g
B   3100 to 3900 g
C   3300 to 3700 g
D   3400 to 3600 g
E   3450 to 3550 g

5.6   The mean birthweight of sample of 25 babies is 3500 g with a standard deviation of 500 g. Thus an approximate 95% confidence interval for the mean birthweight is:

A   3000 to 4000 g
B   3100 to 3900 g
C   3300 to 3700 g
D   3400 to 3600 g
E   3450 to 3550 g

Farndon et al. (2013) report the results of a randomised controlled trial which investigated the effectiveness of salicylic acid plasters (Corn plasters) compared with usual scalpel debridement for treatment of foot corns. One of the secondary outcome measures was the size of the index corn (in mm) measured at 3, 6, 9 and 12 months post-randomisation. Table 5.5 shows the outcome data.

5.7   Table 5.5 reports that the 95% confidence interval for the comparison of mean corn size at 12 months between the corn plaster and scalpel groups is: −1.7 to −0.2 mm.

Which (if any) of the following statements is CORRECT?

A   The above 95% confidence interval definitely contains the true population mean difference in corn size at 12 months between the corn plaster and scalpel groups.
B   The 95% confidence interval is calculated as ±3 standard errors away from the mean difference.

C There is a probability of 0.95 that the population mean difference in corn size at 12 months between the corn plaster and scalpel groups lies between −1.7 and −0.2 mm.

D The 95% confidence interval does not contain the true population mean difference in corn size at 12 months between the corn plaster and scalpel groups.

E The above 95% confidence interval is likely to contain the true population mean difference in corn size at 12 months between the corn plaster and scalpel groups.

Table 5.5 Index corn size, in millimetres, over time by group.

Size of index corn (mm)	Corn plaster (*n* = 101)		Scalpel (*n* = 101)		Mean Difference	95% confidence interval		
	Mean	SD	Mean	SD		Lower	Upper	*P*-value
Baseline	3.9	(1.7)	3.8	(1.8)				
3 months	1.7	(1.5)	2.7	(2.3)	−1.0	−1.5	−0.5	
6 months	1.7	(1.6)	2.4	(2.2)	−0.7	−1.2	−0.2	
9 months	1.7	(1.6)	2.2	(2.1)	−0.5	−1.2	0.1	
12 months	1.3	(1.6)	2.3	(2.2)	−1.0	−1.7	−0.2	0.01

Source: Data from Farndon et al. (2013).

5.8 Table 5.5 reports that the 95% confidence interval for the comparison of mean corn size at six months between the corn plaster and scalpel groups is: −1.2 to −0.2 mm.

Which (if any) of the following statements about the 95% confidence interval is CORRECT?

A There is a probability of 0.05 that the population mean difference in corn size at six months between the corn plaster and scalpel groups lies between −1.2 and −0.2 mm.

B There is a probability of 0.95 that the population mean difference in corn size at six months between the corn plaster and scalpel groups lies between −1.2 and −0.2 mm.

C The 95% confidence interval does not contain the true population mean difference in corn size at six months between the Corn plaster and Scalpel groups.

D The 95% confidence interval contains the true population mean difference in corn size at six months between the corn plaster and scalpel groups.

E If we repeated the study 100 times, we would expect 95 of the resulting 95% confidence intervals to include the population mean difference in corn size at six months between the corn plaster and scalpel groups.

5.9 The PREeMPt study (Keen et al. 2018) aimed to investigate whether or not is was feasible to conduct a randomised controlled trial of pre-transplant exercise (prehabilitation) in patients with multiple myeloma awaiting autologous haematopoietic stem cell transplantation. One of the feasibility outcomes was the recruitment rate defined as the number of participants recruited per month.

The PreEMPt consented and recruited 23 participants in 13 months of recruitment at a single centre, a recruitment rate of 1.8 participants per month.

The approximate standard error of the monthly recruitment rate is:

A 0.37
B 0.28
C 1.50
D 1.81
E 2.05

5.10 The PreEMPt study consented and recruited 23 participants in 13 months of recruitment at a single centre, a recruitment rate of 1.8 participants per month.

The 95% confidence interval for the monthly recruitment rate is:

A −1.2 to 4.8
B −0.7 to 4.2
C 0.5 to 2.0
D 1.1 to 2.5
E 1.5 to 2.8

5.11 One of the secondary aims of the PreEMPt study was to assess the safety of the prehabilitation exercise programme. A serious adverse event was defined as any adverse event or adverse reaction that results in death, is life-threatening, required hospitalisation or prolongation of existing hospitalisation, results in persistent or significant disability or incapacity. There were no serious adverse events observed in the 23 participants during the prehabilitation exercise programme. Calculate a 95% confidence interval for the serious adverse event rate in the PreEMPt study.

The 95% confidence interval for the serious adverse event rate is:

A −14.3 to 14.3%
B 0.0 to 14.3%
C 0.5 to 14.0%
D 1.0 to 12.5%
E 1.5 to 12.5%

6 Hypothesis Testing, *P*-values and Statistical Inference

Medical Statistics: A Textbook for the Health Sciences, Fifth Edition. Stephen J. Walters, Michael J. Campbell, and David Machin.
© 2021 John Wiley & Sons Ltd. Published 2021 by John Wiley & Sons Ltd.
Companion website: www.wiley.com/go/walters/medicalstatistics

Summary

The main aim of statistical analysis is to use the information gained from a sample of individuals to make inferences or form judgements about the parameters (e.g. the mean) of a population of interest. This chapter will discuss two of the basic approaches to statistical analysis: estimation (with confidence intervals (CIs)) and hypothesis testing (with *P*-values). The concepts of the null hypothesis, statistical significance, the use of statistical tests, *P*-values and their relationship to CIs are introduced. The difficulties with the use and mis-interpretation of *P*-values are discussed.

6.1   Introduction

We have seen that, in sampling from a population which can be assumed to have a Normal distribution, the sample mean can be regarded as estimating the corresponding population mean μ. Similarly, s^2 estimates the population variance, σ^2. We therefore describe the distribution of the population with the information given by the sample statistics $\bar{x}$ and s^2. More generally, in comparing two populations, perhaps the population of subjects exposed to a particular hazard and the population of those who were not, two samples are taken, and their respective summary statistics calculated. We might wish to compare the two samples and ask: 'Could they both be regarded as coming from the same population?' That is, does the fact that some subjects have been exposed, and others not, influence the characteristic or variable we are observing? If it does not, then we view the two populations as if they were one with respect to the particular variable under consideration.

6.2   The Null Hypothesis

Statistical analysis is concerned not only with summarising data but also with investigating relationships. An investigator conducting a study usually has a theory in mind; for example, patients with diabetes may have raised blood pressure, or oral contraceptives may cause breast cancer. This theory is known as the study or research hypothesis or research question. However, it is impossible to prove most hypotheses; one can always think of circumstances which have not yet arisen under which a particular hypothesis may or may not hold. Thus, one might hold a theory that all Chinese children have black hair. Unfortunately, despite having observed 1000 or even 1 000 000 Chinese children and checked that they all have black hair this observation would not have proved the hypothesis. On the other hand, if only one fair-haired Chinese child is seen, the theory is disproved. Thus, there is a simpler logical setting for disproving hypotheses than for proving them. The converse of the research hypothesis is the null hypothesis. Examples are: diabetic patients *do not* have raised blood pressure, or oral contraceptives *do not* cause breast cancer. Such a hypothesis is usually phrased in the negative and that is why it is termed the null hypothesis, H_0. The converse of the study hypothesis is the null hypothesis.

Example: Distance Walked On an Endurance Shuttle Walking Test (ESWT) Before and After a Rehabilitation Programme in Patients with COPD (Waterhouse et al. 2010)

Chronic obstructive pulmonary disease (COPD) is the name for a collection of lung diseases including chronic bronchitis, emphysema and chronic obstructive airways disease. The damage to the lungs caused by COPD is permanent, but treatment can help slow down the progression of the condition. Treatments include pulmonary rehabilitation – a specialised programme of exercise and education. The Endurance Shuttle Walk Test (ESWT) is a standardised field test for the assessment of endurance capacity in patients with chronic lung disease. The ESWT is performed on a 10 m long course and allows people to walk at a steady pace equivalent to 85% of their maximal oxygen uptake. Patients are instructed to walk as long as possible at the speed that is dictated by an auditory signal. The test is ended when a patient is more than 0.5 m away from the marker before the signal was given on two successive shuttles, or when the patient has indicated they are too exhausted to carry on walking.

Figure 6.1 shows histograms of the results of ESWTs conducted in 161 patients with COPD recruited into a randomised controlled trial pre- and post- a six-week pulmonary-rehabilitation exercise programme as well as the difference (post − pre).

The research question here was likely to be: does an exercise programme (rehabilitation) change the distance walked of patients with COPD? Do not forget we are interested in the population of COPD patients. However, we have taken a sample of 161 which we study in order to make inferences about the population of interest. In this example the statistical null hypothesis, which is that there is no change in distance walked before and after exercise, is the opposite of the research hypothesis, which is that there is a change in distance walked before and after exercise.

Table 6.1 shows the distance walked during ESWTs pre- and post- an exercise programme in a selection of 13 of the 161 COPD patients. The data in Table 6.1 is an example of paired data since it arises from the same individual at different points in time. This generates a data set in which each data point in the before period is uniquely paired to a data point in the second after sample.

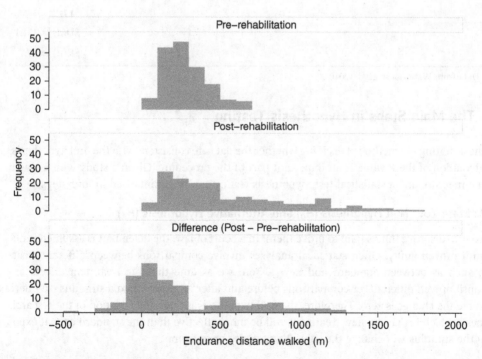

Figure 6.1 Histograms for the distance walked, in metres, on an ESWT in 161 COPD patients pre-, post-rehabilitation and the difference (post − pre) after a six-week pulmonary-rehabilitation exercise programme. (*Source:* data from Waterhouse et al. 2010).

Table 6.1 Distance walked, in metres, on an ESWT in (a sample of 13 out of 161) patients with COPD before and after a six-week duration exercise programme.

Subject (i)	Endurance distance walked (m)		Difference (d_i) (Post − Pre)
	Pre-rehabilitation	Post-rehabilitation	
1	240	480	240
2	460	700	240
3	100	160	60
4	180	240	60
5	240	510	270
6	420	960	540
7	160	170	10
8	560	1780	1220
9	140	260	120
10	320	400	80
159	290	570	280
160	470	1050	580
161	230	300	70
Mean			$\bar{d} = 251.6$
n			171
SD			$SD(d) = 351.1$
SE			$SE(\bar{d}) = 27.7$

Source: Data from Waterhouse et al. (2010).

6.3 The Main Steps in Hypothesis Testing

Hypothesis testing is a method of deciding whether the data are consistent with the null hypothesis. The calculation of the *P*-value is an important part of the procedure. Given a study with a single outcome measure and a statistical test, hypothesis testing can be summarised in four steps.

Step 1: State Your Null Hypothesis (H_0) and Alternative Hypothesis (H_A)

It is easier to disprove things than to prove them. In a court of law, the defendant is assumed innocent until proven guilty. Often statistical analyses involve comparisons between different treatments, such as between standard and new – here we assume that the treatment effects are equal until proven different; or comparisons before and after an exposure to a stimulus or – here we assume the change is zero. Therefore, the null hypothesis is often the negation of the research hypothesis which is that the new treatment will be more effective than the standard or that exposure to the stimulus will change the subject's response or outcome.

Step 2: Choose a Significance Level, α, for Your Test

For consistency we have to specify at the planning stage a value, α, so that once the study is completed and analysed, a *P*-value below this would lead to the null hypothesis (which is specified in step 1) being rejected. Thus, if the *P*-value obtained from a trial is $\leq \alpha$, then one rejects the null hypothesis and concludes that there is a statistically significant difference between treatments. On the other hand, if the *P*-value is $> \alpha$ then one does not reject the null hypothesis. Although the value of α is arbitrary, it is often taken as 0.05 or 5%.

P-value	
Small $\leq \alpha$	Large $> \alpha$
Your results are *unlikely* when the null hypothesis is true.	Your results are *likely* when the null hypothesis is true.

Step 3: Obtain the Probability of Observing Your Results, or Results More Extreme, if the Null Hypothesis is True (*P*-value)

First calculate a test statistic using your data (this reduces your data down to a single number or value). The general formula for a test statistic is:

$$\text{Test Statistic} = \frac{\text{Observed value} - \text{Hypothesised value}}{\text{Standard error (observed value)}}.$$

This test statistic value is then compared to a distribution that we expect if the null hypothesis is true (such as the Normal distribution with mean zero and standard deviation of one, or the *t*, chi-squared or *F*-distributions) to obtain a *P*-value.

Step 4: Use Your *P*-value to Make a Decision About Whether to Reject, or Not Reject, Your Null Hypothesis

We say that our results are statistically significant if the *P*-value is less than the significance level α, which is usually set at 5% or 0.05.

Example: Distance Walked on a 6MWT Before and After a Rehabilitation Programme
The four main steps for hypotheses testing with the distance walked before and after a rehabilitation programme are:

Step 1: State Your Null Hypothesis (*H*₀) and Alternative Hypothesis (*H*ₐ).

H_0: no difference (or change) in the mean distance walked in patients with COPD before and after exercise (note it is the difference in the population that is of interest – we would expect differences in individual patients), i.e. $\delta_{\text{Pair}} = 0$ m.

H_A: there is a difference (or change) in the mean distance walked in patients with COPD before and after exercise (could increase or decrease – two-sided), i.e. $\delta_{\text{Pair}} \neq 0$ m.

Note that in this case the data are paired (measurements on the same individual). Therefore, we are interested in the mean of the difference within an individual, since these differences are independent from one individual to another.

Step 2 Choose a Significance Level, α, for Your Test

Although the value of α is arbitrary, it is often taken as 0.05 or 5%.

Step 3 Obtain the Probability of Observing Your Results, or Results More Extreme, If the Null Hypothesis is True (*P*-value)

First calculate a test statistic using your data (reduce your data down to a single value). The general formula for a test statistic is:

$$\text{Test Statistic} = \frac{\text{Observed mean difference} - \text{Hypothesised mean difference}}{\text{Standard error (mean difference)}} = \frac{\bar{d} - 0}{\text{SE}(\bar{d})}.$$

If the change in distance walked, d, was calculated for each patient and if the null hypothesis is true that there is no effect of exercise on distance walked, then the mean of the $n = 161$ d's should be close to zero. The d's are termed the paired differences and are the basic observations of interest.

Now, if indeed the two populations of distances walked can be assumed each to have approximately Normal distributions, then $\bar{d}$ will also have a Normal distribution. This distribution will have its own mean δ and standard deviation σ, which are estimated by $\bar{d}$ and $\text{SE}(\bar{d})$ respectively. One can even go one step further, if the samples are large enough, and state that the ratio $\bar{d}/\text{SE}(\bar{d})$ will have an approximate Normal distribution with mean δ and a standard deviation of unity. If the null hypothesis were true, this distribution would have mean $\delta = 0$.

In Table 6.1 in the $n = 161$ patients with COPD, the sample paired mean difference in distance walked, $\bar{d}$, is 251.6 m, with a standard deviation, s, of 351.1 m and a standard error of $\text{SE}(\bar{d}) = s/\sqrt{n} = \frac{251.6}{\sqrt{161}} = 27.7$ m. The corresponding test statistic is $z = \frac{251.6 - 0}{27.7} = 9.1$.

The ratio of the mean to its standard error is more than nine standard deviations from the null hypothesis mean of zero. This is a very extreme observation and very unlikely to arise by chance since 99% of observations sampled from a Normal distribution with specified mean and standard deviation will be within three standard deviations of its centre. A value of δ greater than zero seems very plausible. It therefore seems very unlikely that the measurements come from a Normal distribution whose mean is in fact $\delta = 0$. There is strong evidence that δ differs from zero. As a consequence, the notion of no difference or change in outcome suggested by the null hypothesis is rejected. The conclusion is that the exercise programme results in increases in distances walked by COPD patients.

Formally, the test statistic, z, is compared to a distribution that we expect if the null hypothesis is true (such as the Normal distribution with mean zero and standard deviation unity) to obtain a *P*-value. Using Table T1 in the appendix with $Z = 9.10$, a *P*-value <0.001 is obtained (the largest Z-value in the table is 3.59 with a *P*-value <0.0005). So, the probability of observing the test statistic (and our sample data) or more extreme is <0.001 or 1 in 1000, if the null hypothesis (of no change in distance walked) is true. This is a small value, so we are unlikely to observe this data if the null hypothesis is true. It should be noted that when comparing the means of small samples the *t* distribution (which is introduced in Chapter 7) rather than the Normal distribution is usually used.

6.4 Using Your *P*-value to Make a Decision About Whether to Reject, or Not Reject, Your Null Hypothesis

Hypothesis testing is a method of deciding whether the data are consistent with the null hypothesis. The calculation of the *P*-value is an important part of the procedure.

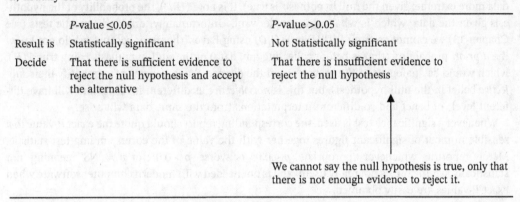

	P-value ≤0.05	P-value >0.05
Result is	Statistically significant	Not Statistically significant
Decide	That there is sufficient evidence to reject the null hypothesis and accept the alternative	That there is insufficient evidence to reject the null hypothesis

We cannot say the null hypothesis is true, only that there is not enough evidence to reject it.

It is important to distinguish between the (pre-set) significance level α and the P-value obtained after the study is completed. If one rejects the null hypothesis when it is in fact true, then one makes what is known as a *Type I error*. The significance level α is the probability of making a Type I error and is set *before* the test is carried out. The P-value is the result observed *after* the study is completed and is based on the observed result.

The term *statistically significant* is spread throughout the published medical literature. It is a common mistake to state that it is the probability that the null hypothesis is true as the null hypothesis is *either* true *or* it is false. The null hypothesis is not, therefore, 'true' or 'false' with a certain probability. However, it is common practice to assign probabilities to events, such as 'the chance of rain tomorrow is 30%'. So, in some ways, the P-value can be thought of as a measure of the strength of the belief in the null hypothesis.

The significance level is usually set at 5% or 0.05. This level is arbitrary and it is ridiculous to interpret the results of a study differently according to whether the P-value obtained was, say 0.055 or 0.045. These P-values should lead to similar conclusions, not diametrically opposed ones and a minor change to the data can easily shift the P-value by this amount or more. Statistical significance does not necessarily mean the result is clinically significant or important.

How to interpret P-values from a single test.

We can think of the P-values as indicating the strength of evidence but always keep in mind the size of the study being considered.

P-value	Interpretation
Greater than 0.10	Little or no evidence of a difference or a relationship[a]
Between 0.05 and 0.10	Very weak evidence of a difference or relationship
Between 0.01 and 0.05	Weak evidence of a difference or a relationship
Less than 0.01:	Strong evidence of a difference or relationship
Less than 0.001:	Very strong evidence of a difference or relationship.

[a]Although we have talked in terms of detecting differences in this chapter, the same principles arise when testing relationships as in Chapter 9 for example.
Source: Adapted from Bland (2000).

In Chapter 4 we discussed different concepts of probability. The *P*-value is a probability, and the concept in this instance is closest to the idea of a repeated sample. If we conducted a large number of similar studies and repeated the test each time, when the null hypothesis is true, then in the long run, the proportion of times the test statistic equals, or is greater than the observed value is the *P*-value.

In terms of the notation of Chapter 4 the *P*-value is equivalent to the probability of the data (*D*), given the null hypothesis is true (*H*), that is, $P(D|H)$ (strictly the probability of the observed data, or data more extreme; given the null hypothesis is true). It is not $P(H|D)$, the probability of the hypothesis given the data, which is what most people want. Unfortunately, unlike diagnostic tests (see Chapter 13) we cannot go from $P(D|H)$ to $P(H|D)$ using Bayes' theorem, because we do not know the *a priori* probability (that is before collecting any data) of the null hypothesis being true $P(H)$, which would be analogous to the prevalence of the disease. Some people try to quantify their *subjective* belief in the null hypothesis, but this is *not objective* as different investigators will have different levels of belief and so different interpretations from the same data will arise.

Whenever a significance test is used, the corresponding report should quote the exact *P*-value to a sensible number of significant figures together with the value of the corresponding test statistic. Merely reporting whichever appropriate, $p < 0.05$ or worse, $p > 0.05$, or $p =$ 'NS' meaning 'not statistically significant', is not really useful and is not needed with modern computer software when exact *P*-values are easily obtained.

Example – Interpreting a *P*-value – Distance Walked Before and After Exercise

In the example of examining the difference in distance walked before and after exercise in 161 patients with COPD the *P*-value was less than 0.001.

What Does *P* < 0.001 Mean?

Your results or ones more extreme are unlikely when the null hypothesis is true.

Is This Result Statistically Significant?

The result is statistically significant because the *P*-value is less than the significance level α set at 5% or 0.05.

You Decide?

That there is sufficient evidence to reject the null hypothesis and accept the alternative hypothesis that there is a difference (an increase) in the mean distance walked of COPD patients before and after rehabilitation.

A common misinterpretation of the *P*-value is that it is the probability of the data having arisen by chance or the probability that the observed effect is not a real one. The distinction between this incorrect definition and the true definition is the absence of the phrase when the null hypothesis is true. The omission of when the null hypothesis is true leads to the incorrect belief that it is possible to evaluate the probability of the observed effect being a real one. The observed effect in the sample is genuine, but we do not know what is true in the population. All we can do with this approach to statistical analysis is to calculate the probability of observing our data (or more extreme data) **when the null hypothesis is true.**

Summary of the Main Steps in Hypothesis Testing

1) State your null hypothesis (H_0).
   (*Statement you are looking to disprove*).
   State your alternative hypothesis (H_A).
2) Choose a *significance level*, α, of the test.
3) Conduct the study, observe the outcome and compute the probability of observing your results, or results more extreme, if the null hypothesis is true (*P*-value).
4) Use your *P*-value to make a decision about whether to reject, or not reject, your null hypothesis.

   That is if the *P*-value is less than or equal to α conclude that the data are not consistent with the null hypothesis. Whereas if the *P*-value is greater than α, do not reject the null hypothesis, and view it as 'not yet disproven'.

6.5   Statistical Power

Type I Error, Test Size and Significance Level

We stated that the second step in hypothesis testing, is to choose a value, α, so that once the study is completed and analysed, a *P*-value below this would lead to the null hypothesis being rejected. Thus, if the *P*-value obtained from a trial is $\leq \alpha$, then one rejects the null hypothesis and concludes that there is a statistically significant difference between treatments. On the other hand, if the *P*-value is $> \alpha$ then one does not reject the null hypothesis. This seems a clear-cut decision with no chance of making a wrong decision. However, as Figure 6.2 shows there are two possible errors when using a *P*-value to make a decision.

Even when the null hypothesis is in fact true there is still a risk of rejecting it. To reject the null hypothesis when it is true is to make a Type I error. Plainly the associated probability of rejecting the null hypothesis when it is true is equal to α. The quantity α is interchangeably termed the test size, significance level or probability of a Type I (or false-positive) error.

Type II Error and Power

A clinical trial of two treatments (intervention and control) could yield an observed difference d that would lead to a *P*-value $> \alpha$ even though the null hypothesis (that the population mean values for the two treatments μ_{Int} and μ_{Con} are equal) is really not true, that is, μ_{Int} is indeed not equal to μ_{Con}. In such a situation, we then accept (more correctly phrased as 'fail to reject') the null hypothesis although it is truly false. This is called a Type II (false-negative) error and the probability of this is denoted by β.

The probability of a Type II error is based on the assumption that the null hypothesis is not true, that is, $\delta = \mu_{Int} - \mu_{Con} \neq 0$. There are clearly many possible values of δ in this instance and each would imply a different alternative hypothesis, H_A, and a different value for the probability β.

The power is defined as one minus the probability of a Type II error, thus the power equals $1 - \beta$. That is, the *power* is the probability of obtaining a 'statistically significant' *P*-value when the null

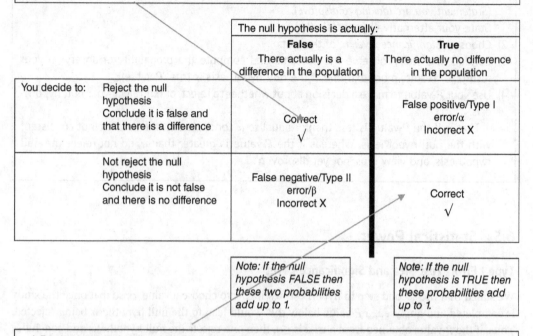

The probability of rejecting the null hypothesis when it is actually false is called the POWER of the study (Power = $1 - \beta$). It is the probability of concluding that there is a difference, when a difference truly exists.

	The null hypothesis is actually:	
	False	**True**
	There actually is a difference in the population	There actually no difference in the population
You decide to: Reject the null hypothesis Conclude it is false and that there is a difference	Correct ✓	False positive/Type I error/α Incorrect X
Not reject the null hypothesis Conclude it is not false and there is no difference	False negative/Type II error/β Incorrect X	Correct ✓

Note: If the null hypothesis FALSE then these two probabilities add up to 1.

Note: If the null hypothesis is TRUE then these probabilities add up to 1.

A P-value is the probability of obtaining your results or results more extreme, **if the null hypothesis is true**. It is the probability of committing a false positive error, that is, of rejecting the null hypothesis when it is fact true.

Figure 6.2 Possible errors arising when performing a hypothesis test.

Table 6.2 Relationship between Type I and Type II errors and significance tests.

Test statistically significant	Difference exists (H_A true)	Difference does not exist (H_0 true)
Yes	Power $(1-\beta)$	Type I error (α)
No	Type II error (β)	

hypothesis is truly false. The relationship between Type I and II errors and significance tests is given in Table 6.2.

These concepts of Type I error and Type II error parallel the concepts of sensitivity and specificity that we will discuss in Chapter 13. The Type I error is equivalent to the false positive rate (1 – specificity) and the Type II error is equivalent to the false negative rate (1 – sensitivity).

6.6 One-sided and Two-sided Tests

The *P*-value is the probability of obtaining a result at least as extreme as the observed result when the null hypothesis is true, and such extreme results can occur by chance equally often in either direction. We allow for this by calculating a two-sided *P*-value. In the vast majority of cases this is the correct procedure. In rare cases it is reasonable to consider that a real difference can occur in only one direction, so that an observed difference in the opposite direction must be due to chance. Here, the alternative hypothesis is restricted to an effect in one direction only, and it is reasonable to calculate a one-sided *P*-value by considering only one tail of the distribution of the test statistic. For a test statistic with a Normal distribution, the usual two-sided 5% cut-off point is 1.96, whereas the corresponding one-sided 5% cut-off value is 1.64.

One-sided tests are seldom appropriate. Even when we have strong prior expectations, for example that a new treatment cannot be worse than an old one, we cannot be sure that we are right. If we could be sure we would not need to conduct the study! If it is felt that a one-sided test really is appropriate, then this decision must be made *before* the data are collected; it must not depend on the observed outcome data from the study itself. In practice, what is often done is that a two-sided *P*-value is quoted, but the result is given more weight, in an informal manner, if the result goes in the direction that was anticipated.

6.7 Confidence Intervals (CIs)

All that we know from a hypothesis test is, for example, that there is a difference in the distance walked of COPD patients before and after exercise. It does not tell us what the difference is or how large the difference is. To answer this, we need to supplement the hypothesis test with an estimate and a CI, which will give us a range of values in which we are confident the true population mean difference will lie.

Simple statements in a study report such as '$p < 0.05$' or '$p = NS$' do not describe the results of a study well, and create an artificial dichotomy between significant and non-significant results. Statistical significance does not necessarily mean the result is clinically significant or of any practical importance. The *P*-value does not relate to the clinical importance of a finding, as it depends to a large extent on the size of the study. Thus, a large study may find small, unimportant, differences that are highly significant and a small study may fail to find important differences.

For example, a study into the effects of alcohol on health (GBD 2016, Alcohol Collaborators 2018) showed a statistically significant risk of drinking slightly more than the UK guidelines of 14 units per week. However as pointed out by David Spiegelhalter (https://medium.com/wintoncentre/the-risks-of-alcohol-again-2ae8cb006a4a) this does not indicate a clinically significant risk. About 914 people in 100 000 would die in a year if they did not drink, and this is raised to 918 in 100 000 for those that drank one alcoholic drink per day. Thus about 4 people in 100 000 would die in a year as a result of drinking one alcoholic drink per day. This is a very low risk, and other risks (such as driving a car) are much more hazardous.

Supplementing the hypothesis test with a CI will indicate the magnitude of the result and this will aid the investigators to decide whether the difference is of interest clinically (see Figure 6.3). The CI gives an estimate of the precision with which a statistic estimates a population value, which is

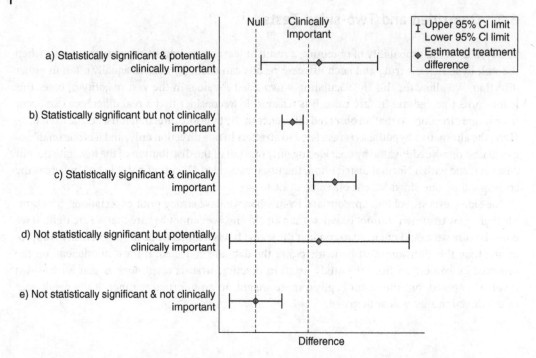

Figure 6.3 Use of confidence intervals (CIs) to help distinguish statistical significance from clinical importance.

useful information for the reader. This does not mean that one should not carry out statistical tests and quote *P*-values, rather that these results should supplement an estimate of an effect and a CI. Many medical journals now require papers to contain CIs where appropriate and not just *P*-values.

Example – Clinical Importance – Change in Distance Walked Before and After Exercise

The mean difference or change in distance walked before and after exercise, in the 161 COPD patients, was 251.6 m with a SD of 352.2 m. The standard error (of the mean difference) is $351.1 / \sqrt{161} = 27.7$ m and so the 95% CI is

$$251.6 - (1.96 \times 27.7) \text{ to } 251.6 + (1.96 \times 27.7)$$

or 197.3 to 305.9.

Therefore, we are 95% confident that the true population mean difference in distance walked lies somewhere between 197 and 306 m, but the best estimate we have is 252 m. Note that when calculating CIs for the mean in small samples, the *t* distribution rather than the Normal distribution is usually used (and this is described in the next chapter).

If we regard an increase or change in distance walked on the ESWT of 100 m or more as a clinically important difference or change in exercise capacity then Figure 6.4a, shows that the above result is both *clinically important* and *statistically significant*; as the CI excludes both the null value (of zero) and the clinically important value of 100 m. If the clinically important difference is changed to say 200 m, then the interpretation of the CIs changes as well. This situation corresponds to

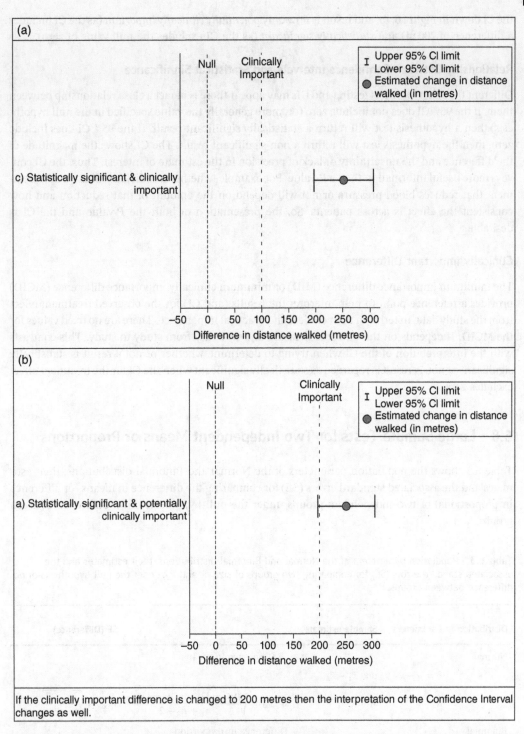

Figure 6.4 Distance walked example: clinical importance and statistical significance. (a) Clinically important difference of 100 m. (b) Clinically important difference of 200 m.

the CI down in Figure 6.4b; and result is now only *potentially clinically important* (as the CI includes a difference of 200 m) and *statistically significant* (as the CI excludes the null value of zero).

Relationship Between Confidence Intervals and Statistical Significance

Different though hypothesis testing and CIs may appear there is in fact a close relationship between them. If the 95% CI does not include zero (or, more generally the value specified in the null hypothesis) then a hypothesis test will return a statistically significant result. If the 95% CI does include zero, then the hypothesis test will return a non-significant result. The CI shows the magnitude of the difference and the uncertainty or lack of precision in the estimate of interest. Thus, the CI conveys more useful information than a *P*-value. For example, whether a clinician will use a new treatment that reduces blood pressure or not will depend on the amount of that reduction and how consistent the effect is across patients. So, the presentation of both the *P*-value and the CI is desirable.

Clinically Important Difference

The minimum importance difference (MID) or minimum clinically importance difference (MCID) provides a reference point to help interpret the results (and CI) for the observed treatment effect from the study data, in terms of their clinical and practical importance. There are no fixed values for the MCID. It depends on the outcome measure and will vary from study to study. This contrasts with the interpretation of the CI when trying to determine whether or not a result is statistically significant or not. A result is regarded as statistically significant when the CI for the treatment effect excludes zero.

6.8 Large Sample Tests for Two Independent Means or Proportions

Table 6.3 shows the population parameters of the Normal and Binomial distributions, their estimates and the associated standard errors (SE) for comparing the difference in means (or difference in proportions) of two independent groups under the null hypothesis of no difference between groups.

Table 6.3 Population parameters of the Normal and Binomial distributions, their estimates and the associated standard errors (SE) for comparing two groups of size n_1 and n_2, under the null hypothesis of no difference between groups.

Distribution	Parameters	Sample estimate		SE (Difference)
Normal		Difference in means		
	$\delta = \mu_1 - \mu_2$	$d = \bar{x}_1 - \bar{x}_2$		
	σ	s_1 and s_2	$s_{Pooled} = \sqrt{\dfrac{(n_1 - 1)s_1^2 + (n_2 - 1)s_2^2}{n_1 + n_2 - 2}}$	$s_{Pooled}\sqrt{\dfrac{1}{n_1} + \dfrac{1}{n_2}}$
Binomial		Difference in proportions		
	$\delta = \pi_1 - \pi_2$	$d = \bar{p}_1 - \bar{p}_2$	$p = \dfrac{n_1 p_1 + n_2 p_2}{n_1 + n_2}$	$\sqrt{p(1-p)\left(\dfrac{1}{n_1} + \dfrac{1}{n_2}\right)}$

Large Sample Z-Test for Comparison of Two Independent Means

In Section 5.6 we described the results of a randomised trial conducted by Farndon et al. (2013) in 189 patients with foot corns to compare a new treatment salicylic acid corn plasters (intervention) with usual scalpel debridement (control). One of the secondary outcomes for the trial was the size of the index corn (in mm) three-months post-randomisation. The sample means $\bar{x}_{Plaster} = 1.7$ mm and $\bar{x}_{Scalpel} = 2.7$ mm estimate the two population mean corn sizes $\mu_{Plaster}$ and $\mu_{Scalpel}$ respectively. In the context of a clinical trial the population usually refers to those patients, present and future, who have the disease or condition and for whom it would be appropriate to treat with either the intervention or control. Now if both approaches are equally effective, $\mu_{Plaster}$ equals $\mu_{Scalpel}$ and the difference between $\bar{x}_{Plaster}$ and $\bar{x}_{Scalpel}$ is only a chance difference. After all, subjects will differ between themselves, so we would not be surprised if differences between $\bar{x}_{Plaster}$ and $\bar{x}_{Scalpel}$ are observed, even if the approaches are identical in their effectiveness. The statistical problem is: when can it be concluded that the difference between $\bar{x}_{Plaster}$ and $\bar{x}_{Scalpel}$ is of sufficient magnitude to suspect that $\mu_{Plaster}$ is not equal to $\mu_{Scalpel}$?

The null hypothesis states that $\mu_{Plaster} = \mu_{Scalpel}$ and this can be alternatively expressed as $\mu_{Plaster} - \mu_{Scalpel} = 0$. The problem is to decide if the observations, as expressed by the sample means and corresponding standard deviations, appear consistent with this hypothesis. Clearly, if $\bar{x}_{Plaster} = \bar{x}_{Scalpel}$ exactly, we would be reasonably convinced that $\mu_{Plaster} = \mu_{Scalpel}$ but what of the actual results given above? To help decide it is necessary to first calculate $d = \bar{x}_{Plaster} - \bar{x}_{Scalpel} = 1.7 - 2.7 = -1.0$ mm and also calculate the corresponding standard deviation of the difference, SD(d) termed SE(d). The formula for the standard error is given in Table 6.3.

The formula given here differs from that given in Table 5.3 which was used when calculating a CI for the true difference between means, δ. The change arises as the standard error is now calculated under the assumption that the two groups have the same population standard deviation, σ. This implies that both s_1 and s_2 are estimating the same quantity and so these are combined into the so-called pooled estimate, s_{Pooled} of Table 6.3. In this case

$$SE_{Pooled}(d) = \sqrt{\frac{(95-1) \times 1.6^2 + (94-1) \times 2.3^2}{95 + 94 - 2} \left(\frac{1}{95} + \frac{1}{94}\right)} = 0.29,$$

which is the same estimate as that given in Section 5.6. Here there is no difference between the two estimates since the two groups are of a similar size. However, if one group were much larger than the other, the two estimates may differ somewhat.

Now, if indeed the two populations of corn sizes can be assumed each to have approximately Normal distributions, then d will also have a Normal distribution. This distribution will have its own mean $\mu_{Plaster-Scalpel}$ and standard deviation $\sigma_{Plaster-Scalpel}$, which are estimated by d and $SE_{Pooled}(d)$ respectively. One can even go one step further, if samples are large enough, and state that the ratio $d/SE_{Pooled}(d)$ will have a Normal distribution with mean $\mu_{Plaster-Scalpel}$ and a standard deviation of unity. If the null hypothesis were true, this distribution would have mean $\delta = 0$.

However, the observed values are $d = -1.0$ mm with $SE_{Pooled}(d) = 0.29$ mm and therefore a ratio of mean to standard error equal to $Z = -1.0/0.29 = -3.47$ or more than three standard deviations from the null hypothesis mean of zero. This is a very extreme observation and very unlikely to arise by chance since 99% of observations sampled from a Normal distribution with specified mean and standard deviation will be within three standard deviations of its centre. Using Table T1 with $Z = 3.47$, a P-value $= 0.0005$ is obtained. A value of δ greater than zero seems very plausible. It therefore seems very unlikely that the measurements come from a Normal distribution whose mean is in fact $\delta = \mu_{Plaster} - \mu_{Scalpel} = 0$. There is strong evidence that $\mu_{Plaster}$ and $\mu_{Scalpel}$ differ perhaps by a substantial amount. As a consequence, the notion of equality of effect of the two treatments suggested by the null hypothesis is rejected. The conclusion is that treatment with salicylic acid plasters (intervention) results in further reductions in corn size at three months post randomisation in patients with foot corns than usual scalpel debridement (control) treatment.

There is no simple, universal rule stating how large the sample size must be to be able to use a Z-test and get an accurate P-value, However, because of the Central Limit Theorem (described in Chapter 5), many test statistics are approximately Normally distributed for large samples. A rule of thumb is that for a single sample there should be at least 30 observations and for two samples at least 30 in each. Therefore, many statistical tests can be conveniently performed as approximate Z-tests if the sample size is large and the population variance is known. If the population variance is unknown (and therefore has to be estimated from the sample itself) and the sample size is not large ($n < 30$ per group), then Student's t-test (described in Chapter 7) may be more appropriate.

Z-test for Comparison of Two Independent Proportions

Provided the sample sizes in the two groups are large, the method of analysis used for comparing the mean distances walked in two groups can be utilised for the comparison of two proportions with minor changes. Thus, the population proportions of success, π_1 and π_2 replace the population means μ_1 and μ_2. Similarly, the sample statistics p_1 and p_2 replace $\bar{x}_1$ and $\bar{x}_2$. However, the standard error is now given by the expression of Table 6.3, which is calculated under the null hypothesis that the two proportions are the same, so that p_1 and p_2 both estimate a common value, π, and so these are combined into the so-called pooled estimate, p_{Pooled} or more briefly p.

Example from the Literature – Haemorrhoidal Artery Ligation Versus Rubber Band Ligation for the Management of Symptomatic Second-degree and Third-degree Haemorrhoids (HubBLe Trial)
The results of randomised controlled trial conducted by Brown et al. (2016) to assess the effect of haemorrhoidal artery ligation (HAL) surgery (intervention) compared with rubber band ligation (RBL) surgery (control) in patients with grade II–III haemorrhoids are summarised in Table 5.4. The primary outcome was recurrence of haemorrhoids at one year. The corresponding proportions of patients who had a haemorrhoid recurrence with 12 months of the surgical treatment is $p_{\text{HAL}} = 48/161 = 0.298$ and $p_{\text{RBL}} = 87/176 = 0.494$. From these data, $d = 0.298 - 0.494 = -0.196$ and, $p = \dfrac{(161 \times 0.298) + (176 \times 0.494)}{161 + 176} = 0.400$, or more simply the total number of patients with a recurrence, $r = 135$ divided by the total number of patients in the trial, $N = 337$. This leads to

$$SE_{\text{Pooled}}(d) = \sqrt{\left[0.400 \times (1 - 0.400)\left(\frac{1}{161} + \frac{1}{176}\right)\right]} = 0.053. \text{ (Compare this with Chapter 5 with}$$

$SE(d) = 0.052$). Finally, $Z = d/SE_{\text{Pooled}}(d) = -0.196/0.053 = 3.67$ (ignoring the sign).

This is a very extreme observation and very unlikely to arise by chance since 99% of observations sampled from a Normal distribution with specified mean and standard deviation will be within three standard deviations of its centre. Using Table T1 with $Z = 3.67$, a P-value $= <0.0003$ is obtained. A value of δ greater than zero seems very plausible. There is strong evidence that π_{HAL} and π_{RBL} differ perhaps by a substantial amount. As a consequence, the notion of equality of effect of the two treatments suggested by the null hypothesis is rejected. The conclusion is that treatment with HAL (Intervention) results in a lower rate of recurrence of haemorrhoids at one year in patients with grade II–III haemorrhoids than RBL (control) treatment.

Key points

- Research questions need to be turned into a statement for which we can find evidence to disprove – the null hypothesis.
- The study data are reduced down to a single probability – the probability of observing our result, or one more extreme, if the null hypothesis is true (*P*-value).
- We use this *P*-value to decide whether to reject or not reject the null hypothesis.
- Remember that 'statistical significance' does not necessarily mean 'clinical significance' or 'clinical or practical importance'.
- CIs should always be quoted with a hypothesis test to give the magnitude and precision of the effect size.

6.9 Issues with *P*-values

There is a huge controversy about the use of *P*-values, and some journals have even banned their use! The main issue is with their being misunderstood and misused. It is our (the authors) belief that *P*-values still have their use, and will continue to appear in the medical literature and so students and researchers need to know about them. The American Statistical Association (Wasserstein and Lazar 2016) issued a statement regarding the use of *P*-values which it is helpful to summarise.

P-values can indicate how incompatible the data are with a specified statistical model. As we have said in this chapter, they do not measure the probability that the studied hypothesis is true, or the probability that the data were produced by random chance alone. Scientific conclusions should not be based only on whether a *P*-value passes a specific threshold. A conclusion does not immediately become 'true' on one side of the divide and 'false' on the other. Researchers should bring many contextual factors into play to derive scientific inferences, including the design of a study, the quality of the measurements, the external evidence for the phenomenon under study, and the validity of assumptions that underlie the data analysis. Pragmatic considerations often require binary 'yes–no' decisions, but this does not mean that *P*-values alone can ensure that a decision is correct or incorrect. The widespread use of 'statistical significance' (generally interpreted as '$P \leq 0.05$') as a licence for making a claim of a scientific finding (or implied truth) leads to considerable distortion of the scientific process.

P-values and related analyses should not be reported selectively. Conducting multiple analyses of the data and reporting only those with certain *P*-values (typically those passing a significance threshold) renders the reported *P*-values essentially uninterpretable. Cherry-picking promising findings, also known by such terms as data dredging, significance chasing, significance questing, selective inference and '*P*-hacking', leads to a spurious excess of statistically significant results in the published literature and should be vigorously avoided. One need not formally carry out multiple statistical tests for this problem to arise: Whenever a researcher chooses what to present based on statistical results, valid interpretation of those results is severely compromised if the reader is not informed of the choice and its basis. Researchers should disclose the number of hypotheses explored during the study, all data collection decisions, all statistical analyses conducted and all *P*-values computed. Valid scientific conclusions based on *P*-values and related statistics cannot be drawn without at least knowing how many and which analyses were conducted, and how those analyses (including *P*-values) were selected for reporting.

A *P*-value, or statistical significance, does not measure the size of an effect or the importance of a result. Statistical significance is not equivalent to scientific, human, or economic significance.

Smaller *P*-values do not necessarily imply the presence of larger or more important effects, and larger *P*-values do not imply a lack of importance or even lack of effect. Any effect, no matter how tiny, can produce a small *P*-value if the sample size or measurement precision is high enough, and large effects may produce unimpressive *P*-values if the sample size is small or measurements are imprecise. Similarly, identical estimated effects will have different *P*-values if the precision of the estimates differs.

By itself, a *P*-value does not provide a good measure of evidence regarding a model or hypothesis. Researchers should recognise that a *P*-value without context or other evidence provides limited information. As we have stated earlier, a *P*-value near 0.05 taken by itself offers only weak evidence against the null hypothesis. Likewise, a relatively large *P*-value does not imply evidence in favour of the null hypothesis; many other hypotheses may be equally or more consistent with the observed data.

6.10 Points When Reading the Literature

1) Have clinical importance and statistical significance been confused?
2) Have CIs of the main results been quoted?
3) How wide is the CI?
4) What clinical implications can be drawn from the interval?
5) Does the CI include any values of particular interest?
6) Is the result medically or biologically plausible and has the statistical significance of the result been considered in isolation, or have other studies of the same effect been taken into account?
7) Can one generalise from the sample to the target population?

6.11 Exercises

6.1 Which (if any) of the following statements about *P*-values is CORRECT?
   A The *P*-value from a hypothesis test is the probability of obtaining your results, or more extreme results.
   B The *P*-value from a hypothesis test is the probability of obtaining your results, or more extreme results, if the null hypothesis is true.
   C If the *P*-value is small then your results are unlikely when the null hypothesis is true.
   D If the *P*-value is large your results are likely when the null hypothesis is true.
   E The *P*-value ranges from 0 to 1.

6.2 Which (if any) of the following statements about the Type I error is CORRECT?
   A The Type I error is the probability of rejecting the null hypothesis when it is true.
   B The Type I error is the probability of a false positive result.
   C The usual cut-off for the Type I error rate in hypothesis tests is 0.05.
   D The Type I error is the probability of rejecting the null hypothesis when it is false.
   E We can reduce the risk of a Type I error by changing the level of statistical significance we demand from 1% to 5%.

6.3 Which (if any) of the following statements about hypothesis testing is CORRECT?

    A With a large sample size you will always calculate a large *P*-value from your hypothesis test.

    B The *P*-value from a hypothesis test is the probability of obtaining your results, or more extreme results, if the null hypothesis were true.

    C With a small sample size you will always calculate a small *P*-value from your hypothesis test.

    D The *P*-value from a hypothesis test tells you what the difference is and how large the difference is.

    E A statistically significant result means the result is clinically significant/practically important.

Farndon et al. (2013) report the results of a randomised controlled trial that investigated the effectiveness of salicylic acid plasters (Corn plasters) compared with usual scalpel debridement for treatment of foot corns. One of the secondary outcome measures was the size of the index corn (in mm) measured at 3, 6, 9 and 12 months post-randomisation. Table 6.4 shows the outcome data.

    You may assume a significance level of 0.05 or 5% has been specified for the various hypothesis tests.

Table 6.4 Index corn size, in millimetres, over time by group.

Size of index corn (mm)	Corn plaster (*n* = 101) Mean	SD	Scalpel (*n* = 101) Mean	SD	Mean Difference	95% CI Lower	Upper	*P*-value
Baseline	3.9	(1.7)	3.8	(1.8)				
3 months	1.7	(1.5)	2.7	(2.3)	−1.0	−1.5	−0.5	
6 months	1.7	(1.6)	2.4	(2.2)	−0.7	−1.2	−0.2	
9 months	1.7	(1.6)	2.2	(2.1)	−0.5	−1.2	0.1	
12 months	1.3	(1.6)	2.3	(2.2)	−1.0	−1.7	−0.2	0.010

6.4 Table 6.4 reports that the *P*-value for the comparison of mean corn size at 12 months between the corn plaster and scalpel groups is $P = 0.010$.

Which, if any of the following statements is CORRECT?

    A The result at 12 months is statistically significant.

    B The probability of getting this difference or more extreme by chance if there had been no difference in population mean outcomes is 0.010.

    C The probability of getting this difference or more extreme is 0.010.

    D There is sufficient evidence to reject the null hypothesis.

    E The results are unlikely when the null hypothesis is true.

6.5 Table 6.4 reports that the 95% CI for the comparison of mean corn size at nine months between the corn plaster and scalpel groups is: −1.2 to 0.1 mm. The research literature suggests that a difference or change in corn size of 1 mm or more would be regarded as clinically or practically important. Therefore the 95% CI shows that the difference in mean corn size at nine months between the corn plaster and scalpel groups is:

A Statistically significant and potentially clinically important.
B Statistically significant and not clinically important.
C Statistically significant and clinically important.
D Not statistically significant but potentially clinically important.
E Not statistically significant and not clinically important.

6.6 Table 6.4 reports that the 95% CI for the comparison of mean corn size at 12 months between the corn plaster and scalpel groups is: −1.7 to −0.2 mm. The research literature suggests that a difference or change in corn size of 1 mm or more would be regarded as clinically or practically important. Therefore the 95% CI shows that the difference in mean corn size at 12 months between the corn plaster and scalpel groups is:

A Statistically significant and potentially clinically important.
B Statistically significant and not clinically important.
C Statistically significant and clinically important.
D Not statistically significant but potentially clinically important.
E Not statistically significant and not clinically important.

6.7 Table 6.4 reports that the 95% CI for the comparison of mean corn size at three months between the corn plaster and scalpel groups is: −1.5 to −0.5 mm. The research literature suggests that a difference or change in corn size of 0.5 mm or more would be regarded as clinically or practically important. Therefore the 95% CI shows that the difference in mean corn size at three months between the corn plaster and scalpel groups is:

A Statistically significant and potentially clinically important.
B Statistically significant and not clinically important.
C Statistically significant and clinically important.
D Not statistically significant but potentially clinically important.
E Not statistically significant and not clinically important.

7   Comparing Two or More Groups with Continuous Data

Medical Statistics: A Textbook for the Health Sciences, Fifth Edition. Stephen J. Walters, Michael J. Campbell, and David Machin.
© 2021 John Wiley & Sons Ltd. Published 2021 by John Wiley & Sons Ltd.
Companion website: www.wiley.com/go/walters/medicalstatistics

Summary

In this chapter we will be putting some of the theory into practice and looking at some of the more basic statistical tests that you will come across in the literature and in your own research. The choice of method of analysis for a problem depends on the comparison to be made and the data to be used. We explain some of the basic methods appropriate for comparing two or more groups or sets of data. These data are described as unpaired or independent when they arise from separate individuals or paired when they arise from the same individual at different points in time. The chapter covers analysis methods for both paired and unpaired data sets, and the methods are valid for small data sets ($n < 30$) given certain other assumptions. In Chapter 6, the methods required large samples to be valid. In this chapter we show the utility of statistics in that we can still make valid inferences with small samples under certain assumptions.

7.1   Introduction

There are often several different approaches to even a simple problem. The methods described here may not be the only methods available but would usually be considered as satisfactory for the purposes for which they are suggested here.

What type of statistical test? – Five key questions to ask

---

1) What are the aims and objectives of the study?
2) What is the hypothesis to be tested?
3) What type of data are the outcome data?
4) How are the outcome data distributed?
5) What is the summary measure for the outcome data?

Given the answers to these five key questions, an appropriate approach to the statistical analysis of the data collected can be decided upon. The type of statistical analysis depends fundamentally on what the main purpose of the study is. In particular, what is the main question to be answered? The data type for the outcome variable will also govern how it is to be analysed, as an analysis appropriate to continuous data would be completely inappropriate for binary or categorical data. The distribution of the outcome variable is also important, as is the summary measure to be used. Highly skewed data require a different analysis compared to that required by data which are Normally distributed.

The choice of method of analysis for a problem depends on the comparison to be made and the data to be used. In particular two common problems in statistical inference are outlined below.

Two common problems in statistical inference

---

1) Comparison of the response for paired observations, for example, the response of one group of patients before and after an exposure to a stimulus or under different conditions.
2) Comparison of independent groups, for example, groups of patients given different treatments.

Before beginning any comparison between groups, it is important to examine the data, using the techniques described in Chapter 2; adequate description of the data should precede and complement the formal statistical analysis. For most studies and for randomised controlled trials in particular, it is good practice to produce a table that describes the initial or baseline characteristics of the sample(s) concerned.

7.2   Comparison of Two Groups of Paired Observations – Continuous Outcomes

One common situation is the comparison of paired data, for example, the response of one group of patients before and after an exposure to a stimulus or under different conditions. When there is more than one group of observations it is vital to distinguish the case where the data are paired from that where the groups are independent. Paired data may arise when the same individuals are studied more than once, usually in different circumstances, or when individuals are paired or matched together. The methods of analysis for paired samples are summarised in Figure 7.1.

The corn plaster study of Farndon et al. (2013) investigated the effectiveness of salicylic acid plasters compared with usual scalpel debridement for treatment of foot corn. One of the secondary clinical outcomes was current levels of self-reported pain, when walking, using a 100 mm visual analogue scale (VAS), scored on a 0 'no pain' to 100 'worst possible pain' at baseline and at a three-month follow-up.

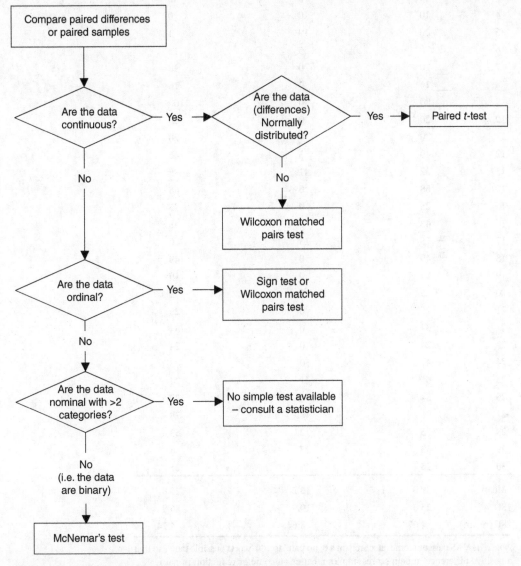

Figure 7.1 Statistical methods for paired data or paired samples.

The VAS pain scores in 30 patients treated with salicylic acid plasters whose index corn resolved at three months are shown in Table 7.1. The table shows the data are paired with each row in the table corresponding to the outcome data for the same patient. We may be interested in seeing if there is a change in pain between baseline and the three-month follow-up in those patients whose foot corn had resolved or healed at three months.

Table 7.1 VAS pain scores, at baseline and three months, in 30 patients treated with salicylic acid plasters whose index corn resolved at three months.

Subject	VAS pain score Baseline	Three-month follow-up	Difference (0–3 m)
1	76	73	3
2	25	25	0
3	40	0	40
4	10	10	0
5	20	19	1
6	70	55	15
7	10	0	10
8	16	0	16
9	100	0	100
10	20	0	20
11	20	0	20
12	49	3	46
13	32	41	−9
14	68	0	68
15	25	0	25
16	43	0	43
17	15	15	0
18	49	0	49
19	19	0	19
20	5	2	3
21	25	0	25
22	34	0	34
23	24	0	24
24	47	50	−3
25	65	41	24
26	34	5	29
27	96	18	78
28	75	12	63
29	33	27	6
30	25	0	25
Mean	39.0	13.2	25.8
SD	25.6	19.9	26.0
SE (mean)	4.67	3.64	4.74

Note: The VAS pain outcome, is scored on a 0 'no pain' to 100 'worst possible pain', so that a positive difference in pain scores implies a better outcome or reduction in pain over time.
Source: data from Farndon et al. (2013).

The VAS pain scores at baseline and three months are both continuous variables and the data are paired as measurements are made on the same individuals at baseline and three months; therefore, interest is in the mean of the paired differences, the data in the last (fourth) column of Table 7.1. If we assume that the paired differences are Normally distributed, then the most appropriate summary measure for the data is the sample paired mean difference in VAS pain score between baseline and three months. The assumption of Normality can be checked by plotting a histogram, of the paired differences; these do not need to be perfect, just roughly symmetrical. At this stage, we shall assume the outcome, is Normally distributed, but we will check this assumption later on. Using the flow diagram of Figure 7.1, the most appropriate hypothesis test appears to be the paired *t*-test (see Box 7.1). In this example a suitable null hypothesis (H_0) is that there is no difference (or change) in mean VAS pain scores between baseline and three-month follow-up, that is, $\delta = 0$. The alternative hypothesis (H_A) is that there is a difference (or change) in mean VAS pain scores between baseline and three-month follow-up, that is $\delta \neq 0$. Do not forget we are interested in the population of patients with foot corns treated with salicylic acid plasters. However, we have taken a sample of 30 that we study in order to make inferences about the population of interest.

There were 30 patients with foot corns and the summary statistics for the VAS pain score outcome at baseline and follow-up for these subjects are shown in the top half of the computer output in Table 7.2. We have a mean difference $\bar{d} = 25.8$ and the $SD(d) = 26.0$, and hence $SD(\bar{d}) = SE(\bar{d}) = 26.0/\sqrt{30} = 4.7$. In this example the data are paired and the degrees of freedom (df)

Box 7.1   Paired *t*-Test

Two groups of paired observations, $x_{11}, x_{12}, ..., x_{1n}$ in Group 1 and $x_{21}, x_{22}, ..., x_{2n}$ in Group 2 such that x_{1i} is paired with x_{2i} and the difference between them, $d_i = x_{1i} - x_{2i}$.

The null hypothesis, H_0, is that the mean change or difference in the population, δ, is zero. The alternative hypothesis (H_A) is that the population mean difference is non-zero, that is $\delta \neq 0$.

Assumptions

1) The d_is are plausibly Normally distributed. It is not essential for the original observations to be Normally distributed.
2) The d_is are independent of each other.

Steps

1) Calculate the differences $d_i = x_{1i} - x_{2i}$, $i = 1$ to n.
2) Calculate the mean $\bar{d}$ and standard deviation, s_d of the differences d_i.
3) Calculate the standard error of the mean difference $SE(\bar{d}) = s_d/\sqrt{n}$.
4) Calculate the test statistic $t = \dfrac{\bar{d}}{SE(\bar{d})}$.
5) Under the null hypothesis, the test statistic, t is distributed as Student's t, with degrees of freedom, $df = n-1$.

Table 7.2 Computer output for paired *t*-test.

Paired samples statistics				
	Mean	N	SD	SE
VAS pain at baseline	39.0	30	25.6	4.7
VAS pain at three-month follow-up	13.2	30	19.9	3.6

Paired Samples *t*-test								
	Paired differences							
				95% confidence interval of the difference				
	Mean	SD	SE	Lower	Upper	t	df	P-value
VAS pain at baseline – VAS pain at three-month follow-up	25.8	26.0	4.7	16.1	35.5	5.438	29	0.00001

The *P*-value or probability of observing the test statistic of 5.438 or more extreme under the null hypothesis is 0.00001. This means that this result is unlikely when the null hypothesis, that $\delta = 0$, is true (of no difference in pain scores). The result is said to be *statistically significant* because the *P*-value is less than the significance level (α) set at 5% and there is sufficient evidence to reject the null hypothesis. The alternative hypothesis that there is a difference or change in pain scores, between baseline and three-month follow-up, is accepted.

Source: data from Farndon et al. (2013).

are one less than the number of patients in the study, that is, $df = n-1 = 30-1 = 29$. The test or *t*-statistic is $t = 25.8/4.7 = 5.44$. This value is then compared to values of the *t*-distribution with $df = 29$ df. From Table T2 in the appendix, this suggests a *P*-value < 0.001. The computer output in Table 7.2 gives a precise *P*-value $= 0.00001$.

The 100 (1-α) % confidence interval (CI) for the mean difference in the population is:

$$\overline{d} - \left[t_{df,\alpha} \times SE(\overline{d}) \right] \quad \text{to} \quad \overline{d} + \left[t_{df,\alpha} \times SE(\overline{d}) \right],$$

where $t_{df,\alpha}$ is taken from the *t* distribution with $df = n-1$ degrees of freedom.

From Table T2 with $df = 29$, $t_{29,0.05} \approx 2.045$, giving the 95% CI for the mean paired difference as

$$25.8 - (2.045 \times 4.7) \text{ to } 25.8 + (2.045 \times 4.7)$$

or 16.1 to 35.5.

The computer output for the comparison of the change in pain scores for these 30 patients at baseline and three months shows that the result is statistically significant (Table 7.2). The VAS pain outcome, is scored on a 0 'no pain' to 100 'worst possible pain', so that a positive difference in pain scores implies a better outcome or reduction in pain over time. The CI of the difference suggests that we are 95% confident that pain has changed (reduced/improved) by between 16 and 36 points over the period and the best estimate is a mean reduction of 26 points.

The assumptions (see Box 7.1) underlying the use of the paired *t*-test are that the paired differences are plausibly Normally distributed. It is a common mistake to assume in such cases that because the basic observations appear not to have Normal distributions, then the methods described here do not apply. However, it is the paired differences, that is, the baseline pain score minus the three-month pain score, that have to be checked for the assumption of a Normal distribution, and not the basic observations. The differences appear not to have a symmetrical distribution, as shown by the histogram in Figure 7.2. If the assumptions underlying the use of the paired *t*-test are not met, then Figure 7.1 suggests that a non-parametric alternative, the Wilcoxon signed rank sum test (see Box 7.2), can be used, to assess whether the differences are centred around zero.

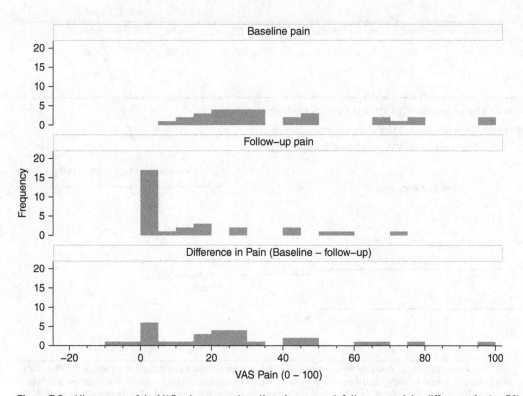

Figure 7.2 Histograms of the VAS pain score at baseline, three-month follow-up and the difference for (*n* = 30) patients with a resolved foot corn, at three months, treated with salicylic acid plasters. (*Source:* data from Farndon et al. 2013).

Wilcoxon (Matched Pairs) Signed Rank Test

This is used when the assumption of Normality of the paired differences underlying the paired t-test is not valid. It is a test of the null hypothesis that the difference between the pairs follows a symmetric distribution around zero; against the alternative hypothesis that the difference between the pairs does not follow a symmetric distribution around zero (see Box 7.2).

The computer output in Table 7.3 using the Wilcoxon signed rank test for the comparison of VAS pain score for these 30 patients between baseline and three months shows that the result is statistically significant with a P-value = 0.00002; and we can reject the null hypothesis that the difference between the pairs follows a symmetric distribution around zero and accept the alternative hypothesis that the difference between the pairs does not follow a symmetric distribution around zero and that there is a difference or change in VAS pain scores between baseline and three months.

Table 7.3 Example computer output for Wilcoxon signed rank test.

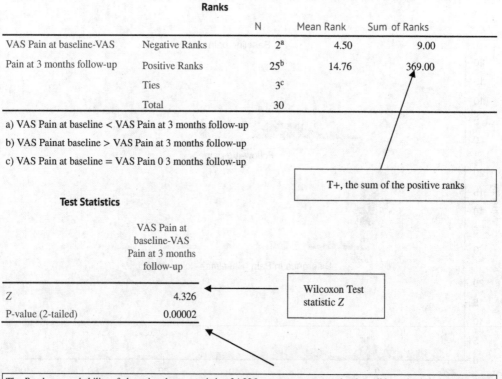

		N	Mean Rank	Sum of Ranks
	Ranks			
VAS Pain at baseline-VAS	Negative Ranks	2[a]	4.50	9.00
Pain at 3 months follow-up	Positive Ranks	25[b]	14.76	369.00
	Ties	3[c]		
	Total	30		

a) VAS Pain at baseline < VAS Pain at 3 months follow-up
b) VAS Painat baseline > VAS Pain at 3 months follow-up
c) VAS Pain at baseline = VAS Pain 0 3 months follow-up

T+, the sum of the positive ranks

Test Statistics

	VAS Pain at baseline-VAS Pain at 3 months follow-up
Z	4.326
P-value (2-tailed)	0.00002

Wilcoxon Test statistic Z

The *P-value* or probability of observing the test statistic of 4.326 or more extreme under the null hypothesis is 0.00002. This means that this result is unlikely when the null hypothesis is true (of no difference in pain scores between baseline and three months). The result is said to be *statistically significant* because the *P-value* is less than the significance level (α) set at 5% or 0.05 and there is sufficient evidence to reject the null hypothesis. The alternative hypothesis that there is a difference or change in VAS Pain scores between baseline and 3-months, is accepted.

Source: data from Farndon et al. (2013).

Box 7.2   Wilcoxon (Matched Pairs) Signed Rank Test

Two groups of paired observations, $x_{11}, x_{12}, ..., x_{1n}$ in Group 1 and $x_{21}, x_{22}, ..., x_{2n}$ in Group 2 such that x_{1i} is paired with x_{2i} and the difference between them, $d_i = x_{1i} - x_{2i}$. The null hypothesis, H_0, is that the difference between the pairs follows a symmetric distribution around zero; and the alternative hypothesis, H_A, is that the difference between the pairs does not follow a symmetric distribution around zero.

Assumptions

1) The data are paired.
2) The paired differences, the d_is are independent of each other.
3) The data are measured at least on an ordinal scale.

Steps

1) Calculate the differences $d_i = x_{1i} - x_{2i}$, $i = 1$ to n.
2) Ignoring the signs of the differences, rank them in order of increasing magnitude from 1 to n', with zero values being ignored (so n' is the number of non-zero differences, and so may be less than the original sample size n). If some of the observations are numerically equal, they are given tied ranks equal to the mean of the ranks which would otherwise have been used.
3) Calculate, T^+, the sum of the ranks of the positive values. The standard error of T^+ is $\sqrt{\dfrac{n'(n' + 1)(2n' + 1)}{24}}$ and the hypothesised or expected value of T^+ under the null hypothesis is $n'(n' + 1)/4$.
4) Calculate the test statistic $Z = \dfrac{T^+ - \left(\dfrac{n'(n' + 1)}{4}\right)}{\sqrt{\dfrac{[n'(n' + 1)(2n' + 1)]}{24}}}$
5) Under the null hypothesis, Z has an approximately Normal distribution, with mean 0 and standard deviation 1.

In our example and formulation, we are testing for symmetry of the paired differences around zero and using the Wilcoxon signed rank test for symmetry. It is a test of the null hypothesis that the difference between the pairs follows a symmetric distribution around zero; against the alternative hypothesis that the difference between the pairs does not follow a symmetric distribution around zero. This does not preclude a symmetric distribution around a different value than zero. Li and Johnson (2014) show that if you can assume the distribution of the paired differences is symmetric you can use the Wilcoxon signed rank test as a more specific test for the median, m, (taking a specific or known constant value, m_0, under the null hypothesis (i.e. H_0: $m = m_o$, against the alternative hypothesis that the median does not equal this value (H_A: $m \neq m_0$).

7.3   Comparison of Two Independent Groups – Continuous Outcomes

This section describes the statistical methods available for comparing two independent groups, when we have a continuous outcome. The Behavioural Activation Therapy for Depression after Stroke (BEADS) trial was a parallel group feasibility multi-centre randomised controlled trial in patients with post-stroke depression. The aim of the BEADS trial was to evaluate the feasibility of undertaking a full trial comparing behavioural activation (BA) to usual stroke care for four months for patients with post-stroke depression (Thomas et al. 2019). Trial participants were randomly allocated to receive BA therapy (intervention) in addition to usual care or usual care (UC) alone (control). The primary clinical outcome measure was the Patient Health Questionnaire-9 (PHQ-9) measured at six-month post-randomisation. The PHQ-9 is a nine-item self-completed questionnaire used as a screening and diagnostic tool for mental health disorders, scored on a 0 to 27 scale with higher scores indicating more depressive symptoms. If the values for one or two of the nine items are missing then they can be substituted with the average score of the non-missing items. Questionnaires with more than two missing values should be disregarded. Table 7.4 shows the PHQ-9 scores (after calculation with substitution for missing items) at six-month post-randomisation in 39 patients with post-stroke depression by intervention group.

One of the main questions of interest in the BEADS trial was whether there was a difference in PHQ-9 depression scores between the BA and the UC groups six-month post-randomisation. As the PHQ-9

Table 7.4 PHQ-9 scores at six-month post-randomisation in 39 patients with post-stroke depression by intervention group.

	BA (*n* = 18)	UC (*n* = 21)
	15.0	11.6
	6.0	19.0
	6.0	20.0
	20.6	8.0
	14.0	16.0
	5.0	10.0
	6.0	13.0
	2.0	15.0
	23.0	10.0
	3.0	14.0
	6.0	7.0
	3.0	18.0
	10.0	10.0
	7.0	10.0
	12.0	15.0
	5.0	17.0
	15.0	27.0
	23.0	22.0
		17.0
		8.0
		14.0
Mean	10.09	14.36
SD	6.88	5.11
SE	1.62	1.12

outcome generates quantitative data and there are two independent groups, assuming the data are Normally distributed in each of the two groups, then the most appropriate summary measure for the data is the sample mean and the best comparative summary measure is the difference in mean PHQ-9 scores between the two groups. Under these assumptions, the flow diagram of Figure 7.3

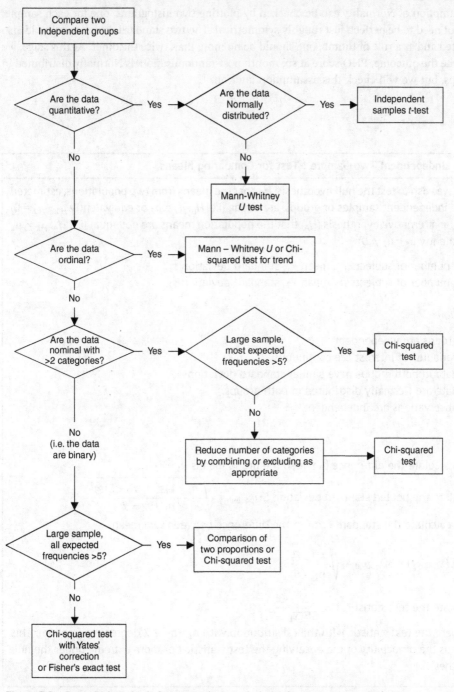

Figure 7.3 Statistical methods for comparing two independent groups or samples.

suggests that the two independent samples t-test should be used (see Box 7.3). The independent samples t-test is used to test for a difference in the mean values of a continuous variable between two groups.

When conducting any statistical analysis it is important to check that the assumptions that underpin the chosen method are valid. The assumptions underlying the two independent samples t-test are outlined below.

The assumption of Normality can be checked by plotting two histograms, one for each sample; these do not need to be perfect, just roughly symmetrical. The two standard deviations should also be calculated and as a rule of thumb, one should be no more than twice the other. At this stage, we shall assume the outcome, PHQ-score at six-month post-randomisation, is Normally distributed in both groups, but we will check this assumption later on.

Box 7.3   Independent Two-Sample t-Test for Comparing Means

Suppose we wish to test the null hypothesis, H_0, that the means from two populations, estimated from two independent samples or groups, are equal, (i.e. H_0: $\mu_1 = \mu_2$ or equivalently $\mu_1 - \mu_2 = 0$) against the alternative hypothesis (H_A) that the population means are not equal (i.e. H_A: $\mu_1 \neq \mu_2$ or equivalently $\mu_1 - \mu_2 \neq 0$).

Group 1: number of subjects n_1, mean $\bar{x}_1$, standard deviation s_1,
Group 2: number of subjects n_2, mean $\bar{x}_2$, standard deviation s_2.

Assumptions

1) The groups are independent.
2) The variables of interest are continuous.
3) The data in both groups have similar standard deviations.
4) The data are Normally distributed in both groups.
5) The observations are independent.

Steps

1) First calculate the difference between the group means $\bar{x}_1 - \bar{x}_2$

2) Calculate the pooled standard deviation $SD_{pooled} = \sqrt{\dfrac{(n_1 - 1)s_1^2 + (n_2 - 1)s_2^2}{n_1 + n_2 - 2}}$.

3) Then calculate the standard error of the difference between two means

$$SE(\bar{x}_1 - \bar{x}_2) = SD_{pooled} \times \sqrt{\frac{1}{n_1} + \frac{1}{n_2}}.$$

4) Calculate the test statistic. $t = \dfrac{\bar{x}_1 - \bar{x}_2}{SE(\bar{x}_1 - \bar{x}_2)}$.

5) Compare the test statistic with the t distribution with $n_1 + n_2 - 2$ degrees of freedom. This gives us the probability of the observing the test statistic t or more extreme under the null hypothesis.

In this example a suitable null hypothesis (H_0) is that there is no difference in mean PHQ-9 scores, at six-month post-randomisation, between BA and UC groups, that is, $\mu_{BA}-\mu_{UC} = 0$. The alternative hypothesis (H_A) is that there is a difference in mean PHQ-9 scores between BA and UC groups, i.e. $\mu_{BA}-\mu_{UC} \neq 0$.

The summary statistics for the PHQ-9 outcome at six-month post-randomisation for the UC and BA groups are shown in the top half of the computer output in Table 7.5. We have a mean difference between the groups (UC mean – BA mean), $\bar{x}_1 - \bar{x}_2 = 14.4 - 10.1 = 4.3$ points and the standard error of this mean difference $SE(\bar{x}_1 - \bar{x}_2) = 1.92$. Since the PHQ-9 outcome is scored on a 0 to 27 scale with higher scores indicating more depressive symptoms; the patients in the UC group have on average a higher (or worse) score than patients in the BA group. In this example the degrees of freedom are, $df = n_1 + n_2 - 2$ or $21 + 18 - 2 = 37$. The test statistic is $t = 4.3/1.9 = 2.22$. This value is then compared to values of the t-distribution with $df = 37$. From Table T2, the closest tabulated value with $df = 37$ is between 0.03 and 0.04 suggesting a P-value of somewhere between 0.03 and 0.04. This is clearly less than 0.05. The computer output in Table 7.5 shows that the exact P-value = 0.033.

Table 7.5 Computer output from the two independent samples t-test.

	Group statistics				
	Group	**N**	**Mean**	**SD**	**SE**
PHQ-9 score at six months	UC	21	14.4	5.1	1.1
	BA	18	10.1	6.9	1.6

The standard deviations for the two groups are different; but broadly similar. As a rough estimate, one should be no more than twice the other. The ratio of the two SDs, i.e. 6.9/5.1 = 1.4, is less than 2.

	Independent samples t-test						
				t-test for equality of means			
						95% CI of the difference	
	t	**df**	***P*-value**	**Difference in means**	**SE Difference**	**Lower**	**Upper**
PHQ-9 score at six months	2.221	37	0.033	4.3	1.9	0.4	8.2

The P-value is 0.033. Thus the results are unlikely when the null hypothesis (that there is no difference between the groups is true). The result is said to be statistically significant because the P-value is less than the significance level (α) set at 5% or 0.05 and there is sufficient evidence to reject the null hypothesis and accept the alternative hypothesis, that there is a difference in mean PHQ-9 scores at six-month post-randomisation between the intervention and control groups.

Source: data from Thomas et al. (2016).

The $100(1 - \alpha)\%$ CI for the mean difference in the population is:

$$(\bar{x}_1 - \bar{x}_2) - [t_{df,\alpha} \times SE(\bar{x}_1 - \bar{x}_2)] \ to \ (\bar{x}_1 - \bar{x}_2) + [t_{df,\alpha} \times SE(\bar{x}_1 - \bar{x}_2)],$$

where $t_{df,\alpha}$ is taken from the t distribution with $df = n_1 + n_2 - 2$. For a 95% CI $t_{37, \, 0.05} = 2.026$. Thus giving the 95% CI for the mean difference as:

$$4.3 - (2.026 \times 1.9) \ to \ 4.3 + (2.026 \times 1.9) \ or \ 0.4 \ to \ 8.2.$$

Table 7.5 shows the computer output for comparing mean PHQ-9 scores between the two groups using two independent samples t-test. It can be seen that there is a significant difference between the groups; the 95% CI for the difference suggests that that patients in the BA group have between 0.4 and 8.2 lower (or better) PHQ-9 scores than patients in the UC group and the best estimate is a mean difference of 4.3 points lower.

When conducting any statistical analysis it is important to check that the assumptions that underpin the chosen method are valid. For two independent samples t-test, the assumption that the outcome is Normally distributed in each group can be checked by plotting two histograms, one for each sample. Figure 7.4 shows two histograms for the PHQ-9 outcome. The outcome in both groups is clearly not Normally distributed. Hence in these circumstances it looks like the two-independent samples t-test is not the most appropriate test. The flow diagram of Figure 7.3, suggests that the Mann–Whitney U test may be a more suitable alternative (see Box 7.4).

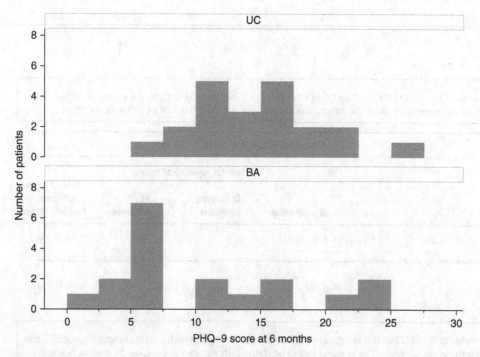

Figure 7.4 Histograms of six-month PHQ-9 score by the intervention group ($N = 39$). (*Source:* data from Thomas et al. 2016).

Mann–Whitney *U* Test

When the assumptions underlying the *t*-test are not met, then the non-parametric equivalent, the Mann–Whitney *U* test, may be used (see Box 7.4). There are two derivations of the test, one due to Wilcoxon and the other to Mann and Whitney. It is better to call the method the Mann–Whitney *U* test to avoid confusion with the paired test due to Wilcoxon. The test requires all the observations (n_1 in Group 1 and n_2 in Group 2) to be ranked as if they were from a single sample. We can now use two alternative test statistics, *U* and *W*. The statistic *W* (due to Wilcoxon) is simply the sum of the ranks in one of the groups and is easier to calculate by hand. The statistic *U* (due to Mann and Whitney) is more complicated. The observations are ranked together in order of increasing magnitude. There are $n_1 n_2$ pairs of ranks from the two groups; of these *U* is the number of all possible pairs of observations comprising one from each group for which the rank value in the first group exceeds the rank value in the second group. Any pairs for which the ranks are the same count ½ a unit towards *U*.

Whilst the independent samples *t*-test is specifically a test of the null hypothesis that the groups have the same mean value, the Mann–Whitney *U* test is a more general test of the null hypothesis that the distribution of the outcome variable in the two groups is the same; it is possible for the outcome data in the two groups to have similar measures of central tendency or location, such as mean and medians, but different distributions.

Box 7.4   Mann–Whitney *U* Test

Suppose we wish to test the null hypothesis, H_0, that two samples come from the same population (i.e. that two independent samples are from populations with the same distribution). The alternative hypothesis, H_A, is that the distributions are not equal. The data are at least ordinal and from two independent groups of size n_1 and n_2 respectively.

Assumptions

1) The groups are independent.
2) The variables of interest are at least ordinal (can be ranked).
3) The observations are independent.

Steps

1) First combine the two groups and rank the entire data set in increasing order (smallest observation to the largest). If some of the observations are numerically equal, they are given tied ranks equal to the mean of the ranks which would otherwise have been used.
2) Sum the ranks for one of the groups. Let *W* be the sum of the ranks for the n_1 observations in this group. The standard error of *W* is $\sqrt{\dfrac{n_1 n_2 (n_1 + n_2 + 1)}{12}}$ and the expected or hypothesised value of *W* under the null hypothesis is $\dfrac{1}{2} n_1 (n_1 + n_2 + 1)$.

Box 7.4 (Continued)

3) If there are no ties or only a few ties, calculate the test statistic

$$Z = \frac{W - \left(\frac{n_1(n_1 + n_2 + 1)}{2}\right)}{\sqrt{\frac{[n_1 n_2 (n_1 + n_2 + 1)]}{12}}}.$$

4) Under the null hypothesis that the two samples come from the same population, the test statistic, Z, is approximately Normally distributed with mean zero, and standard deviation of 1, and can be referred to Table T1 to calculate a P-value.

Many text books give special tables for the Mann–Whitney U test, when sample sizes are small, that is when n_1 and n_2 are less than 20. However, the above expression is usually sufficient. The formula is not very accurate if there any many ties in the data. When there are ties in the data the denominator or standard error formula is modified to $\sqrt{\frac{n_1 n_2}{12n(n-1)} \left[n^3 - n - \sum_t (t^3 - t)\right]}$, where n is the combined total sample size (i.e. $n = n_1 + n_2$ and t being the number of observations with a particular tied value or rank; and the summations being taken over all groups of tied observations (Armitage et al. 2002).

The output from the Mann–Whitney U test in Table 7.6 shows sufficient evidence to reject the null hypothesis and accept the alternative hypothesis that there is a difference in the distribution of PHQ-9 scores at six-month post-randomisation between the BA and UC groups; with patients in the BA group having the lower ranked scores (the better outcome – fewer depressive symptoms) than patients in the UC group.

However, this example illustrates that the t-test is very robust to violations of the assumptions of Normality and equal variances, particularly for moderate to large sample sizes, as the P-values and conclusions, from both the t-test and Mann–Whitney test are the same, despite the non-Normal distribution of the data.

Discrete Count Data

In the majority of cases it is reasonable to treat discrete count data, such as number of children in a family or number of visits to a general practice clinic in a year, as if they were approximately Normally distributed, at least as far as the statistical analysis goes. Ideally, there should be a large number of different possible values, but in practice this is not always necessary. However, where ordered categories are numbered such as stage of disease or social class, the temptation to treat these numbers as statistically meaningful must be resisted. For example, it is not sensible to calculate the average social class or stage of cancer, and in such cases the data should be treated in statistical analyses as if they are ordered categories.

Table 7.6 Computer Output for Mann–Whitney U test.

	Ranks			
	Randomisation group	N	Mean rank	Sum of ranks
PHQ-9 score at six months	UC	21	23.9	502.5
	BA	18	15.4	277.5
	Total	39		

Test Statistics	
	PHQ-9 score at six months
Mann–Whitney U	106.5
Wilcoxon W	277.5
Z	-2.33^a
P-value (two-tailed)	0.020

P-value: probability of observing the statistic, W or U, under the null hypothesis. As the value of 0.020 is less than the significance level (α) set at 0.05 or 5% this means that the result obtained is unlikely when the null hypothesis is true. Thus there is sufficient evidence to reject the null hypothesis and accept the alternative hypothesis that there is a difference in the distribution of PHQ-9 scores at six-month post-randomisation between groups.

^{a} Corrected for ties.

7.4 Comparing More than Two Groups

The methods outlined above can be extended to more than two groups. For the independent samples t-test, the analogous method for more than two groups is called Analysis of Variance (ANOVA) and the assumptions underlying it are similar. The non-parametric equivalent for the method of ANOVA when there are more than two groups is called the Kruskal–Wallis test. A fuller explanation of these methods is shown in the technical details section of this chapter.

For example, consider the data presented in Table 7.7 on 171 young male cancer survivors. This data is taken was taken from a cross-sectional, observational study of male cancer cases and controls (Greenfield et al. 2007). Table 7.7 describes the mean general health, as measured by the SF-36, of four different types of cancer survivors: germ cell (testicular); lymphoma; leukaemia, and other. Suppose we wish to compare the mean quality of life or general health across the four different cancer groups. We could perform a series of six hypothesis tests, using the t-test or the Mann–Whitney test described previously, to compare the means in each pair of groups. However, this may result in a high Type I error rate, because of the large number of

Table 7.7 Self-reported quality of life, SF-36 general health, by cancer type in 171 men aged 20–45.

Cancer type	Mean	SD	n
Leukaemia	73.7	21.1	11
Germ cell (testicular)	69.2	23.4	66
Other	61.9	26.1	24
Lymphoma	55.5	24.2	70
Total	62.9	24.7	171

The SF-36 general health outcome is measured on a 0 (poor quality of life) to 100 (good) scale.
Source: data from Greenfield et al. (2007).

comparisons, and this may mean that we draw incorrect conclusions from the test. Therefore, it may be preferable to carry out a single global test to determine whether the means differ in any of the groups.

One-way Analysis of Variance

One-way ANOVA separates the total variability in the data into several components. One component is the variability in the data that can be attributed to differences between the individuals from the different groups. This is known as the *between-group* variation. A second component is the random variation between the individuals within each group. This is known as the *within-group* variation, although it is sometimes referred to as the *unexplained* or *residual* variation. The components are measured using variances (see Chapter 2), hence the name ANOVA. Under the null hypothesis that the group means are the same, the between-group variance will be similar to the within-group variance. If, however, there are differences between the groups, then the between-group variance will be larger than the within-group variance. The ANOVA test statistic or *F* test is based on the ratio of these two variances.

The calculations involved in ANOVA are complex (see Box 7.5) and are best left to a computer. Most computer packages will output the values directly in an ANOVA table, which will usually include the *F*-ratio and a *P*-value.

Table 7.8 shows the computer output for comparing general health between the four cancer groups using a one-way ANOVA. The *F*-statistic, of 4.453, shows that the between group variation is about four times that of the within group variation. When compared to the *F*-distribution on 3 and 167 degrees of freedom this results in a *P*-value of 0.005. This is statistically significant so we can reject the null hypothesis and accept the alternative hypothesis that at least one cancer group has a different mean general health score from the other three groups.

If we obtain a significant result, at this initial stage, we may consider performing a series of specific pairwise post hoc comparisons. We can use one of a number of special tests devised for this purpose or we can use the two independent samples *t*-test (described previously) adjusted for multiple hypothesis testing. We can also calculate a CI for each individual group mean.

Table 7.8 Computer output from the one-way ANOVA.

	SF-36v2 General Health (0–100)				
	Sum of squares	**df**	**Mean square**	**F**	**P-value**
Between groups	7708.007	3	2569.336	4.453	0.005
Within groups	96346.625	167	576.926		
Total	104054.632	170			

P-value: probability of observing the *F*-statistic under the null hypothesis that all four group means in the population are equal. As the value of 0.005 is less than the significance level (α) set at 005 or 5% this means that the result obtained is unlikely when the null hypothesis is true. Thus there is sufficient evidence to reject the null hypothesis and accept the alternative hypothesis that at least one cancer group has a different mean General Health score from the other three groups.

Although the independent samples *t*-test and ANOVA appear to be different methods of statistical analysis, they will give the same results when there are only two groups. Like the *t*-test, ANOVA is relatively robust to moderate departures from Normality. It is not as robust to unequal variances. Therefore, before carrying out the analysis we should check for Normality and whether the variances are similar by graphical methods (histograms, dot plots, box, and whisker plots) described in Chapter 2 or by simply eyeballing the standard deviations. The descriptive statistics in Table 7.7 suggests that standard deviations are broadly similar across the four cancer groups. If the assumptions are not satisfied, we can either transform the data or use the non-parametric equivalent of one-way ANOVA, the Kruskal–Wallis test.

The Kruskal–Wallis Test

This is a non-parametric extension of the Mann–Whitney *U* test. Under the null hypothesis of no differences in the distributions between the groups, the sums of the ranks in each of the groups should be comparable after allowing for any differences in sample size. The steps for performing a Kruskal–Wallis test are described in Box 7.6 in the technical details section at the end of this chapter.

Table 7.9 shows the computer output for the Kruskal–Wallis test. The Kruskal–Wallis test statistic is 12.88 (with allowance for tied ranks) this is very similar to the value of 12.84 using the formulae in Box 7.2 with no allowance for ties, suggesting the effect of tying in the ranks is negligible. The conclusions from the analysis are very similar to those from the ANOVA example in Table 7.8: the differences are statistically significant. Thus there is sufficient evidence to reject the null hypothesis and accept the alternative hypothesis that each cancer type group does not have the same distribution of SF-36 general health scores.

Table 7.9 Computer output from the Kruskal–Wallis test.

		Ranks		
	Cancer type	N	Mean rank	Sum of ranks
SF-36v2 general health (0–100)	Germ cell (testicular)	66	98.53	6503
	Lymphoma	70	71.11	4978
	Leukaemia	11	108.45	1193
	Other	24	84.67	2032
	Total	171		

Kruskal-Wallis Test Statistic

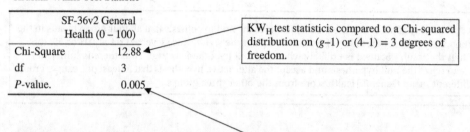

	SF-36v2 General Health (0 – 100)
Chi-Square	12.88
df	3
P-value.	0.005

KW_H test statisticis compared to a Chi-squared distribution on $(g-1)$ or $(4-1) = 3$ degrees of freedom.

P-value: probability of observing the statistic, under the null hypothesis that each group has the same distribution of values in the population. As the value of 0.005 is less than the significance level (α) set at 0.05 or 5% this means that the resultobtained is unlikely when the null hypothesis is true. Thus there is sufficient evidence to reject the null hypothesis and accept the alternative hypothesis that each cancer type group does not have the same distribution of SF-36 general health scores.

7.5 Non-Normal Distributions

Non-parametric Tests

Non-parametric methods such as the Wilcoxon signed rank test and the Mann–Whitney U test described here provide alternative data analysis techniques without assuming anything about the shape of the data, i.e. they do not assume an underlying distribution for the data. Hence non-parametric methods often referred to as 'distribution free' methods. Non-parametric techniques are usually based on the ordered or ranked values of the observations in the sample and not the actual data. Non-parametric methods are used when:

1) Data does not seem to follow any particular shape or distribution (for example, the Normal distribution);
2) Assumptions underlying parametric tests not met;
3) A plot of the data appears to be very skewed;
4) There are potential outliers in the dataset (an outlier is a data value that is distant from the other values in the dataset).

It is important to note that it is the test that is non-parametric, NOT the data. Non-parametric methods should not be considered as an alternative way to find significant *P*-values!

Why Not Always Use Non-parametric Tests?

It can be argued that since non-parametric tests can always be used – why not use them always! The argument has much appeal but can be answered albeit in somewhat technical terms. It turns out that if a non-parametric test is used when the data follow a Normal distribution, then the calculated *P*-value will always exceed that that would be obtained using the *t*-test. Thus one is less likely to declare a result significant using a non-parametric test than using a parametric test with the same data. In these circumstances the non-parametric test is termed less powerful, although the loss of power is often not very great. This is because the more assumptions one is prepared to make about the data the more precisely one can investigate hypotheses. The corresponding non-parametric CIs will also be wider and more difficult to calculate, although help with this is provided by Altman et al. (2000, Chapter 5).

However, the overwhelming argument against the routine use of non-parametric procedures is that they are not flexible enough. For example, they do not easily allow for analyses such as multiple regression (see Chapter 9), which take into account other characteristics of the groups being compared.

There is also some misunderstanding about the flexibility of parametric tests. For example, for the data summarised in Figure 7.4, it is clearly indicated that a Normal distribution for the outcome, PHQ-9 score, does not seem reasonable for either of the BA or control groups. However, this does not in itself invalidate the use of the *t*-test. We are interested in comparing the sample means of the two groups and the Central Limit Theorem, which we described in Chapter 5, ensures that the sample means will be approximately Normally distributed, when the sample size is sufficiently large. Generally, if n is greater than 25, these approximations to Normality for sample means will be good. Furthermore the work of Heeren and D'Agostino (1987) and Sullivan and D'Agostino (2003) supports the robustness of the two independent samples *t*-test even when applied to three-, four-, and five-point ordinal scaled data using assigned scores, in sample sizes as small as 20 subjects per group.

7.6 Degrees of Freedom

The number of degrees of freedom, df, depends on two factors: first the number of groups we wish to compare and secondly the number of parameters we need to estimate to calculate the standard deviation of the contrast of interest. When comparing two means, there are degrees of freedom for between-groups, there are also degrees of freedom for estimating σ. How the degrees of freedom are calculated depends on the particular problem. For a paired situation $df =$ (number of subjects minus one); for an unpaired two-sample situation $df =$ (total number of subjects minus two), in the case of equal group sizes this is $n-1$ for each group. Thus the *t*-test has implicitly two sets of degrees of freedom attached to it. The first, a degree of freedom for between-groups, the second one for within-groups. However, the first of these degrees of freedom is not usually explicitly referred to as it is always unity. The *t*-test can be used for small or large samples providing the relevant assumptions are met. An alternative to the *t*-test for large samples (described in Chapter 6 is the *Z*-test). The *Z*-test is similar to the *t*-test, but since in this case σ is assumed known effectively the within-group degrees of freedom are infinite and so these also are seldom explicitly referred to. There is no simple, universal rule stating how large the sample size must be to be able to use a *Z*-test and get an accurate

P-value A rule of thumb is that for a single sample there should be at least 100 observations and for two samples at least 50 in each.

7.7 Points When Reading the Literature

1) Have clinical importance and statistical significance been confused?
2) Has the sample size been taken into account when determining the choice of statistical tests; that is, are small-sample tests used when appropriate?
3) Is it reasonable to assume that the quantitative variables have a Normal distribution?
4) Have paired tests been utilised in the appropriate places?
5) Have CIs of the main results been quoted?
6) Is the result medically or biologically plausible and has the statistical significance of the result been considered in isolation, or have other studies of the same effect been taken into account?
7) Be careful of paired tests comparing baseline with outcome, as described in Section 7.1, if they form part of a clinical trial. Simply because an outcome changes does not mean that the change is due to the intervention. One has to compare changes between different groups
8) Recall a Mann-Whitney test does not test for differences in medians

7.8 Technical Details

Student's *t*-Distribution

In discussing the Z-test in Chapter 6 two assumptions were made. The first is that the variable under consideration follows an approximately Normal distribution, and secondly that samples from the respective population have always been relatively large. However, it is intuitively obvious that with small samples one can make less precise statements about population parameters than one can with large samples. Thus, it is necessary to recognise that if samples are small $\bar{x}$ and s will not always be necessarily close to μ and σ respectively. How does the sample size influence the calculations? Inone way sample size is already taken into account through the calculation of the standard deviation of the mean, $\mathrm{SE}(\bar{x})$, when dividing by $\sqrt{n}$, the square-root of the sample size. In small samples, however, s may be a poor estimator of σ (the population standard deviation), and one consequence is that although $\bar{x}$ will still have a Normal distribution, it can no longer be assumed the ratio, $Z = \bar{x}/\mathrm{SE}(\bar{x})$, will.

As a consequence it is necessary to modify the calculation of both the P-value and a CI. For the CI z_α is replaced by t_α, in the expression given for a CI for the difference between two means in Section 6.2, to obtain

$$\bar{d} - \left\{ t_{df,\alpha} \times \mathrm{SE}(\bar{d}) \right\} \text{ to } \bar{d} + \left\{ t_{df,\alpha} \times \mathrm{SE}(\bar{d}) \right\},$$

while the expression for Z is relabelled, $t = \dfrac{\bar{d}}{\mathrm{SE}(\bar{d})}$. This is known as Student's t-statistic. Under the null hypothesis of no difference in the means t is assumed to be distributed as Student's t-distribution rather than as a Normal distribution.

In the expression for the CI the particular value for t_α, depends not only on α but also on the number of degrees of freedom, *df*, on which σ is estimated. We explain how to calculate degrees of freedom in Section 7.8. Table T2 gives some values of t_α for different values of *df* and α.

Examination of the bottom row of Table T2 shows that with $df = \infty$, that is with very large degrees of freedom, the same value for t_α is obtained as for z_α in Table T1 for each value of α. However, the values of t_α get larger as the df get smaller. This reflects the increasing uncertainty concerning the estimate of σ as sample sizes get smaller.

Welch's *t*-Test

In statistics, Welch's *t*-test, or unequal variances *t*-test, is a modification of a Student's *t*-test that is used to test the hypothesis that two populations have equal means. It is named for its creator, Bernard Lewis Welch, and is an adaptation of Student's *t*-test, and is more reliable when the two samples have unequal variances and/or unequal sample sizes. The modification is to the degrees of freedom used in the test, which tends to increase the test's power for samples with unequal variance. The null hypothesis for the test is that the means are equal. The alternate hypothesis for the test is that means are not equal.

Welch's *t*-test, unlike Student's *t*-test, does not have the assumption of equal variance (however, both tests have the assumption of Normality). When two groups have equal sample sizes and variances, Welch's tends to give the same result as Student's. However, when sample sizes and variances are unequal, Welch's test tends to perform better.

Welch's *t*-test defines the test statistic t by the following formula: $t = \dfrac{\bar{x}_1 - \bar{x}_2}{\sqrt{\dfrac{s_1^2}{n_1} + \dfrac{s_2^2}{n_2}}}$.

The degrees of freedom associated with this statistic are approximated using the Welch–Satterthwaite equation: $df = \dfrac{\left(\dfrac{s_1^2}{n_1} + \dfrac{s_2^2}{n_2}\right)^2}{\dfrac{1}{n_1-1}\left(\dfrac{s_1^2}{n_1}\right)^2 + \dfrac{1}{n_2-1}\left(\dfrac{s_2^2}{n_2}\right)^2}$.

The approximate degrees of freedom are rounded to the nearest integer.

Table 7.10 shows the computer output for comparing mean PHQ-9 scores between the two groups using two independent samples *t*-test and the Welch test. The standard deviations for the two groups are different; but broadly similar, and the ratio of the two SDs, is $6.9/5.1 = 1.4$. The degrees of freedom for the Welch test are 31 compared to 37 for the *t*-test. The results of the two tests are very similar and both tests lead to similar conclusions that there is a significant difference between the groups, although the CI is wider for the Welch test. The 95% CI for the difference (from the Welch test and SE of the difference) suggests that that patients in the BA group have between 0.3 and 8.3 lower (or better) PHQ-9 scores than patients in the UC group and the best estimate is a mean difference of 4.3 points lower.

Wilcoxon Signed Rank Sum Test

Table 7.11 shows the ranks of the differences in order of increasing magnitude (ignoring the three zero values). The number of non-zero differences, n' is 27 (and this is less than the original sample size of $n = 30$). Table 7.11 also has a column with a sign for whether the differences are positive or negative. The sum of the 25 positive ranks, T^+, is 369.

Table 7.10 Computer output from the two independent samples *t*-test and Welch test.

	Group	N	Mean	SD	SE
PHQ-9 score at six months	UC	21	14.4	5.1	1.1
	BA	18	10.1	6.9	1.6

	t	df	P-value	Difference in means	SE difference	95% CI of the difference Lower	Upper
t-test (equal variances assumed)	2.22	37	0.033	4.27	1.92	0.37	8.17
Welch test (equal variances not assumed)	2.17	30.996	0.038	4.27	1.97	0.26	8.29

The value of the test statistic for the Welch test is 2.17 this is compared to the *t*-distribution on 31 degrees of freedom, which results in a *P*-value of 0.038. Thus the results are unlikely when the null hypothesis (that there is no difference between the groups is true). The result is said to be statistically significant because the *P*-value is less than the significance level (α) set at 5% or 0.05 and there is sufficient evidence to reject the null hypothesis and accept the alternative hypothesis, that there is a difference in mean PHQ-9 scores at six-month post-randomisation between the BA and UC groups.

The Wilcoxon signed rank sum test statistic is $Z = \dfrac{T^+ - \left(\dfrac{n'(n'+1)}{4}\right)}{\sqrt{\dfrac{[n'(n'+1)(2n'+1)]}{24}}} =$

$\dfrac{369 - \left(\dfrac{27(27+1)}{4}\right)}{\sqrt{\dfrac{27(27+1)(2 \times 27+1)}{24}}} = \dfrac{180}{41.62} = 4.32.$

Under the null hypothesis, Z has an approximately Normal distribution. The *P*-value or probability of observing the test statistic of 4.32 or more extreme under the null hypothesis is 0.00002. This means that this result is unlikely when the null hypothesis is true (of no difference in pain scores between baseline and three months).

Mann–Whitney *U* Test

Table 7.12 shows the ranks of the 39 PHQ-9 scores in order of increasing magnitude. Table 7.12 also has a separate column with the ranks for thus patients in the BA group. For whether the differences are positive or negative. The sum of the 18 ranks in the BA group, W, is 277.5. The Mann–Whitney U test statistic, with no adjustment for ties, is:

$Z = \dfrac{W - \left(\dfrac{n_1(n_1+n_2+1)}{2}\right)}{\sqrt{\dfrac{[n_1 n_2(n_1+n_2+1)]}{12}}} = \dfrac{277.5 - \left(\dfrac{18 \times (18+21+1)}{2}\right)}{\sqrt{\dfrac{18 \times 21 \times (18+21+1)}{12}}} = \dfrac{277.5 - 360}{35.50} = -2.324.$

Table 7.11 Ranked differences in VAS pain scores between baseline and three months, in 30 patients treated with salicylic acid plasters whose index corn resolved at three months.

Subject	Difference (0–3 m)	Rank	Sign	Positive ranks	Negative ranks
1	3	3	+	3	
2	0		+		
3	40	20	+	20	
4	0		+		
5	1	1	+	1	
6	15	8	+	8	
7	10	7	+	7	
8	16	9	+	9	
9	100	27	+	27	
10	20	11.5	+	11.5	
11	20	11.5	+	11.5	
12	46	22	+	22	
13	−9	6	−		6
14	68	25	+	25	
15	25	16	+	16	
16	43	21	+	21	
17	0		+		
18	49	23	+	23	
19	19	10	+	10	
20	3	3	+	3	
21	25	16	+	16	
22	34	19	+	19	
23	24	13.5	+	13.5	
24	−3	3	−		3
25	24	13.5	+	13.5	
26	29	18	+	18	
27	78	26	+	26	
28	63	24	+	24	
29	6	5	+	5	
30	25	16	+	16	
	Sum	378		369	9

Source: data from Farndon et al. (2013).

Table 7.12 Ranked PHQ-9 scores at six-month post-randomisation in 39 patients with post-stroke depression by group.

PHQ-9 score	Group	Rank	Tied rank	Ranks in BA group
2.0	BA	1	1	1
3.0	BA	2	2.5	2.5
3.0	BA	3	2.5	2.5
5.0	BA	4	4.5	4.5
5.0	BA	5	4.5	4.5
6.0	BA	6	7.5	7.5
6.0	BA	7	7.5	7.5
6.0	BA	8	7.5	7.5
6.0	BA	9	7.5	7.5
7.0	BA	10	10.5	10.5
7.0	Control	11	10.5	
8.0	Control	12	12.5	
8.0	Control	13	12.5	
10.0	BA	14	16	16
10.0	Control	15	16	
10.0	Control	16	16	
10.0	Control	17	16	
10.0	Control	18	16	
11.6	Control	19	19	
12.0	BA	20	20	20
13.0	Control	21	21	
14.0	BA	22	23	23
14.0	Control	23	23	
14.0	Control	24	23	
15.0	BA	25	26.5	26.5
15.0	BA	26	26.5	26.5
15.0	Control	27	26.5	
15.0	Control	28	26.5	
16.0	Control	29	29	
17.0	Control	30	30.5	
17.0	Control	31	30.5	
18.0	Control	32	32	
19.0	Control	33	33	
20.0	Control	34	34	
20.6	BA	35	35	35
22.0	Control	36	36	
23.0	BA	37	37.5	37.5
23.0	BA	38	37.5	37.5
27.0	Control	39	39	
			Sum	277.5

Source: data from Thomas et al. (2019).

Table 7.13 Tied PHQ-9 scores at six-month post-randomisation in 28 patients.

Tied PHQ-9 scores	Number of ties t	t^3	$t^3 - t$
3.0	2	8	6
5.0	2	8	6
6.0	4	64	60
7.0	2	8	6
8.0	2	8	6
10.0	5	125	120
14.0	3	27	24
15.0	4	64	60
17.0	2	8	6
23.0	2	8	6
Sum	28		300

Source: data from Thomas et al. (2019).

Under the null hypothesis, Z, has an approximate Normal distribution. The P-value or probability of observing this test statistic of -2.324 or more extreme under the null hypothesis is 0.02.

Table 7.13 shows there are 10 tied PHQ-9 scores from 28 of the 39 trial participants. If we use the modified denominator or standard error formula for ties, then the denominator for the MW test statistic is changed to $\sqrt{\dfrac{n_1 n_2}{12 n(n-1)} \left[n^3 - n - \sum_t (t^3 - t) \right]} =$

$\sqrt{\dfrac{18 \times 21}{12 \times 39 \times (39-1)} \left[39^3 - 39 - 300 \right]} = 35.41$. Compared this to a value of 35.50 with no allowance for ties.

The Mann–Whitney U test statistic, with adjustment for ties, is:

$$Z = \frac{277.5 - 360}{35.41} = -2.330.$$

The P-value or probability of observing this test statistic of -2.330 (compared to -2.324 with no allowance for ties) or more extreme under the null hypothesis is 0.0198 (compared to a P-value of 0.02 with no allowance for ties). Thus even with quite a large number of tied values and ranks in the data the adjustment for tied values has very little impact on the Mann–Whitney test statistic value.

Comparing More than Two Groups

One-way Analysis of Variance

Box 7.5 describes the calculations for a one-way ANOVA.

The calculations involved in ANOVA are complex (see Box 7.5) and are best left to a computer. Most computer packages will output the values directly in an ANOVA table, which will usually include the F-ratio and a P-value.

Box 7.5 One-way Analysis of Variance (ANOVA)

Suppose there are g ($g \geqslant 2$) independent groups of observations on a variable y and let y_{ij} denote the jth observation in the ith group. The sample size, means and standard deviations in each group are n_i, $\bar{y}_i$ and s_i respectively (i = 1, 2,..., g) The total sample size is $N = n_1 + n_2 + ... + n_g = \sum_{i=1}^{g} n_i$. We wish to test the null hypothesis, H_0, that all the group means in the population are equal against the alternative hypothesis, H_A, that at least one group mean in the population differs from the others.

Assumptions

1) The groups are independent.
2) The variable of interest is quantitative.
3) The data in the groups have similar variances or standard deviations.
4) The data are Normally distributed in each group.

Steps

1) Calculate:

   $\bar{y}_i$ = mean of observations in the ith group;

   $S_i = \sum_{i=1}^{n_i} y_i^2$ = sum of squares of observations in the ith group;

   $T = \sum_{i=1}^{g} n_i \bar{y}_i$ = sum of all observations;

   $S = \sum_{i=1}^{g} S_i$ = sum of squares of all observations.

2) Calculate the overall or total variability of the data about its overall mean, $\bar{y}$, called the *total sum of squares* $SS_{Total} = \sum_{i,j} (y_{ij} - \bar{y})^2 = S - \frac{T^2}{N}$.

3) Calculate the within-group variability called the *within-groups sum of squares* $SS_{Within} = S - \sum_{i=1}^{g} n_i \bar{y}_i^2$.

4) Calculate the *between-group variability* or the between groups sum of squares $SS_{Between} = \sum_{i=1}^{g} n_i \bar{y}_i^2 - T^2/N$.

5) Calculate the mean squares ($MS_{Between}$ and MS_{Within}) by dividing the sums of squares by the degrees of freedom.

6) Calculate the variance ratio (VR) or F test statistic by dividing the $MS_{Between}$ by MS_{Within}.

7) Compare the test statistic with the F distribution with $(g - 1, N - g)$ degrees of freedom in the numerator and denominator, respectively (see Table T4). This gives us the probability of the observing the test statistic F or more extreme under the null hypothesis.

Table 7.14 One-way ANOVA table to compare g group means.

Source of variation	Sums of squares (SS)	Degrees of freedom (df)	Mean square (MS) or variances	Variance ratio F
Between Groups	$SS_{Between} = \sum_{i=1}^{g} n_i \bar{y}_i^2 - \dfrac{T^2}{N}$	$g-1$	$MS_{Between} = \dfrac{SS_{Between}}{g-1}$	$F = \dfrac{MS_{Between}}{MS_{Within}}$
Within Groups	$SS_{Within} = S - \sum_{i=1}^{g} n_i \bar{y}_i^2$	$N-g$	$MS_{Within} = \dfrac{SS_{Within}}{N-g}$	
Total	$SS_{Total} = S - \dfrac{T^2}{N}$	$N-1$		

If we obtain a significant result, at this initial stage, we may consider performing a series of specific pairwise post hoc comparisons. We can use one of a number of special tests devised for this purpose or we can use the two independent samples t-test (described previously) adjusted for multiple hypothesis testing (see Chapter 16). We can also calculate a CI for each individual group mean. Note that we use a pooled estimate of the variance of the values from all the groups when calculating CIs and performing t-tests. Most software packages refer to this estimate of the variance as the residual variance or the residual mean square. It is found in the ANOVA table. The square root of the within groups mean square is the residual standard deviation. The example in Table 7.14 shows a residual variance of 576.9 or residual standard deviation of $\sqrt{576.9} = 24.0$.

Although independent sample t-test and ANOVA appear to be different, they will give the same results when there are only two groups. Like the t-test, ANOVA is relatively robust to moderate departures from Normality. It is not as robust to unequal variances. If the assumptions are not satisfied, we can either transform the data or use the non-parametric equivalent of one-way ANOVA, the Kruskal–Wallis test.

The Kruskal–Wallis Test

This is a non-parametric extension of the Mann–Whitney U test. Under the null hypothesis of no differences in the distributions between the groups, the sums of the ranks in each of the groups should be comparable after allowing for any differences in sample size. The steps for performing a Kruskal–Wallis test are described in Box 7.6.

Box 7.6   Kruskal–Wallis Test

Suppose we wish to test the null hypothesis, H_0, that g ($g >= 2$) samples or groups come from the same population. That is, each group has the same distribution of values in the population, against the alternative hypothesis, H_A, each group does not have the same distribution of values in the population. The data are at least ordinal and from g independent groups of size $n_1, n_2 ... n_g$ respectively. The total sample size is $N = \sum_{i=1}^{g} n_i$, where n_i is the number of observations in group i.

Assumptions

1) The groups are independent.
2) The variables of interest are at least ordinal (can be ranked).

Box 7.6 (Continued)

Steps

1) First combine the data in all *g* groups and rank the entire data set, of *N* values, in increasing order (smallest observation to the largest) from 1 to *N*. If some of the observations are numerically equal, they are given tied ranks equal to the mean of the ranks which would otherwise have been used.

2) Separately sum the ranks for each of the *g* groups. Let R_i be the sum of the ranks for the n_i observations in group *i*.

3) If there are no ties or only a few ties, calculate the Kruskal–Wallis *H* test statistic

$$KW_H = \frac{12}{N(N+1)} \sum_{i=1}^{g} \frac{R_i^2}{n_i} - 3(N+1).$$

4) Under the null hypothesis that the *g* samples come from the same population, the test statistic, KW follows a Chi-squared distribution with (*g*-1) *df* and can be referred to Table T3 in the appendix to calculate a *P*-value.

The formula is not very accurate if there any many ties in the data. The reader is referred to Armitage et al. (2002) in such situations.

7.9 Exercises

The self-reported, physical functioning, as measured by the EORTC QLQ-C30 questionnaire, in eight patients with multiple myeloma awaiting autologous haematopoietic stem cell transplantation before and after a six-week duration pre-transplant exercise programme (prehabilitation) are shown in Table 7.15 (Keen et al. 2018). The EORTC QLQ-C30 physical functioning scale is scored on 0 to 100 scale with higher scores representing a high/healthy level of functioning.

Table 7.15 Self-reported, physical functioning scores, in eight patients with multiple myeloma awaiting autologous haematopoietic stem cell transplantation before and after a six-week duration pre-transplant exercise programme.

Subject (*i*)	EORTC QLQ-C30 physical function scale score	
	Before	**After**
1	40.0	60.0
2	66.7	80.0
3	100.0	100.0
4	80.0	100.0
5	53.3	86.7
6	80.0	90.3
7	53.3	60.0
8	20.0	46.7
Mean	61.7	78.0

Source: data from Keen et al. (2018).

7.1 For the data in Table 7.15, suppose we wish to compare the difference in EORTC QLQ-C30 physical function domain scores before and after exercise. Which ONE of the following statistical methods would be most appropriate to compare physical function scores before and after exercise?

    A Two independent samples *t*-test

    B Paired *t*-test

    C Mann–Whitney *U* test

    D Chi-squared test

    E One-way ANOVA

7.2 For the data in Table 7.15, the mean difference in EORTC QLQ-C30 physical function domain scores before and after exercise is:

    A −9.0

    B −1.0

    C 16.3

    D 61.7

    E 78.0

7.3 For the data in Table 7.15, the standard error of the mean difference in EORTC QLQ-C30 physical function domain scores before and after exercise is:

    A 3.9

    B 4.8

    C 7.1

    D 9.0

    E 25.4

7.4 Calculate the 95% CI for the difference in mean EORTC QLQ-C30 physical function domain scores before and after exercise for the data reported in Table 7.15.

    A −5.6 to 18.1

    B −9.0 to 9.0

    C −9.6 to 7.6

    D 7.2 to 25.4

    E 1.0 to 17.0

7.5 What are the degrees of freedom (*df*) for the *t*-test for comparing the mean difference in EORTC QLQ-C30 physical function domain scores before and after exercise for the data in Table 7.15?

    A 6

    B 7

    C 8

    D 38

    E 39

7.6 Calculate the value of the test statistic for the *t*-test for comparing the mean difference in EORTC QLQ-C30 physical function domain scores before and after exercise for the data in Table 7.14.

A 0.23
B 1.0
C 1.1
D 4.2
E 4.8

7.7 The *P*-value from the *t*-test for comparing the mean difference in EORTC QLQ-C30 physical function domain scores before and after exercise for the data in Table 7.14 is?
A <0.01
B Between 0.02 and 0.05
C Between 0.05 and 0.10
D Between 0.10 and 0.20
E >0.20

Table 7.16 EQ-5D VAS score at six-month post-randomisation by group in 39 stroke patients with depression.

Participant	BA (*n* = 18)	Control (*n* = 21)
1	30	45
2	70	70
3	30	45
4	75	60
5	27	50
6	30	78
7	80	30
8	50	35
9	50	70
10	70	50
11	65	80
12	75	40
13	45	55
14	80	30
15	80	30
16	70	30
17	45	40
18	30	40
19		50
20		70
21		40
Mean	55.67	49.43
SD	20.26	16.24
SE	4.77	3.54

Source: data from the BEADs trial; Thomas et al. (2019).

The BEADS trial (Thomas et al, 2019) was a parallel group feasibility multi-centre randomised controlled trial in patients with post-stroke depression. The aim of the BEADS trial was to evaluate the feasibility of undertaking a full trial comparing BA to usual stroke care for four months for patients with post-stroke depression. Trial participants were randomly allocated to receive BA therapy in addition to usual care or usual care alone (control). One of the secondary outcome measures was the EQ-5D VAS measured at six-month post-randomisation. The EQ-5D VAS records the patient's self-rated health on a vertical VAS, scored on a 0 (worst imaginable health state) to 100 (best imaginable health state) scale.

7.8 The mean EQ-5D VAS outcomes in Table 7.16 were compared between the BA and control groups using a two independent samples *t*-test.

Which of the following IS NOT an assumption for the two independent samples *t*-test?

A Two independent groups

B Continuous outcome data

C Outcome data in both groups is Normally distributed

D The standard deviation of the outcome is similar in both groups

E The standard error of the mean is similar in both groups

7.9 For the data in Table 7.16, the difference in mean EQ-5D VAS scores at six months between the BA and control groups is:

A −9.0

B −1.0

C 5.0

D 6.2

E 10

7.10 What are the *degrees of freedom (df)* for the two independent samples *t*-test for the six-month post-randomisation outcome reported in Table 7.16?

A 18

B 21

C 37

D 38

E 39

7.11 Calculate the *standard error of the difference between two means*, for the two independent samples *t*-test, for the six-month post-randomisation EQ-5D VAS outcome for the data reported in Table 7.16?

A 3.5

B 4.8

C 5.8

D 12

E 13

7.12 Calculate the value of the *test statistic* for the difference in means between the BA and control treated groups for the two independent samples *t*-test for the six-month post-randomisation EQ-5D VAS outcome reported in Table 7.16?

The test statistic value is:

A 0.23
B 1.0
C 1.1
D 4.0
E 4.8

7.13 The *P-value* from the two independent samples *t*-test for the six-month post-randomisation EQ-5D VAS outcome reported in Table 7.16 is?

A <0.01
B Between 0.02 and 0.05
C Between 0.05 and 0.10
D Between 0.10 and 0.20
E >0.20

7.14 Calculate the *95% CI for the difference in means* between the BA and control treated groups for the two independent samples *t*-test for the six-month post-randomisation EQ-5D VAS outcome reported in Table 7.16.

A −5.6 to 18.0
B −9.0 to 9.0
C −9.6 to 7.6
D −3.6 to 13.6
E 1.0 to 17.0

8   Comparing Groups of Binary and Categorical Data

Medical Statistics: A Textbook for the Health Sciences, Fifth Edition. Stephen J. Walters, Michael J. Campbell, and David Machin.
© 2021 John Wiley & Sons Ltd. Published 2021 by John Wiley & Sons Ltd.
Companion website: www.wiley.com/go/walters/medicalstatistics

Summary

In this chapter we will explain some of the basic methods appropriate for analysing and comparing categorical outcome data. We consider the comparison of two independent groups such as groups of patients given different treatments and the comparison of paired data, for example, the response of one group of patients before and after an exposure to a stimulus or under different conditions.

8.1 Introduction

This chapter outlines some of the basic methods appropriate for analysing and comparing categorical outcome data. We shall illustrate some of various statistical tests by using data from the HubBLE trial, referred to in Chapters 5 and 6, which aimed to compare haemorrhoidal artery ligation (HAL) surgery (intervention) with rubber band ligation (RBL) surgery (control) in patients with grade II–III haemorrhoids (Brown et al. 2016). In this trial, 337 patients were randomly allocated to HAL (161) or RBL (176) surgery. HAL is an operation designed to reduce the blood flow to the haemorrhoid; the vessels supplying blood are located and stitched closed to block the blood supply, which causes the haemorrhoid to shrink over the following days and weeks. RBL involves the surgeon placing a very tight elastic band around the base of the haemorrhoid to cut off the blood supply. The haemorrhoids should then fall off within about a week of having the treatment. Patients were treated and followed up for 12 months. The primary outcome was whether the haemorrhoid recurred 12 months after the procedure, and this fact was derived from the patient's self-reported assessment in combination with their GP and hospital records.

8.2 Comparison of Two Independent Groups – Binary Outcomes

In the HubBle trial the outcome is binary, and the surgeons wished to know whether there was a difference between the HAL and RBL groups in the proportions whose haemorrhoid recurred within one year of follow-up. With two independent groups (HAL and RBL) and a binary (haemorrhoid recurred versus not recurred) rather than a continuous outcome, the data can be cross-tabulated as in Table 5.2 and again in the top part of the computer output in Table 8.1. This is an example of a 2×2 contingency table with two rows (for treatment) and two columns (for outcome), that is, four cells in total. The most appropriate summary measure is the difference in the proportions in the two groups of haemorrhoid recurrence at 12 months.

Figure 7.3 shows that there are several different approaches to analysing these data. One approach which we outlined in Chapter 6 would be to compare the proportions whose haemorrhoid has recurred at a 12-month follow-up in the two groups. In this example a suitable null hypothesis (H_0), is that there is no difference in outcomes, the proportion of patients whose haemorrhoid has recurred at 12 months between HAL and RBL groups, that is, $\pi_{HAL} - \pi_{RBL} = 0$. The alternative hypothesis (H_A) is that there is a difference in the proportion of patients whose haemorrhoid has recurred at 12 months, that is, $\pi_{HAL} - \pi_{RBL} \neq 0$. Note that we are interested in the difference in the population of patients with grade II–III haemorrhoids and we have taken a sample of patients that we study in order to make inferences about the population of interest.

In general, the corresponding hypothesis test assumes that there is a common proportion, π, estimated by $p = \dfrac{(n_1 p_1 + n_2 p_2)}{(n_1 + n_2)}$ and standard error (SE) for the difference in proportions is estimated by $SE(p_1 - p_2) = \sqrt{p(1-p)\left(\dfrac{1}{n_1} + \dfrac{1}{n_2}\right)}$ (see Table 6.4). From this the test statistic:

$Z = (p_1 - p_2)/SE(p_1 - p_2)$ is computed and Z is assumed to follow a standard Normal distribution.

This value is then compared to what would be expected under the null hypothesis of no difference, in order to get a P-value. The computer output in the top half of Table 8.1 implies: $n_1 = 161$, $p_1 = 48/161 = 0.298$; $n_2 = 176$, $p_2 = 87/176 = 0.494$ and $p_1 - p_2 = -0.196$ or 0.196 ignoring the sign.

Table 8.1 Computer output for the chi-squared test for the HubBle trial data.

			Randomised treatment group		
			HAL	RBL	Total
Haemorrhoid recurrence 12 months after procedure?	No	Count	113	89	202
		% within group	70.2%	50.6%	59.9%
	Yes	Count	48	87	135
		% within group	29.8%	49.4%	40.1%
Total		Count	161	176	337
		% within group	100.0%	100.0%	100.0%

Chi-Square Tests

	Value	df	P-value	Exact P-value
Pearson Chi-Square	13.48[a]	1	<0.001	
Continuity Correction[b]	12.67	1	<0.001	
Fisher's Exact Test				<0.001
N of Valid Cases	337			

a) 0 cells (0.0%) have expected count less than 5. The minimum expected count is 64.50.

b) Computed only for a 2×2 table

The P-value of < 0.001 indicates that the results obtained are unlikely if the null hypothesis (of no association between the rows and columns of the contingency table above) is true. Thus there is sufficient evidence to reject the null hypothesis and the results are said to be statistically significant.

See Box 8.1 to calculate the expected counts from a 2×2 table

In a 2×2 table when expected cell counts are less than 5, or any are less than 1 even Yates' correction does not work and thus Fisher's exact test is used.

To improve the approximation for a 2 x 2 table, Yates' correction for continuity is sometimes applied.

This suggests that the Chi-squared test is valid as all the expected counts are greater than 5.

Note: In a 2×2 table any count <5 is sufficient to invoke Yates' continuity correction.
Source: data from Brown et al. (2016).

$$p = \frac{(n_1 p_1 + n_2 p_2)}{(n_1 + n_2)} = \frac{[(161 \times 0.298) + (176 \times 0.494)]}{(161 + 176)} = \frac{(135)}{337} = 0.401$$

and $SE(p_1 - p_2) = \sqrt{p(1-p)\left(\frac{1}{n_1} + \frac{1}{n_2}\right)} = \sqrt{0.401(1-0.401)\left(\frac{1}{161} + \frac{1}{176}\right)} = 0.053.$

The test statistics is: $Z = (p_1 - p_2)/SE(p_1 - p_2) = 0.196/0.053 = 3.67$ and the probability of observing the test statistic $Z = 3.67$ or more extreme under the null hypothesis, using the standard Normal distribution Table T1 in the appendix, is <0.001. This means the results are unlikely if the null hypothesis is true and that there is sufficient evidence to reject the null hypothesis. Therefore, there is reliable evidence of a difference in haemorrhoid recurrence rates at 12 months between the HAL and RBL treated patient groups.

The 95% confidence interval (CI) for the difference in proportions is:

$$(p_1 - p_2) \pm [1.96 \times SE(p_1 - p_2)].$$

For the calculation of the confidence interval, we do not need to make any assumptions about there being a common proportion π and use the formula in Table 6.4 for the $SE(p_1 - p_2)$:

$$SE(p_1 - p_2) = \sqrt{\frac{p_1(1-p_1)}{n_1} + \frac{p_2(1-p_2)}{n_2}} = \sqrt{\frac{0.298 \times 0.702}{161} + \frac{0.494 \times 0.506}{171}} = 0.052.$$

The 95% confidence interval (CI) for the difference in proportions is:

$$(-0.196) - [1.96 \times 0.052] \text{ to } (-0.196) + [1.96 \times 0.052] \text{ or } -0.298 \text{ to } -0.094.$$

Therefore, we are 95% confident that the true population difference in the proportion of patients whose haemorrhoid has recurred at 12 months, between the HAL intervention and RBL control treated groups, lies somewhere between −29.8% and −9.4%, but our best estimate is −19.6% (i.e. the HAL treated group has the lower recurrence rate).

Figure 7.3, also shows that alternative approach to the comparisons of two proportions, assuming a large sample and all expected counts are at least five, is the chi-squared test. The null hypothesis is that the two classifications (group and haemorrhoid recurrence status at 12 months) are unrelated in the relevant population (patients with grade II–III haemorrhoids). More generally the null hypothesis, H_0, for a contingency table is that there is no association between the row and column variables in the table, that is, they are independent. The general alternative hypothesis, H_A, is that there is an association between the row and column variables in the contingency table and so they are *not* independent or unrelated. For the chi-squared test to be valid three key assumptions need to be met, as outlined in Box 8.1.

Under the null hypothesis, both treatments will have the same effect and we would expect the same proportion of recurrent haemorrhoids at 12 months. We can calculate what proportion this would be, and the expected cell counts, based on the expected proportion of recurrent haemorrhoids at 12 months. We base them on the overall counts we have observed in the study.

The best estimate of the common haemorrhoid recurrence rate at 12 months is the one for the total study, that is 135/337 = 40.1%. We can use this to calculate the expected number of haemorrhoid recurrences for each group, and the expected number with no haemorrhoid recurrence for each group. With 161 patients following HAL, we expect 40.1% of their haemorrhoids to have

---

Box 8.1   Chi-squared Test for Association in $r \times c$ Contingency Tables

Suppose we wish to test the null hypothesis, for an $r \times c$ contingency table, that there is no association between the row and column variables in the table, i.e. they are independent.

Assumptions

1) Two independent unordered categorical variables that form an $r \times c$ contingency table.
2) At least 80% of expected cell counts >5.
3) All expected cell counts >1.

Steps

1) Calculate the expected frequency (E_{ij}) for the observation in row i and column j of the $r \times c$ contingency table:

$$E_{ij} = \frac{\text{Row total } (R_i) \times \text{Column total } (C_j)}{N}, \text{ where } N \text{ is the total sample size.}$$

2) For each cell in the table calculate the difference between the observed value and the expected value ($O_{ij} - E_{ij}$).
3) Square each difference and divide the resultant quantity by the expected value $(O_{ij} - E_{ij})^2/E_{ij}$.
4) Sum all of these to get a single number, the χ^2 statistic.

$$\chi^2 = \sum_{i=1}^{r} \sum_{j=1}^{c} \frac{(O_{ij} - E_{ij})^2}{E_{ij}} = \sum \frac{(O - E)^2}{E}$$

5) Compare this number with tables of the chi-squared distribution with the following degrees of freedom: df = (number of rows − 1) × (number of columns − 1).

---

recurred by 12 months, which is 64.5. With 176 patients following RBL, we expect 40.1% of their haemorrhoids to have recurred by 12 months, which is 70.5. The observed (O) and expected (E) cell counts are shown in Table 8.2. It is worth noting that we only need to calculate *one* of the expected counts. All the others follow because for each row and column the sum of the expected counts must equal the sum of the observed counts. Thus, there is only one degree of freedom. For a 2×3 table we have to calculate *two* expected counts and the rest follow. In general, for r rows and c columns the degrees of freedom are $(r − 1) \times (c − 1)$.

Table 8.3 shows more details of the calculations and how we compare what we have observed (O) with what we would have expected (E) under the null hypothesis of no association. If what we have observed is very different from what we would have expected, then the null hypothesis is unlikely.

The value of $\sum \frac{(O-E)^2}{E} = 13.48$ and this is given in Table 8.1 as 'Pearson chi-square'. This value can be compared with Table T3 for the chi-squared distribution with df = (no. of rows − 1)×

Table 8.2 Observed and expected cell counts for the HubBle trial data.

		Randomised treatment				
		HAL		RBL		Total
		O	*E*	*O*	*E*	
Recurrent	No	113	**96.5**	89	**105.5**	202
haemorrhoids	Yes	48	**64.5**	87	**70.5**	135
Total		161	**161.0**	176	**176.0**	337

Source: data from Brown et al. (2016).

Table 8.3 Calculation of the chi-squared statistic for HubBle trial data.

	O	*E*	*O − E*	*(O − E)²/E*
HAL intervention/recurred	48	64.5	−16.5	4.22
HAL intervention/not recurred	113	96.5	16.5	2.82
RBL control/recurred	87	70.5	16.5	3.86
RBL control/not recurred	89	105.5	−16.5	2.58
Total	337	337.0	0	13.48

Source: data from Brown et al. (2016).

(number of columns − 1) = (2−1) × (2−1) = 1. Under the null hypothesis of no association the probability of observing this value of the test statistic X^2 or more, is *P*-value <0.001.

If more than 20% of expected cell counts are less than five then the test statistic does not approximate a chi-squared distribution. If any expected cell counts are <1 then we cannot use the chi-squared distribution. In large contingency tables we may have to combine categories to make fewer but containing larger patient numbers (providing it is meaningful). The bottom half of Table 8.1 shows the typical computer output for a chi-squared test. In this example it appears that the uncorrected chi-squared test is valid as all the expected counts are greater than five.

A χ^2 distribution is a continuous distribution, and the X^2 statistic is calculated from discrete count data. It can be shown in 2 × 2 tables the observed value of X^2 (calculated from count data) can be made closer to the true χ^2 value (under the null hypothesis) using *Yates' continuity correction*, χ^2_{CC}. This simply involves subtracting 0.5 from the absolute value for the difference between the observed and expected cell values so that: $\chi^2_{CC} = \sum \frac{(|O-E|-0.5)^2}{E}$.

$$\chi^2_{CC} = \frac{(|48-64.5|-0.5)^2}{64.5} + \frac{(|113-96.5|-0.5)^2}{96.5} + \frac{(|87-70.5|-0.5)^2}{70.5} + \frac{(|89-105.5|-0.5)^2}{105.5}$$

$$\chi^2_{CC} = \frac{(16.0)^2}{64.5} + \frac{(16.0)^2}{96.5} + \frac{(16.0)^2}{70.5} + \frac{(16.0)^2}{105.5} = 12.67.$$

Again, this value can be compared with Table T3 for the chi-squared distribution with $df = 1$. Under the null hypothesis of no association, the probability of observing this value of the test statistic or more, is less than 0.001.

Fisher's Exact Test

In a 2×2 table, when all the expected cell counts are smaller than 5, or any <1, even Yates' correction does not yield a good approximation to the true distribution. In this situation we can use Fisher's exact test which deals with 2×2 tables with very small expected frequencies. To understand this we need to go back to definitions of basic probability and estimate the probability of falsely rejecting the null hypothesis directly, based on all the possible tables, or more extreme, than we could have observed. This is very time-consuming by hand! Fortunately, most computer packages will calculate Fisher's exact test for all 2×2 tables, as the output in Table 8.1 shows. A fuller explanation of how to derive Fisher's exact test is given in the technical details section at the end of this chapter.

Chi-squared Test for Trend in a 2 × c Table

An important class of tables are $2 \times c$ tables, where the multi-level factor has c ordered levels. For example, patients might score their pain on an integer scale from 1 to 5 on one of two treatments. In this case the chi-squared test is very inefficient, because it fails to take account of the ordering and one should use the chi-squared test for trend. A fuller explanation of the chi-squared test for trend in a $2 \times c$ table is given in the technical details section at the end of this chapter.

8.3   Comparing Risks

There is yet another method of comparing 2×2 tables – comparison of two groups with respect to the risk of some event. We calculate the proportion having the outcome in each group, and so the ratio of these proportions is a measure of the raised risk in one group compared to another – the relative risk.

Table 8.4 shows that the risk of the haemorrhoid recurring by 12 months in the HAL group is $a/(a + c) = 48/161$ or 0.298 and in the RBL group it is $b/(b + d) = 87/176$ or 0.494. The relative of risk of the haemorrhoid recurring (RRHAL vs RBL) is 0.298/0.494 = 0.603. That is the risk of the haemorrhoid recurring at 12 months in the HAL group is 0.6 times that of recurring in the RBL group (i.e. the haemorrhoid is less likely to recur in the HAL group). This means a relative risk reduction of $1 - 0.6 = 0.4$ or a 40% reduction in the relative risk of recurrence with HAL compared to RBL. A confidence interval can be calculated for the relative risk estimate (using the methodology described in the technical details of this chapter). The 95% CI for the RR estimate is 0.46 to 0.80. As the RR <1, and since the CI the confidence interval does not include 1, haemorrhoid recurrences are significantly less likely (at the 5% level) with HAL than with RBL.

Comparing Groups Via the Odds Ratio

Chapter 3 showed that for a 2×2 table, the odds ratio (OR) is defined as $OR_{\text{Int vs Con}} = \dfrac{a}{c} / \dfrac{b}{d} = \dfrac{ad}{bc}$. A confidence interval can be obtained in a similar manner to the relative risk. Table 8.1 shows that the odds of the haemorrhoid recurring with HAL is $a/c = 48/113$ or 0.425 and that with

Table 8.4 Haemorrhoid recurrence rates, in HAL (haemorrhoidal artery ligation) and RBL (rubber band ligation) groups, at 12 months after the surgical procedure in patients with grade II–III haemorrhoids.

Haemorrhoid Recurrence	HAL intervention n		RBL control n	
Yes	48	(a)	87	(b)
No	113	(c)	89	(d)
Total	161	($a + c$)	176	($b + d$)

Source: data from Brown et al. (2016).

RBL is $b/d = 87/89$ or 0.978. The OR of the haemorrhoid recurring is $OR_{HAL\ vs\ RBL} = 0.425/0.978 = 0.435$. That is the odds of the haemorrhoid recurring at 12 months with HAL group is 0.4 times that of the odds of the haemorrhoid recurring with RBL. A confidence interval can be calculated for the OR estimate. The 95% CI for the OR estimate is 0.28 to 0.68. As the interval does not include 1, which indicates equal risk (or odds) in the two groups, we can infer that there is a difference in the risk (odds) of haemorrhoids recurring at 12 months between the two treatments.

In general, if the RR (the relative risk) or the OR (the odds ratio) equals one, or the 95% confidence interval includes one, then there is no statistically significant difference between treatment and control groups. If the RR >1, and the CI does not include 1, events are significantly more likely in the treatment than the control group. If the RR <1, and the CI does not include 1, events are significantly less likely in the treatment than the control group.

8.4 Comparison of Two Groups of Paired Observations – Categorical Outcomes

Just as for continuous data, we require a special analysis if paired or matched data are involved. As we have indicated previously, these can arise from the response of one group of patients before and after an exposure to a stimulus or under different conditions. Sometimes patients may be treated with two different treatments A and B and the outcomes (+ or −) from the two treatments compared. In this case the data and proportions are paired and the usual chi-squared test is inappropriate. The test of paired proportions is known as McNemar's test.

Consider the data in Table 8.5, which gives the results from a study by Bentur et al. (2009) in which airway hyper-responsiveness (AHR) status – an indication of pulmonary complications – was measured in 21 children before and after stem cell transplantation (SCT). The incidence of AHR increased from 2 out of 21 (10%) children before to 8 out of 21 (38%) after SCT.

In Table 8.5 there are four matched pairs:

Pair 1: Both with AHR before and after SCT (e);
Pair 2: Both with no AHR before and after SCT (h);
Pair 3: AHR before SCT but no AHR after SCT (f);
Pair 4: No AHR before SCT but AHR after SCT (g).

If all matched pairs were like pairs 1 and 2 we would be unable to answer the question: 'does SCT result in a greater risk of AHR?' It is only the discordant pairs 3 and 4, cells f and g, that provide

Table 8.5 Airway hyper-responsiveness (AHR) status before and after stem cell transplantation (SCT) in 21 children.

Before SCT			After SCT AHR		
			AHR	No AHR	Total
AHR	AHR		1 (e)	1 (f)	2
	No AHR		7 (g)	12 (h)	19
	Total		8	13	21

Source: data from Bentur et al. (2009).

relevant information in that the children differ in their response. If there were many more matched pairs like pair 3 than pair 4, we would have evidence against the null hypothesis, and answer the above question in the affirmative. If there were about the same number of matched pairs like pairs 3 and 4, we would answer the above question in the negative. If there were many more matched pairs like pair 3 than pair 4, we would have evidence that SCT exerts a protective effect.

In this example an appropriate null hypothesis is that the population proportions with AHR are the same before and after SCT; with the alternative hypothesis being that one proportion exceeds the other. If the null hypothesis is true we would expect the values of f and g to be equal. Given that we have $f + g$ discordant pairs, we would expect half to be pair 3 (AHR before SCT but no AHR after SCT). Thus $O_1 = f$ whilst $E_1 = (f + g)/2$ and $O_2 = g$ whilst $E_2 = (f + g)/2$. A chi-squared test using the general expression for χ^2 given in Section 8.2 leads to $\chi^2_{\text{McNemar}} = \dfrac{(f - g)^2}{f + g}$.

For the data of Bentur et al. (2009) we have $\chi^2_{\text{McNemar}} = \dfrac{(1 - 7)^2}{1 + 7} = 4.50$. We compare this with the tabulated values of χ^2 with $df = 1$ in Table T3. This indicates that P is between 0.04 and 0.03. A more precise P-value is 0.0339.

McNemar's test may be adjusted for small values of either f or g, to $\chi^2_{\text{McNemar\_CC}} = \dfrac{(|f - g| - 1)^2}{f + g}$. The correction of -1 makes little difference to the calculations in large samples. However, the data of Bentur et al. (2009) is a small sample of 21 pairs and the continuity corrected test $\chi^2_{\text{McNemar\_CC}} = \dfrac{(|1 - 7| - 1)^2}{1 + 7} = 3.125$. When compared with the tabulated values of χ^2 with $df = 1$ in Table T3. This indicates that P-value between 0.1 and 0.05 and a more precise P-value is 0.077 and so we do not have enough evidence to reject the null hypothesis. An exact test for paired data, equivalent to Fisher's exact test for unpaired data, is described in the technical details. The exact test gives a P-value of 0.07 which is similar to using McNemar's test with the correction. From the last two tests we would conclude there is no strong evidence to reject the null hypothesis.

8.5 Degrees of Freedom

In general, there are two way of calculating the degrees of freedom (*df*): one depends on the number of groups to be compared and the second on the number of parameters that need to be estimated in order to calculate the standard deviation of the contrast of interest. How the degrees of freedom are calculated depends on the particular problem concerned.

For the χ^2 test for the comparison of two proportions there are two groups to compare; hence $df = 1$ for the between-groups comparison. However, in this case the second calculation is not required as once a proportion is estimated for each group, a direct estimate of the SE of each is obtained as $\sqrt{[p(1 - p)/n]}$. Therefore, no further parameters are to be estimated and so there is no second df required. This is because the Binomial distribution, for a particular n, is completely determined by the value of p.

In contrast, the t-test has implicitly two sets of degrees of freedom attached to it. As for the χ^2 test, and as only two groups are compared in this situation the first is $df = 1$. However, although one parameter to be estimated is the mean of each group a second parameter (the standard deviation, σ) is required before the SE can be calculated. This necessitates the second (within groups) type of $df =$ (number of subjects minus two) which, in the case of independent groups of equal size, implies $df = 2(n - 1)$. Nevertheless, the first of these degrees of freedom is not usually explicitly referred to as it is always unity. The Z-test is similar to the t-test, but since in this case σ is assumed known effectively the within-groups degrees of freedom are infinite and so these df too are seldom explicitly referred to. For the paired t-test situation the $df = (n - 1)$.

8.6 Points When Reading the Literature

1) Have clinical importance and statistical significance been confused?
2) Has the sample size been taken into account when determining the choice of statistical tests; that is, are small-sample tests used when appropriate?
3) Have paired tests been utilised if the data are matched or paired?
4) Have confidence intervals of the main results been quoted?
5) Is the result medically or biologically plausible and has the statistical significance of the result been considered in isolation, or have other studies of the same effect been taken into account?

8.7 Technical Details

Fisher's Exact Test

If any expected value in a 2×2 table is less than about 5, the P-value given by the chi-squared test is not strictly valid.

Given the notation of Table 8.6, the probability of observing the particular table is $\dfrac{m!n!r!s!}{N!a!b!c!d!}$, where $n!$ means $1 \times 2 \times 3 \times \ldots \times (n - 1) \times n$ and where $0!$ and $1!$ are both taken to be unity. We next calculate the probability of other tables that can be identified that have the same marginal totals, m, n, r, s and also give as much or more evidence for an association between the factors. These probabilities are then summed and for a two-sided test we double the probability so obtained.

Table 8.6 Notation for unmatched 2 × 2 table. Number of subjects classified by factors A and B.

		Factor A		
		Present	Absent	Total
Factor B	**Present**	a	b	m
	Absent	c	d	n
Total		r	s	N

Worked Example: Calculation of Fisher's Exact Test

Van Nood et al. (2013) studied patients with *Clostridium difficile* (*C. difficile*) infections, which cause persistent diarrhoea. They randomly assigned patients to receive standard vancomycin (V) therapy for 14 days; or an initial *V* for 4 days, followed by bowel lavage and subsequent infusion of a solution of donor faeces (DF) through a nasoduodenal tube (donor-Faeces infusion, VF group). The primary end point was the resolution of diarrhoea associated with *C. difficile* infection without relapse after 10 weeks. The percentage of people who were cured (diarrhoea resolved) in the VF group was 81% (13 out of 16) and 31% (4 out of 13) in V. They used Fisher's exact probability test to analyse the data.

The null hypothesis is that the relative proportions of one variable are independent of the second variable; in other words, the proportions at one variable are the same for different values of the second variable. In the *C. difficile* example, the null hypothesis is that the probability of getting cured is the same whether you receive a VF or V.

The probability of observing this table, is

$$P(i) = \frac{12!17!16!13!}{29!3!9!13!4!} = 0.0077154.$$

The OR for the diarrhoea being resolved for the VF group compared to V is $(13 \times 9)/(4 \times 3) = 9.75$. There are 12 'sick' patients with unresolved diarrhoea and 3 of these are in the VF group. There are three further rearrangements of the table with 2, 1, or 0 sick (unresolved diarrhoea) patients in the VF group which give greater ORs for an association between the outcome and group. These are given in Table 8.8.

The probability associated with Table 8.7 is $P(i) = 0.0077154$ with those of Table 8.8 are $P(ii) = 0.0006613$, $P(iii) = 0.0000240$ and $P(iv) = 0.0000003$. Thus the total probability is $0.0077154 + 0.0006613 + 0.0000240 + 0.0000003 = 0.00840$. This is multiplied by two, to obtain that for a two-sided test, to give the associated P-value $= 0.01680$. On this basis, we can reject the null hypothesis and accept the alternative hypothesis that patients with *C. difficile* are more likely to be cured if they receive a VF compared to V alone.

One problem with the method of multiplying the one-sided P-value by two to get the two-sided P-value is that the probability of the observed table appears twice. The *mid-P*-value calculates only half the probability of the observed table in the one-sided P-value, thus one-sided $P = 0.0077154/2 + 0.0006613 + 0.0000240 + 0.0000003 = 0.0045433$ and two-sided $P = 0.0090866$. The mid-P approach is generally preferable (Fagerland et al. 2017, p. 28).

Chi-squared Test for Trend (2 × *c* Table)

An important class of tables are 2 × *c* tables, where the multi-level factor has ordered levels. For example, patients might score their pain on an integer scale from 1 to 5 on one of two treatments. In

Table 8.7 Resolution of diarrhoea associated with *C. difficile* infection without relapse after 10 weeks in patients randomised to vancomycin (V) alone or with donor-faeces infusion (VF) treatments.

| Outcome Diarrhoea resolved | Treatment group | | Total |
	VF	V	
No	3	9	12
Yes	13	4	17
Total	16	13	29

Source: data from van Nood et al. (2013).

Table 8.8 Tables with more extreme ways of distributing the 12 patients still with unresolved diarrhoea.

| | Diarrhoea | Treatment group | | Totals | |
		VF	V		
Table (ii)	No	2	10	12	OR = 23.3
	Yes	14	3	17	
	Total	16	13	29	
Table (iii)	No	1	11	12	OR = 82.5
	Yes	15	2	17	
	Total	16	13	29	
Table (iv)	No	0	12	12	OR = ∞
	Yes	16	1	17	
	Total	16	13	29	

this case the chi-squared test is very inefficient, because it fails to take account of the ordering and one should use the chi-squared test for trend. In this test one must assign scores to the ordered outcome. So long as the scores reflect the ordering, the actual values affect the result little.

Chi-squared Test for Trend in $2 \times c$ Contingency Tables

Suppose we wish to test the null hypothesis, for a $2 \times c$ contingency table, that there is:

H_0: No linear trend in a set of ordered proportions;
H_A: Linear trend in a set of ordered proportions.

Assumptions

One binary categorical variable and one ordered categorical variable that form a $2 \times c$ contingency table with the notation below.

Consider the notation in Table 8.9 and the example and the following steps for calculating the chi-squared test for trend.

Steps

1) Assign a score x_i to each of the c_i ordered categories.
2) Calculate the proportions $p_i = a_i/n_i$ in each ordered category.
3) Calculate the overall proportion $\bar{p} = \dfrac{\sum\limits_{i=1}^{c} a_i}{N}$ and $\bar{q} = 1 - \bar{p}$.
4) And the summations $\sum\limits_{i=1}^{c} a_i x_i$, $\sum\limits_{i=1}^{c} n_i x_i$, $\sum\limits_{i=1}^{c} n_i x_i^2$.
5) Calculate

$$T_{xp} = \sum_{i=1}^{c} n_i (p_i - \bar{p})(x_i - \bar{x}) = \sum_{i=1}^{c} a_i x_i - \frac{\sum\limits_{i=1}^{c} a_i \sum\limits_{i=1}^{c} n_i x_i}{N}$$

$$\text{and } T_{xx} = \sum_{i=1}^{c} n_i x_i^2 - \frac{\left(\sum\limits_{i=1}^{c} n_i x_i\right)^2}{N}.$$

6) Finally calculate, the χ^2_{Trend} statistic.

$$X^2_{\text{Trend}} = \frac{T_{xp}^2}{(T_{xx}\bar{p}\bar{q})}.$$

7) Compare this number with tables of the chi-squared distribution with one degree of freedom.

Koletsi and Pandis (2016) were interested in whether the frequency of using oral mouth rinse was associated with the presence or absence of gingivitis in 131 orthodontic patients. They compared the distribution of a binary variable (the presence or absence of gingivitis) across the levels of an ordered categorical variable (the frequency of mouth rinse use). The data are shown in Table 8.9. The research question was whether the proportion of patients with gingivitis increases or decreases across the mouth rinse groups. In this example the null hypothesis is no linear trend in the population proportions with gingivitis according to the frequency of mouth wash usage.

Table 8.9 Presence or absence of gingivitis according to mouth rinse schedule.

Presence of gingivitis	Mouth rinse usage per week				
	Once	Twice	Each day	Total	
Yes (a_i)	16	9	2	27	$= \sum a_i$
No	29	36	39	104	
Total (n_i)	45	45	41	131	N
$p_i = a_i/n_i$	0.3556	0.2000	0.0488	0.2061	$\bar{p}$
Score (x_i)	1	2	3		
$a_i x_i$	16	18	6	40	$= \sum a_i x_i$
$n_i x_i$	45	90	123	258	$= \sum n_i x_i$
$n_i x_i^2$	45	180	369	594	$= \sum n_i x_i^2$

Source: data from Koletsi and Pandis (2016).

Table 8.10 Contingency tables for calculation of the exact test.

		(i) After AHR	(i) After No AHR	(ii) After AHR	(ii) After No AHR
Before	AHR	1	1	1	0
	No AHR	7	12	8	12

With the notation given in Table 8.9, $T_{xp} = 40 - (27 \times 258)/131 = -13.18$, $T_{xx} = 594 - (258)^2/131 = 85.88$ and $\chi^2_{\text{trend}} = (-13.18)^2/(85.88 \times 0.2061 \times 0.7939) = 12.36$. From Table T3, we find P-value <0.001. A more precise P-value is $P = 0.0004$. Thus, we can reject the null hypothesis and accept the alternative that the presence of gingivitis declines as the mouth rinse usage increases. Note that the scoring in Table 8.10 is 1, 2, 3 and yet the frequencies (usage per week) are 1, 2, 7 (days). In general, it can be shown that the results are robust to other scoring systems and the default linear system works well (Walters 2004).

Exact Test for Small Samples with Paired Binary Outcomes

The exact test requires the calculation of $P = \dfrac{(f+g)!}{f!g!} \left(\dfrac{1}{2}\right)^{f+g}$ for the table observed and those indicating a stronger association with the same total $f + g$ of discordant pairs. These probabilities are then summed and for a two-sided test we double the probability so obtained.

Example

In the matched case–control study of Bentur et al. (2009) the two tables for calculation are:

Giving $P(i) = \dfrac{8!}{1!7!} \left(\dfrac{1}{2}\right)^8 = 0.03125$ and $P(ii) = \dfrac{8!}{0!8!} \left(\dfrac{1}{2}\right)^8 = 0.00391$.

Thus, the total probability is $0.03125 + 0.00391 = 0.03516$. For a two-sided test P-value $= 2 \times 0.03516 = 0.0703$. This is very close to the value P-value $= 0.0771$ calculated in Section 8.5 using a McNemar's test with Yates's correction.

An approximate 95% confidence interval for the true difference in proportions can be calculated as follows. First calculate $p_1 = (e + f)/N$ and $p_2 = (e + g)/N$ the difference between them is $p_1 - p_2 = \dfrac{(f - g)}{N}$. The SE for the difference $p_1 - p_2$ is given by $\text{SE}(p_1 - p_2) = \dfrac{\sqrt{f + g - \{(f - g)^2/N\}}}{N}$. Hence, the 95% confidence interval for the true difference in proportion is

$$(p_1 - p_2) - \{1.96 \times \text{SE}(p_1 - p_2)\} \text{ to } (p_1 - p_2) + \{1.96 \times \text{SE}(p_1 - p_2)\}.$$

Confidence Interval for a Relative Risk

Given the notation of Table 8.6 the SE of the natural logarithm of the relative risk for large samples is given by

$$SE(\log RR) = \sqrt{\left(\frac{1}{a} - \frac{1}{a+c} + \frac{1}{b} - \frac{1}{b+d}\right)}.$$

The reason for computing the SE on the logarithmic scale is that this is more likely to be Normally distributed than the RR itself. It is important to note that when transformed back to the original scale, the confidence interval so obtained will be asymmetric about the RR. There will be a shorter distance from the lower confidence limit to the RR than from the RR to the upper confidence limit. The sampling distribution of the log(RR) is the Normal distribution, so we can construct a 95% CI for log(RR) as

$$\log(RR) - \{1.96 \times SE(\log RR)\} \text{ to } \log(RR) + \{1.96 \times SE(\log RR)\}.$$

Worked Example

From the data of Table 8.8 the natural logarithm of the RR estimate of 0.603 is log(RR) = log (0.603) = −0.506 and the SE of the natural logarithm of the RR is:

$$SE(\log RR) = \sqrt{\left(\frac{1}{48} - \frac{1}{161} + \frac{1}{87} - \frac{1}{176}\right)} = 0.143.$$

Thus a 95% CI for log(RR) is −0.506− (1.96 × 0.143) to −0.506 + (1.96 × 0.143) or −0.786 to −0.225.

Thus the 95% CI for the RR is from $e^{-0.786}$ to $e^{-0.225}$ which is 0.46 to 0.80. As the interval excludes 1, which would indicate equal risk (or odds) in the two groups, we can infer that there is a difference in the risk (odds) haemorrhoids recurring at 12 months between the two treatment groups.

CI for an Odds Ratio

Using the notation of Table 8.8 the SE of the natural logarithm of the OR, in large samples, is given by

$$SE(\log OR) = \sqrt{\frac{1}{a} + \frac{1}{b} + \frac{1}{c} + \frac{1}{d}}.$$

The sampling distribution of the log(OR) is the Normal distribution, so we can construct a 95% CI for log(OR) as:

$$\log(OR) - \{1.96 \times SE(\log OR)\} \text{ to } \log(OR) + \{1.96 \times SE(\log OR)\}.$$

Worked Example

For the data of Table 8.8 the natural logarithm of the OR estimate of 0.435 is log OR = log (0.435) = −0.833, whilst

$$SE(\log OR) = \sqrt{\left(\frac{1}{48} + \frac{1}{87} + \frac{1}{113} + \frac{1}{89}\right)} = 0.229.$$

Thus a 95% CI for log(OR) is −0.833 − (1.96 × 0.229) to −0.833 + (1.96 × 0.229) or −1.282 to −0.385.

Thus the 95% CI for the OR is from $e^{-1.282}$ to $e^{-0.385}$, or 0.277 to 0.681.

The corresponding a 95% CI for the OR is 0.28 to 0.68. As the interval excludes 1, which indicates equal risk (or odds) in the two groups, we can infer that there is a difference in the risk (odds) of haemorrhoids recurring at 12 months between the two treatment groups.

8.8 Exercises

Farndon et al. (2013) report the results of a randomised controlled trial that investigated the effectiveness of corn plasters compared with usual scalpel debridement for treatment of foot corns. One of the secondary outcome measures was the size of the index corn (in mm) measured at 6, 9, and 12 month post-randomisation. Table 8.11 shows the outcome data.

Assume a significance level of 0.05 or 5% has been specified for the various hypothesis tests.

Table 8.11 Number of patients examined and the number and proportion with the index corn healed over time from randomisation by treatment group.

	Corn plaster	Scalpel
Randomised (*n*)	101	101
Examination post-randomisation (months)		
6	27/74	24/80
9	18/55	22/64
12	20/43	16/51

Source: data from Farndon et al. (2013).

8.1 From the data in Table 8.11 what is the proportion of participants in the corn plaster group who had a completely healed corn at six-month post-randomisation?
  A 0.30
  B 0.36
  C 0.64
  D 0.70
  E 0.90

8.2 From the data in Table 8.11 what is the proportion of participants in the scalpel group who had a completely healed index corn at six-month post-randomisation?
  A 0.30
  B 0.37
  C 0.64
  D 0.70
  E 0.90

8.3 From the data in Table 8.11, what is the difference in response (proportion of participants who had a completely healed index corn at six-month post-randomisation) between the corn plaster and scalpel groups?
  A −0.135
  B −0.075
  C 0.04
  D 0.065
  E 0.135

8.4 From the data in Table 8.11 calculate a 95% confidence interval for the difference in response (proportion of participants who had a completely healed index corn at six-months post-randomisation) between the corn plaster and scalpel groups?
A −0.07 to 0.07
B −0.05 to 0.10
C −0.08 to 0.21
D −0.02 to 0.20
E   0.08 to 0.21

8.5 Which of the following statements IS NOT an assumption of the Pearson chi-squared test for a contingency table in order for it to be valid?
A The data comprise two unordered categorical variables.
B At least 80% of the expected cell counts should be >5.
C All expected cell counts should be ≥1.
D All the observed cell counts should be ≥1.
E The null hypothesis is that there is no association between the row and column variables.

8.6 For the completely healed index corn at six-month post-randomisation outcome and data in Table 8.11 calculate the chi-squared test statistic (without continuity correction) to compare the proportions with a healed index corn in the corn plaster and scalpel groups.
A 0.036
B 0.730
C 1.667
D 2.263
E 3.894

8.7 For the completely healed index corn at six-month post-randomisation outcome and data in Table 8.11 calculate the degrees of freedom for the chi-squared test statistic.
A 1
B 2
C 3
D 4
E 5

8.8 The *P*-value from the chi-squared test for comparing the completely healed index corn at six-months post-randomisation outcome and data in Table 8.11 is?
A <0.01
B Between 0.02 and 0.05
C Between 0.05 and 0.10
D Between 0.10 and 0.20
E >0.20

8.9 From the data in Table 8.11 the 95% confidence interval for the difference in proportions with a completely healed index corn at 12-months post-randomisation between the corn plaster and scalpel treated groups is:

−0.04 to 0.33.

Which of the following statements about the above 95% confidence interval is INCORRECT?

A The above 95% confidence interval contains the true population difference in proportions with a completely healed index corn at 12-month post-randomisation between the corn plaster and scalpel treated groups.

B The 95% confidence interval for the difference in proportions with completely healed index corn at 12-month post-randomisation is calculated as ± 1.96 SEs away from the difference in proportions completely healed index corn at 12-months post-randomisation between the corn plaster and scalpel treated groups.

C If we repeated the study 100 times we would expect 95 of the resulting 95% confidence intervals to include the population difference in proportions with a completely healed index corn at 12-month post-randomisation between the corn plaster and scalpel treated groups

D The 95% confidence interval is consistent with there being no difference in the population between the corn plaster and scalpel treated groups in the proportions with a completely healed index corn at 12-month post-randomisation.

E The above 95% confidence interval is likely to contain the true population difference in proportions with a completely healed index corn at 12-month post-randomisation between the corn plaster and scalpel treated groups.

9   Correlation and Linear Regression

Medical Statistics: A Textbook for the Health Sciences, Fifth Edition. Stephen J. Walters, Michael J. Campbell, and David Machin.
© 2021 John Wiley & Sons Ltd. Published 2021 by John Wiley & Sons Ltd.
Companion website: www.wiley.com/go/walters/medicalstatistics

Summary

Correlation and linear regression are techniques for dealing with the relationship between two or more continuous variables. In correlation we are looking for a linear association between two variables, and the strength of the association is summarised by the correlation coefficient. In regression we are looking for a dependence of one variable, the dependent variable, on another, the independent variable. In regression the independent variable may be called the predictor variable and is plotted on the horizontal axis of a scatter plot, and the dependent variable is called the outcome variable and is plotted on the vertical axis of a scatter plot. The relationship is summarised by a regression equation defined by of a slope and an intercept. In linear regression the slope represents the amount the dependent variable increases with unit increase in the independent variable, and the intercept represents the value of the dependent variable when the independent variable takes the value zero. In multiple regression we are interested in the simultaneous relationship between one dependent variable and a number of independent variables.

9.1   Introduction

Many statistical analyses are undertaken to examine the relationship between two continuous variables within a group of subjects. Two of the main purposes of such analyses are:

1) To assess whether the two variables are associated. We do not need to designate one variable as independent and one variable as dependent; we are just interested in whether they are linearly associated and the strength of the association.
2) To enable the value of one variable to be predicted from any known value of the other variable. One variable is regarded as a response to the other predictor variable and the value of the predictor variable is used to predict what the response would be.

For the first of these, the statistical method for assessing the association between two continuous variables is known as *correlation*, whilst the technique for the second, prediction of one continuous variable from another is known as *regression*. Correlation and regression are often presented together and it is easy to get the impression that they are inseparable. In fact, they have distinct purposes and it is relatively rare that one is genuinely interested in performing both analyses on the same set of data. However, when preparing to analyse data using either technique it is always important to construct a scatter plot of the values of the two variables against each other. By drawing a scatter plot it is possible to see whether or not there is any visual evidence of a straight line or linear association between the two variables.

Example – Systolic and Diastolic Blood Pressure

Figure 9.1 shows the relationship between systolic and diastolic blood pressure in 96 patients with carotid artery disease, aged 42–89 prior to surgery (Sivaguru et al. 1998). Systolic pressure is the maximum pressure your heart exerts whilst beating and diastolic pressure is the pressure in your arteries between heart beats. Here one is interested in the association between these two variables and a scatter plot shows this nicely. From Figure 9.1, there appears to be a linear

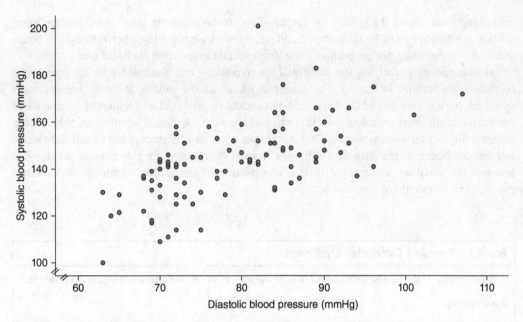

Figure 9.1 Scatter diagram of the relationship between systolic and diastolic blood pressure in 96 patients with carotid artery disease, aged 42–89 prior to surgery. (*Source:* data from Sivaguru et al. 1998).

relationship between systolic and diastolic blood pressure, with higher values of diastolic blood pressure being associated with higher values of systolic blood pressure. How can we summarise this relationship simply? We could calculate the correlation coefficient which is a measure of the linear association between two variables. It is used when you are not interested in predicting the value of one variable for a given value of the other variable, but would like to know how strongly they are related. Any observed relationship is not necessarily assumed to be a causal one – it may be caused by other factors. For correlation systolic and diastolic blood pressures can be plotted on either axis.

Rather than waste space, the scales on either the horizontal or vertical axes or both axes can be truncated to reflect the actual range of observations for the two variables in the sample. In these circumstances, as Figure 9.1 illustrates, it is good practice to notch or score the truncated axis with two parallel line symbols '//' to indicate that the origin or zero value for the axis has been omitted.

9.2 Correlation

In order to examine whether there is an association between the two variables of diastolic and systolic blood pressure, the correlation coefficient can be calculated. At this point, no assumptions are made about whether the relationship is causal, i.e. whether one variable is influencing the value of the other variable. The standard method (often ascribed to Karl Pearson [1857–1936]) leads to a statistic called *r* (see Box 9.1). In essence *r* is a measure of the scatter of the points around an underlying linear trend: the greater the spread of points the lower the correlation. Pearson's correlation coefficient r must be between -1 and $+1$, with -1 representing a perfect negative correlation, $+1$ representing perfect positive correlation and 0 representing no linear trend.

The assumptions underlying the validity of the hypothesis test associated with the correlation coefficient are outlined in Box 9.1. The easiest way to check the validity of the hypothesis test is by examining a scatter plot of the data. This plot should be produced as a matter of routine when correlation coefficients are calculated, as it will give a good indication of whether the relationship between the two variables is roughly linear and thus whether it is appropriate to calculate a correlation coefficient. If the data do not have a Normal distribution, or a non-linear relationship between the variables is suspected then a non-parametric correlation coefficient, Spearman's rho (ρ_s), can be calculated (see Box 9.2).

Box 9.1   Pearson's Correlation Coefficient

The correlation coefficient can be calculated for any data set with two continuous variables.

Assumptions

1) There is a linear relationship between the variables.
2) For a valid hypothesis test the two variables are observed on a random sample of individuals and the data for at least one of the variables should have a Normal distribution in the population.
3) For the calculation of a valid confidence interval for the correlation coefficient both variables should have a Normal distribution.

Steps
Given a set of n pairs of observations $(x_1, y_1), (x_2, y_2), ..., (x_n, y_n)$, with means $\bar{x}$ and $\bar{y}$ respectively then the Pearson correlation coefficient, r, is given by

$$r = \frac{\sum_{i=1}^{n}(y_i - \bar{y})(x_i - \bar{x})}{\sqrt{\sum_{i=1}^{n}(y_i - \bar{y})^2 \sum_{i=1}^{n}(x_i - \bar{x})^2}}.$$

Hypothesis test for ρ
The null hypothesis, H_0, is that population correlation, ρ, (the Greek letter rho) is zero, against the alternative hypothesis, H_A, that the population correlation does not equal zero. To test whether r is significantly different from zero, calculate the standard error $SE(r) = \sqrt{\frac{(1-r^2)}{(n-2)}}$, and the test statistic:

$$t = \frac{r}{\sqrt{(1-r^2)/(n-2)}}.$$

Compare the test statistic with the t-distribution with degrees of freedom (df) = $n-2$.

Box 9.1 (Continued)

Confidence interval for ρ

To find a confidence interval for the population value of ρ we have to use a transformation of r known as the tanh transformation, to get a quantity Z that has an approximately Normal distribution.

The transformed value, Z, is given by $Z = \frac{1}{2} \log_e \left(\frac{1+r}{1-r} \right)$ which has SE $= 1/\sqrt{(n-3)}$ where n is the sample size.

For a 100(1 − α)% confidence interval we then find

$$Z_{lower} = Z - \frac{z_{1-\alpha/2}}{\sqrt{n-3}} \text{ to } Z_{upper} = Z + \frac{z_{1-\alpha/2}}{\sqrt{n-3}}.$$

Where $z_{1-\alpha/2}$ is the appropriate value from the standard Normal distribution for the 100(1 − α/2) percentile.

The values of Z_{lower} and Z_{upper} need to be transformed back to the original scale to give a 100 (1 − α)% confidence interval for the population correlation coefficient as

$$\frac{e^{2Z_{lower}} - 1}{e^{2Z_{lower}} + 1} \text{ to } \frac{e^{2Z_{upper}} - 1}{e^{2Z_{upper}} + 1}.$$

The correlation coefficient is a dimensionless quantity ranging from −1 to +1. A positive correlation is one in which both variables increase together. A negative correlation is one in which one variable increases as the other decreases. When variables are exactly linearly related, then the correlation coefficient equals either +1 or −1. Values for different strengths of association are shown in Figures 9.2a to c.

The correlation coefficient is unaffected by the units of measurement. Thus, if one is assessing the strength of association between, say, weight and height it does not matter whether weight is measured in kilogrammes or pounds, or height measured in metres, centimetres or feet or inches, as the correlation coefficient remains unaffected.

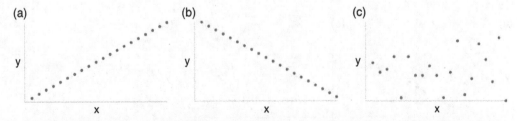

Figure 9.2 Scatter plots showing data sets with different correlations: (a) r = +1 perfect positive linear association, (b) r = −1 perfect positive linear association, (c) r = 0 uncorrelated (no linear association).

When Not to Use the Correlation Coefficient

To determine whether the correlation coefficient is an appropriate measure of association, a first step should always be to look at a plot of the raw data. The situations where it might not be appropriate to use the correlation coefficient are:

i) The correlation coefficient should not be used if the relationship is non-linear.

Figure 9.3a shows a situation in which y is related to x by means of the equation $y = a + bx + cx^2$. In this case it is possible to predict y exactly for each value of x. There is therefore a perfect association between x and y. However, it turns out that r is not equal to one. This is because the expression for y involves an x^2 term, or what is known as a quadratic term, and so the relationship is non-linear as is clear from the figure. Figure 9.3b shows a situation in which y is also clearly strongly associated with x and yet the correlation coefficient is zero. Such an example may arise if y represented overall mortality of a groups of people and x some average measure of obesity for the group. Very thin and obese people both have higher mortality than people with average weight for their height so an overall correlation coefficient for the groups representative of a population is likely to be close to zero.

In the situations depicted by both Figures 9.3a and b there is clearly a close relationship between y and x, but it is not linear. In situations such as these, one should abandon trying to find a single summary statistic of the relationship.

ii) The correlation coefficient should be used with caution in the presence of outliers.

For example, Figure 9.3c shows a situation in which one observation is well outside the main body of the data. This observation has a great deal of influence on the estimated value of the correlation coefficient. Since it is so extreme it is possible that this observation in fact comes from a different population from the others. If this case is excluded from the data set, the correlation coefficient becomes close to zero for the remainder.

iii) The correlation coefficient should be used with caution when the variables are measured over more than one distinct group.

One situation where this may occur is if the blood pressure observations, are made on a group of patients with hypertension (high blood pressure), and also in a group of healthy controls. Such studies may result in two distinct clusters of points with zero correlation within each cluster but when combined produce the same effect as the outlier in Figure 9.3c.

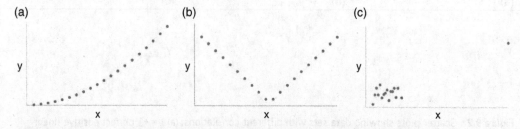

Figure 9.3 Examples where the use of the correlation coefficient is not appropriate. (a) Non-linear association, (b) non-linear association, (c) outliers and/or more than one distinct group.

iv) The correlation coefficient should not be used in situations where one of the variables is determined in advance.

For example, if one were measuring responses to different doses of a drug, one would not summarise the relationship with a correlation coefficient. It can be shown that the choice of the particular drug dose levels used by the experimenter will result in different correlation coefficients, even though the underlying dose–response relationship is fixed. Thus, if the dose range chosen to investigate is narrow estimates of the correlation will tend to be small whilst if the doses are very disparate the estimates will tend to be large.

Example – Correlation Between Systolic and Diastolic Blood Pressure

In Figure 9.1 we are not really interested in causation, that is whether a high systolic blood pressure causes a high diastolic blood pressure; but rather, is a high systolic blood pressure associated with a high diastolic blood pressure? Using the data in Figure 9.1 and the calculation in Box 9.1 we find the sample correlation coefficient is 0.62.

Having plotted the data, and established that it is plausible the two variables are associated linearly, we have to decide whether the observed correlation could have arisen by chance, since even if there were no association between the variables, the calculated correlation coefficient is extremely unlikely to be exactly zero. The associated statistical test of the null hypothesis $\rho = 0$ is described in Box 9.1.

For the data from Figure 9.1, the number of observations $n = 96$, $r = 0.62$, $SE(r) = \sqrt{\dfrac{1 - 0.62^2}{96 - 2}} = 0.08$ and the test is $t = r/SE(r) = 0.62/0.08. = 7.66$ with $df = 94$. From tables of the t-distribution Table T2 in the appendix, $t_{94, \, 0.001} = 3.397$, hence the P-value is less than 0.001. This means that with 96 observations a correlation of 0.62 (or one more extreme), is very unlikely when the null hypothesis (of no or zero correlation in the population) is true. The result is statistically significant because the P-value is less than the significance level (α) set at 5% or 0.05; and we decide that there is sufficient evidence to reject the null hypothesis and therefore accept there is enough evidence to say there is an association between systolic and diastolic blood pressure, and from the scatter plot that it is plausibly linear. The 95% confidence interval calculated as in Box 9.1 is 0.48 to 0.73, so there are quite a wide range of plausible correlation values associated with these data.

Assumptions Underlying the Test of Significance

The assumption underlying the test of significance of a correlation coefficient is that the observations are random samples, and at least one of the two variables has a Normal distribution. Outlying points, away from the main body of the data, suggest a variable may not have a Normal distribution and hence invalidate the test of significance. In this case, it may be better to replace the recorded value of each variable by their ranks. That is replace the continuous variable, say the x_i of individual i, by its corresponding rank position amongst the n individuals in the study. The rank having a value of between 1, if the observation was the smallest of the group, to n if it was the largest. The correlation coefficient is then calculated in the same manner but with the ranks for each variable replacing the original observation pair for each subject. When it is calculated from the ranks of the data it is known as the *Spearman rank* correlation coefficient (Box 9.2) and the assumption of Normality is no longer required.

Box 9.2   Spearman's Rank Correlation Coefficient

The Spearman's rank-order correlation is the non-parametric version of the Pearson product–moment correlation. Spearman's correlation coefficient, measures the strength and direction of association between two ranked variables.

Suppose we have a set of n pairs of observations (x_1, y_1), (x_2, y_2), ..., (x_n, y_n) and we require a measure of association between the two variables when their relationship is non-linear but monotonic. A monotonic relationship is a relationship that does one of the following: (i) as the value of one variable increases, so does the value of the other variable; or (ii) as the value of one variable increases, the other variable value decreases.

Assumptions

Both variables, x or y, are measured on at least an ordinal scale and can be ranked.

Neither x nor y need be Normally distributed.

Steps

To estimate the population value of Spearman's rank correlation coefficient ρ_s, by its sample value, r_s:

1) Rank the x observations in order of increasing magnitude from 1 to n. If some of the observations are numerically equal, they are given tied ranks equal to the mean of the ranks which would otherwise have been used.

2) Rank the y observations in order of increasing magnitude from 1 to n. If some of the observations are numerically equal, they are given tied ranks equal to the mean of the ranks which would otherwise have been used.

3) Spearman's rank correlation, r_s, is calculated from Pearson's correlation coefficient (see Box 9.1) on the *ranks* of the data.

4) An alternative, and easier to calculate, formula is

$$r_{\text{Spearman}} = 1 - \frac{6 \sum d_i^2}{n^3 - n}$$

where d_i is the difference in ranks for the ith individual.

Example – Spearman and Pearson Correlation Coefficients – Systolic and Diastolic Blood Pressure

For the 96 patients with carotid artery disease prior to surgery the Spearman's rank correlation coefficient between systolic and diastolic blood pressure, r_s, was calculated to be 0.65. This is very similar to Pearson's correlation coefficient estimate, r, of 0.62.

The Pearson correlation coefficient between systolic and diastolic blood pressure is 0.62 and this is statistically significant ($P < 0.001$). However, it is important to note that if the sample size is large, as in this example, then the null hypothesis, H_0, (that population correlation ρ is zero) may be rejected even if the sample estimate, r is quite close to zero. Alternatively, even if r is large, H_0 may not be rejected if the sample size is small. Table 9.1 illustrates the relationship between sample size and value of correlation coefficient which becomes significant at the 5% level. With a sample size of 100 a correlation of 0.20 or more will result in a P-value for the hypothesis test of less than 0.05. For this reason, it is particularly important to look at the absolute value of the correlation

Table 9.1 Relationship between sample size and value of correlation coefficient which becomes statistically significant at the 5% level.

Sample size	Value at which the correlation coefficient becomes significant at the 5% level
10	0.63
20	0.44
50	0.28
100	0.20
150	0.16

Table 9.2 Interpretation of the values of the sample estimate of the correlation coefficient.

$|r| \geq 0.8$ very strong relationship

$0.6 \leq |r| < 0.8$ strong relationship

$0.4 \leq |r| < 0.6$ moderate relationship

$0.2 \leq |r| < 0.4$ weak relationship

$|r| < 0.2$ very weak relationship

$|r|$ denotes the modulus or absolute value of r (i.e. ignoring the sign in front of the correlation coefficient).

coefficient r and Table 9.2, which provides a guide to interpreting the value of the observed correlation in the sample. In this example, the correlation of 0.62 suggests strong relationship between systolic and diastolic blood pressure.

Another helpful way to interpret the correlation coefficient is to calculate r^2, the proportion of the total variance of one variable explained by its linear relationship with the other variable. Note r^2 is the percentage of variance of one variable 'explained' by the other. For example, $r = 0.62$, and $P < 0.001$ for a sample size of 96, but the relationship, between systolic and diastolic blood pressure, is only explaining 38% ($= 0.62^2 \times 100$) of the variability of one variable by the other.

9.3 Linear Regression

The Regression Line

Often it is of interest to quantify the relationship between two continuous variables, x and y, and given the value of one variable for an individual, to predict the value of the other variable. This is not possible from the correlation coefficient as it simply indicates the strength of the association as a single number; in order to describe the relationship between the values of the two variables, a technique called regression is used. In regression, we assume that a change in the *independent* variable (x) will lead directly to a change in the *dependent* variable (y). Thus, in contrast to when we considered correlation, x and y here have a different status. Often, we are interested in predicting y for a given value of x and it would not be logical in these circumstances to believe that y caused x. It is conventional to plot the dependent variable on the vertical or *y*-axis and the independent variable on the horizontal or *x*-axis.

Suppose for example that we are interested in predicting the birthweight of a new born baby from the gestational age of the baby. Gestational age is the common term used during pregnancy to describe how far along the pregnancy is. It is measured in weeks, from the first day of the woman's last menstrual cycle to the current date. If we make the reasonable assumption that gestation is influencing birthweight, rather than the other way around then we may want to quantify the relationship between birthweight and gestational age, and predict on average what the birthweight would be, given a particular gestation using regression. Gestation is regarded as the dependent or *x* variable. Other names are the predictor or explanatory variable and it should be plotted on the horizontal axis of the scatter plot. Birthweight is regarded as the dependent or *y* variable. Other names are the outcome or response variable and is plotted on the vertical axis of the scatter plot (Figure 9.4).

The equation

$$y = \alpha + \beta x$$

is defined as the population linear regression equation, where α is the *intercept*, and β is the *regression coefficient*. As we have done earlier, the Greek letters are used to show that these are *population parameters*. The regression equation is an example of what is often termed a *model* with which one attempts to model or describe the relationship between *y* and *x*. On a graph, α is the value of the equation when $x = 0$ and β is the *slope* of the line. When *x* increases by one unit, *y* will change by β units.

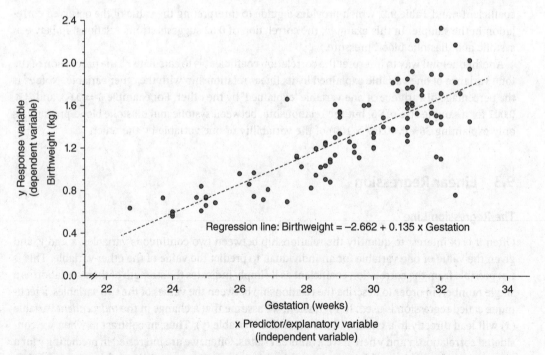

Figure 9.4 A scatterplot of birthweight and gestation in 98 preterm infants with the corresponding fitted regression line. (*Source:* data from Simpson 2004).

Given a series of n pairs of observations (x_1, y_1), (x_2, y_2) ... (x_n, y_n), in which we believe that y is linearly related to x, what is the best method of estimating α and β? We think of the parameters α and β as characteristics of a population and we require estimates of these parameters calculated from a sample taken from the population. We label these sample estimates a and b respectively. If we had estimates for a and b then, for any subject i with value x_i, we could predict their y_i by $Y_i = a + bx_i$. Here we denote the predicted value of y from the regression equation with a capital Y to distinguish it from the observed value. Clearly, we would like to choose a and b so that y_i and Y_i are close and hence make our prediction error as small as possible. This can be done by choosing a and b to minimise the sum $\sum(y_i - Y_i)^2$. This leads us to call a and b the *least-squares estimates* of the *population parameters* α and β. The model now becomes $y_i = \alpha + \beta x_i + \varepsilon_i$. The ε_i are usually assumed to be Normally distributed and to have an average value of zero. They are the amount that the observed value differs from that predicted by the model, and represent the variation not explained by fitting the straight line to the data.

All sample estimates like b have an inherent variability, estimated by SE(b). To calculate the degrees of freedom associated with the standard error, given n independent pairs of observations, two degrees of freedom are removed for the two parameters α and β that have been estimated: thus $df = n-2$.

Box 9.3   Linear Regression

The equation which estimates the simple linear regression line is:

$$y = a + bx, \tag{9.1}$$

where a and b are called the regression coefficients. a is the *intercept* (the value of the dependent y variable, when the independent x variable is equal to zero) and b is the *slope* or *gradient* (the average change in the dependent y variable for a unit change in the x variable).

Estimated linear regression line showing the intercept, a, and the slope, b

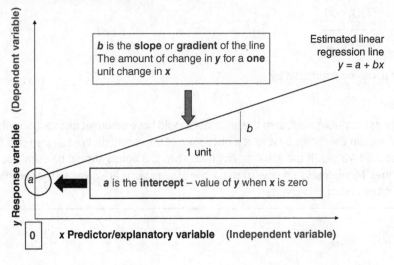

Box 9.3 (Continued)

Assumptions

1) The values of the response variable *y* should have a Normal distribution for each value of the explanatory variable *x*.
2) The variance (or standard deviation) of *y* should be the same at each value of *x*, i.e. there should be no evidence that as the value of *y* changes, the spread of the *x* values changes.
3) The relationship between the two variables should be linear.
4) The observations in the sample are independent.
5) The variable x can be measured without error. (This is a difficult and almost impossible assumption to check and satisfy! The x variable is rarely measured without any error. We have to assume this error is small. Providing this is the case, then this is likely to have little effect on the model and the conclusions from the model.)

We perform a regression analysis using a sample of observations and obtain *a* and *b* the sample estimates of the true population parameters α and β. The population regression model is $y = \alpha + \beta x$. The coefficients *a* and *b* are the sample estimates determined by the *method of least squares* (often called *ordinary least squares*, OLS) in such a way that the fit of the line $Y = a + bx$ to the points in the scatter diagram is best. (We denote the expected or predicted value of y from the regression equation given the value of x with a capital Y). We determine the *line of best fit* by considering the *residuals*. The residuals are the vertical distance from each data point on the scatter diagram to the regression line, i.e. residual = observed *y* – fitted *Y*. The line of best fit is chosen so that the sum of the squared residuals is a minimum. For simple linear regression the coefficients *a* and *b* can be calculated using the steps below.

Steps
Given a set of *n* pairs of observations $(x_1, y_1), (x_2, y_2), ..., (x_n, y_n)$, with means $\bar{x}$ and $\bar{y}$ respectively (with $i = 1$ to n).

The estimated slope, *b*, is given by

$$b = \frac{\sum_{i=1}^{n}(x_i - \bar{x})(y_i - \bar{y})}{\sum_{i=1}^{n}(x_i - \bar{x})^2}$$

The intercept *a*, can be estimated by

$$a = \bar{y} - b\bar{x}.$$

If the first three assumptions hold, then the residuals should have a Normal distribution with a mean of zero. So we can check this by way of a histogram of the residuals. We can also plot the residuals against the *x* values. If the assumptions hold, then the points should be evenly scattered at all *x* values. More details on how to check the assumptions are given in the technical details section at the end of this chapter.

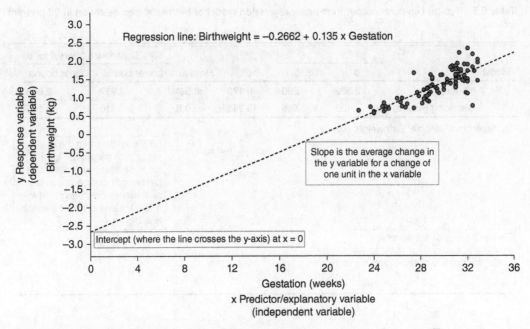

Figure 9.5 A scatterplot of birthweight and gestation in 98 preterm infants with zero shown on the x-axis to illustrate the intercept. (*Source:* data from Simpson 2004).

Regression slopes can be used to predict the response of a new patient with a particular value of the predictor/explanatory/independent variable. However, it is important that the regression model is not used to predict outside of the range of observations. In addition, it should not be assumed that just because an equation has been produced it means that x causes y.

Example – Linear Regression – Birthweight and Gestation

Simpson (2004) describes a prospective study, in which 98 preterm infants were given a series of tests shortly after they were born, in an attempt to predict their outcome after one year. The birthweight (in kilogrammes) of the baby was recorded as well as gestation (in weeks), sex and type of delivery (normal or non-normal) and the maternal age (in years) of the mother. The data of birthweight and gestation are plotted in Figure 9.4. It is logical to believe that increasing gestation may affect birthweight, and not the other way around. There appears to be a linear relationship between birthweight and gestation; with increasing gestation associated with a heavier birthweight.

Table 9.3 gives a typical computer output and shows that the linear regression equation is

$$\text{Birthweight (kg)} = -2.662 + 0.135 \times \text{Gestation (weeks)},$$

where $a = -2.662$ is the estimate of the intercept and $b = 0.135$ is the estimate of the slope, i.e. for every unit increase (or week) in gestation there is an additional expected 0.135 kg increase in birthweight. When gestation is zero, the predicted birthweight is -2.662 kg, a result that is not physiologically possible. This illustrates the pitfalls when extrapolating beyond the range of the observed gestation data. The intercept is needed for the prediction equation but its associated

Table 9.3 Typical computer output from linear regression model of birthweight on gestation in 98 preterm infants.

Model		b	SE(b)	t	P-value	95% Confidence Interval for b Lower bound	Upper bound
1	Intercept	−2.662	.290	−9.179	<0.001	−3.237	−2.086
	Gestation (weeks)	.135	.010	13.748	<0.001	.116	.155

a. Dependent Variable: Birthweight (kg)

> 95% confident that the true population parameter for the slope or relationship between birthweight and gestation lies somewhere between 0.116 to 0.155 kg, and our best estimate is 0.135 kg.

> The probability of the observing this slope coefficient or more extreme under the null hypothesis, (that $\beta = 0$), is <0.001.

P-value and confidence interval, which are routinely produced by packages, should be ignored and not reproduced in publications, since they are not that helpful.

If we extend the range of the horizontal x-axis to include a value of zero, and the regression line to cross the y-axis at x = 0, then Figure 9.5 shows the intercept for the regression line is around −2.7 kg. Figure 9.6 shows the estimate of the slope, that is, for every unit increase (or week) in gestation there is an additional 0.135 kg increase in birthweight.

Tests of Significance and Confidence Intervals

To test the hypothesis that there is no association between birthweight and gestation, we compare $t = b/SE(b)$ with a t-statistic with $df = n − 2$.

Example – Linear Regression – Birthweight and Gestational Age – Hypothesis Test and Confidence Interval

The corresponding test for significance for the slope is given by calculating $t = 0.135/0.010 = 13.748$. Referring this value to the t-distribution with $df = 96$ gives $P < 0.001$.

A 95% CI for β with $n–2$ df is given by

$$b − t_{n−2,0.05} \times SE(b) \text{ to } b + t_{n−2,0.05} \times SE(b).$$

From the t-distribution with $df = 96$ and a 5% significance value we obtain $t_{96, 0.05} = 1.985$. Thus the 95% CI for β is given by

$$0.135 − (1.985 \times 0.010) \text{ to } 0.135 + (1.985 \times 0.010),$$

or 0.115 to 0.155. In this example as $df = 96$ is large the Normal distribution could be used instead of the t-distribution and 1.96 used as the multiplier for the standard error instead of 1.985.

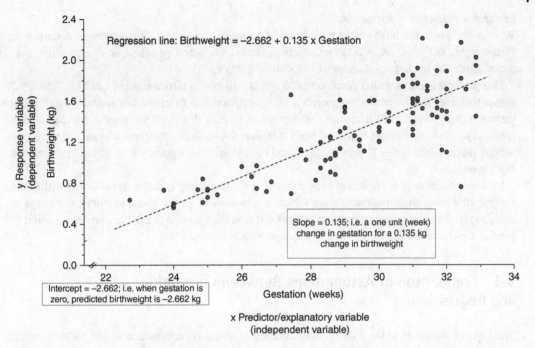

Figure 9.6 A scatterplot of birthweight and gestation in 98 preterm infants with the corresponding fitted regression line. (*Source:* data from Simpson 2004).

Do the Assumptions Matter?

The art in statistics occurs when deciding how far the assumptions can be stretched without providing a seriously misleading summary and when the procedure should be abandoned altogether and other methods tried. In general, lack of Normality of the residuals is unlikely to affect seriously the estimates of a regression equation, although it may affect the standard errors and the size of the P-value. Similarly, a lack of constant variance of the residuals is unlikely to seriously affect the estimates, but again will have some influence on the final P-value. In either case the advice would be to proceed, but with caution, particularly if the P-value is close to some critical value such as 0.05.

The lack of linearity is more serious, and would suggest either a transformation of y or x before fitting the regression equation, or a model involving quadratic (squared) or higher terms of x using multiple regression (see Section 9.5). The most common transformation is the logarithmic.

Lack of independence of the residuals can also be serious. If the data form a time sequence, or if the data involve repeated measures on individuals, a correct analysis may be difficult and expert advice should be sought.

Regression and Prediction

Regression slopes can be used to predict the value of the dependent variable with a particular value of the predictor/explanatory/independent variable.

Example – Prediction – Birthweight

What is the predicted birthweight for a baby of 30 weeks' gestation? The regression equation is: Birthweight (kg) = −2.662 + 0.135 × Gestation(weeks). So, when gestation is 30 weeks the: predicted Birthweight (kg) = −2.662 + (0.135 × 30) = 1.388 kg.

This predicts a foetus with a gestation of 30 weeks will have a birthweight of 1.388 kg. Figure 9.7 shows this graphically, where we project a vertical dotted line from the horizontal x-axis from a gestation of 30 weeks until it crosses the regression line; at this point we draw a horizontal line (parallel to the x-axis) across to the left until it crosses the vertical y-axis; and we read off the birthweight value on the scale. This is the predicted birthweight for a gestation of 30 weeks; given the regression line.

In these situations, it is important to be aware that the prediction equation is valid only within the range of the independent variable from which it was derived. In the above example, the range of gestation in the sample was from 22 to 33 weeks. It would be unwise to use the derived equation to predict a birthweight of a baby whose gestation was 20 weeks.

9.4 Comparison of Assumptions Between Correlation and Regression

The tests of significance for a correlation coefficient and a regression coefficient yield identical *t*-statistics and *P*-values for a particular data set.

It is one of the nice coincidences in statistics that two completely different sets of assumptions lead to the same test of significance. This would seem logical since one would not expect to have a significant correlation in the absence of a significant regression effect. Unfortunately, this has often led to a confusion between correlation and regression. The major difference in assumptions is that in regression there is no stipulation about the distribution of the independent variable *x*. It is often

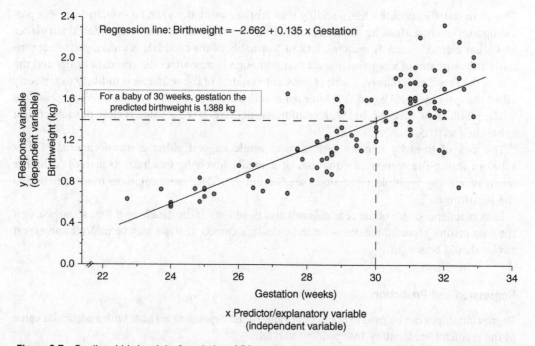

Figure 9.7 Predicted birthweight for a baby of 30 weeks' gestation. (*Source:* data from Simpson 2004).

the case that the x's are determined by the experimenter. In an anaemia survey one might choose fixed numbers of women in specified age groups; in a laboratory survey one might be interested in the responses of patients to fixed levels of a drug chosen by the experimenter. Moreover, choosing fixed values for the x's violates the assumption underlying the correlation coefficient, namely that the x's (as well as the y's) have a Normal distribution. The Spearman correlation coefficient may be more robust in such circumstances.

In contrast it is perfectly valid in regression problems to have x variables that can take only two values (say) 0 and 1. These are clearly very far from being Normally distributed.

It is worth noting that the test of significance of a regression coefficient when x is a binary 0/1 variable is equivalent to the t-test for the difference between two means. One mean is the mean value of y for those subjects with $x = 0$ and the other the mean value of y for those with $x = 1$. This result is useful because computer packages that can carry out regression can also be used to do t-tests.

9.5 Multiple Regression

The Multiple Regression Equation

Life is rarely simple, and outcome variables in medical research are usually affected by a multitude of factors. Sometimes there is more than one possible explanatory variable influencing the outcome variable. Fortunately, the simple linear regression situation with one independent variable is easily extended to multiple regression. Multiple linear regression can be used to investigate the influence of several explanatory variables simultaneously on the outcome.

There are three main reasons for carrying out a multiple regression analysis.

1) To investigate the extent to which one or more explanatory variables are linearly related to the y variable after adjusting for other variables that may be related to it.
2) To identify any explanatory variables that may be associated with the y variable.
3) To predict the value of the y variable from the explanatory x variables.

The assumptions for multiple linear regression are the same as for simple linear regression (see Box 9.2). We just replace the single 'x' variable with several 'x's'. The assumptions can be checked in the same way (see Technical details section at the end of this chapter).

In that case the corresponding multiple linear regression model is

$$y = \beta_0 + \beta_1 x_1 + \beta_2 x_2 + \ldots + \beta_p x_p + \varepsilon$$

where x_1 is the first independent variable, x_2 is the second, and so on up to the pth independent variable x_p.

The term β_0 is the intercept or constant term. It is the value of y when all the independent variables are zero. With just one independent variable, it is commonly labelled α, as we have done earlier. The regression coefficients β_0, β_1, ..., β_p are again estimated by minimising the sum of the squares of the differences from the observed and predicted outcome variables, y and Y. Although the variables x_1, ..., x_p are termed the independent variables, as we have said earlier this is a misnomer since they need not be independent of one another. Although it is not essential that investigators understand the computational details of multiple regression, it is such a commonly used technique that they will need to be able to understand both computer output from a multiple regression calculation and read papers which use the results of multiple regression.

Suppose we are interested in the effect of several explanatory variables, $x_1, x_2, ..., x_p$, on the response variable y. The estimated multiple regression equation, with p explanatory variables, would be:

$$y = b_0 + b_1x_1 + b_2x_2 + ... + b_px_p$$

Here x_p is the pth explanatory variable or covariate. Y is the estimated/predicted/expected mean or fitted value of y given a particular set of values of $x_1, x_2, ..., x_p$; b_0, is the estimated intercept and is a constant term and is the value of Y when all the x_p's are zero. The b_p's are the estimated regression coefficients. That is b_1 represents the amount by which y increases on average if we increase x_1 by one unit, but keep all the other x_p's constant (or adjust or control for them).

Examples of Uses of Multiple Regression

1) *To investigate the extent to which one or more explanatory variables are linearly related to the y variable after adjusting for other variables that may be related to it.*

   Suppose an investigator wished to test whether, on average, male babies have a different birthweight than female babies. The mean and standard deviation of birthweight for the 53 female babies are 1.22 kg and 0.44 kg, and for the 45 male babies 1.41 kg and 0.38 kg.

   A two independent groups t-test as described in Chapter 7 yields a difference between the male and female birthweights of 0.19 kg ($t = 2.237$, $df = 96$, $P = 0.028$), which is significant. We already know that gestation is associated with birthweight. Therefore, if there were a difference in gestation between male and female babies then this might account for the difference observed in birthweights between them and not the sex status of the baby itself.

   However, sex of the baby can be added to a multiple regression, which includes gestational age, by use of a dummy variable. Such a variable takes the value 1 if the baby is male and 0 if the baby is female. The output from a multiple regression programme is given in Table 9.4. Note that the size of the coefficient associated with gestation (0.133) has reduced slightly from the 0.135 of Table 9.3. This is because gestation and sex are being fitted simultaneously. The interpretation of the coefficient associated with the variable sex is that, allowing or adjusting for gestation, the birthweights of male babies are 0.105 kg heavier than female babies. The corresponding 95% confidence interval for β_{Sex} with $df = 95$ is

$$0.105 - t_{95,0.05} \times 0.05 \text{ to } 0.105 + t_{95,0.05} \times 0.05$$

or 0.006 to 0.203. This interval just excludes zero, and so the conclusion made previously that there was a non-zero difference in birthweight between male and female babies of the same gestation is still valid, although the lower limit is compatible with a very small difference or increase in birthweight of 0.006 kg (or 6 g) for male babies and the upper limit an increase in birthweight of 0.203 kg (or 200 g) and the point estimate is an increase of 0.105 kg.

Table 9.4 Output obtained from a multiple regression of birthweight on gestational age and sex of the baby.

Variable	Coefficients				95% CI for b	
	b	SE (b)	t	P-value	Lower	Upper
Constant	−2.635	0.285	−9.239	<0.001	−3.201	−2.069
Gestation (weeks)	0.133	0.010	13.623	<0.001	0.113	0.152
Sex (0 = female, 1 = male)	0.105	0.050	2.107	0.038	0.006	0.203

Source: data from Simpson (2004).

Table 9.5 Estimated regression coefficients from the multiple linear regression model to predict birthweight (in kg) from maternal age, gestation, sex and delivery type in 98 new babies.

Explanatory variables	Regression coefficient			95% CI for *b*	
	b	SE(*b*)	*P*-value	Lower	Upper
Intercept	−3.005	0.312	<0.001	3.625	−2.384
Maternal age (years)	0.002	0.004	0.588	0.006	0.01
Gestation (weeks)	0.141	0.01	<0.001	0.122	0.16
Sex (0 = female, 1 = male)	0.117	0.048	0.016	0.022	0.212
Delivery (0 = non-normal, 1 = normal)	0.164	0.05	0.002	0.064	0.264

Source: data from Simpson (2004).

2) To identify any explanatory variables that may be associated with the y variable.

In the pre-term birthweight example, apart from gestation, the sex of the baby, type of delivery and maternal age may have a role to play influencing birthweight. These explanatory variables may be fitted into the model to examine what their influence on birthweight is, over and above that exerted by gestation alone. For the birthweight data the estimated multiple regression equation would be:

Birthweight = b_0 + b_1Age + b_2Gestation + b_3Sex + b_4Delivery

Table 9.5 shows the estimated regression coefficients, b_1, b_2, b_3, and b_4 for maternal age, gestation, sex and delivery respectively, and their associated confidence intervals and P-values. It appears that gestation, sex and delivery are significantly associated with birthweight. Maternal age is not significantly associated with birthweight.

3) *To predict the value of the y variable from the explanatory x variables.*

We can use the multiple regression equation to predict the value of the y variable given the values of the explanatory x values. For example, what is the predicted birthweight for a baby girl of 30 weeks' gestation born with a normal delivery to a mother aged 40? Using the multiple regression equation (of Table 9.5):

Birthweight (kg) = − 3.005 + 0.002age + 0.141Gestation + 0.117Sex + 0.164Delivery.

Then

Birthweight (kg) = − 3.005 + (0.002 x 40) + (0.141 x 30) + (0.117 x 0) + (0.164 x 1)
= 1.422 kg.

9.6 Correlation is not Causation

One of the most common errors in the medical literature is to assume that simply because two variables are correlated, therefore one causes the other. Amusing examples include the positive correlation between the mortality rate in Victorian England and the number of Church of England marriages, and the negative correlation between monthly deaths from ischaemic heart disease and monthly ice-cream sales. In each case here, the fallacy is obvious because all the variables are time-related. In the former example, both the mortality rate and the number of Church of England marriages went down during the nineteenth century, in the latter example, deaths from ischaemic heart disease are higher in winter when ice-cream sales are at their lowest. However, it is always worth trying to think of other variables, confounding factors, which may be related to both of the variables under study. Further details on assessing causation are given in Chapter 14.

Association Between Two Variables: Correlation or Regression?

Correlation is used to denote association between two quantitative variables. The degree of association is estimated using the correlation coefficient. It measures the level of linear association between the two variables. Regression quantifies the relationship between two quantitative variables. It involves estimating the best straight line with which to summarise the association. The relationship is represented by an equation, the regression equation. It is useful when we want to describe the relationship between the variables, or even predict a value of one variable for a given value of the other.

Regression is more informative than correlation. Correlation simply quantifies the degree of linear association (or not) between two variables. However, it is often more useful to describe the relationship between the two variables, or even predict a value of one variable for a given value of the other and this is done using regression. If it is sensible to assume that one variable may be causing a response in the other then regression analysis should be used.

9.7   Points When Reading the Literature

1) When a correlation coefficient is calculated, is the relationship likely to be linear?
2) Are the variables likely to be Normally distributed?
3) Is a plot of the data in the paper? (This is a common omission.)
4) If a significant correlation is obtained and the causation inferred, could there be a third factor, not measured, which is jointly correlated with the other two, and so accounts for their association?
5) Remember correlation does not necessarily imply causation.
6) If a scatter plot is given to support a linear regression, is the variability of the points about the line roughly the same over the range of the independent variable? If not, then perhaps some transformation of the variables is necessary before computing the regression line.
7) If predictions are given, are any made outside the range of the observed values of the independent variable?
8) Sometimes logistic regression (see Chapter 10) is carried out when a continuous dependent variable is dichotomised. For example, low birthweight (LBW) is defined by the World Health Organization as a birthweight of an infant of 2.49 kg or less, regardless of gestational age. Normal weight at term delivery is 2.5 to 4.2 kg. So, birthweight could be dichotomised to 'LBW' or 'Normal'. It is important that the cut point is not derived by direct examination of the data for example to find a 'gap' in the data which maximises the discrimination between the selected groups as this can lead to biased results. It is best if there are a priori grounds for choosing a particular cut point.

9.8   Technical Details

Table 9.6 lists some of the statistical methods available for examining the relationships between two variables measured on the same sample of subjects.

Table 9.6 Statistical methods for relationships between two variables measured on the same sample of subjects.

y response/dependent variable	x Predictor/explanatory/independent variable				
	Continuous, Normal	Continuous, non-Normal	Ordinal	Nominal	Binary
Continuous, Normal	Regression Correlation: (Pearson's r)	Regression Rank correlation: (Spearman's r_s)	Rank Correlation: (Spearman's r_s)	One-way analysis of variance	Independent samples t-test
Continuous, non-Normal		Regression Rank correlation: (Spearman's r_s)	Rank correlation: (Spearman's r_s)	Kruskal–Wallis test	Mann–Whitney U test
Ordinal			Rank Correlation (Spearman's r_s)	Kruskal-Wallis test	Mann–Whitney U test Chi-squared test for trend
Nominal				Chi-squared test	Chi-squared test
Binary					Chi-squared test Fisher's exact test

Correlation Coefficient

Worked Example – Correlation Coefficient

The distance walked, in metres, on a 6 minutes walking test (6MWT) in 13 patients with multiple myeloma awaiting autologous haematopoietic stem cell transplantation before and after a 6-week duration pre-transplant exercise programme (prehabilitation) are shown in Table 9.7 (Keen et al. 2018). What is the correlation between the baseline and follow-up distance walked?

Thus, $n = 13$, $\bar{y} = 451.8\,\mathrm{m}$, $\bar{x} = 346.8\,\mathrm{m}$, $\Sigma(y-\bar{y})^2 = 78\,058.3$, $\Sigma(x-\bar{x})^2 = 122\,113.7$, $\Sigma(x-\bar{x})(y-\bar{y}) = 69\,492.5$ and so the Pearson correlation coefficient is:

$$r = \frac{\sum\limits_{i=1}^{n}(y_i - \bar{y})(x_i - \bar{x})}{\sqrt{\sum\limits_{i=1}^{n}(y_i - \bar{y})^2 \sum\limits_{i=1}^{n}(x_i - \bar{x})^2}} = \frac{69492.5}{\sqrt{78058.3 \times 122113.7}} = 0.712.$$

From Table 9.3 this correlation value can be interpreted as evidence of a 'strong relationship'. $SE(r) = \sqrt{\{(1-0.712^2\})/11\}} = 0.212$ and $t = 0.712/0.212 = 3.361$.

From Table T2, with $df = 13-2 = 11$, $t_{11,\,0.01} = 3.106$, $t_{11,\,0.001} = 4.437$, hence $0.001 < P < 0.01$; computer output gives $P = 0.006$. Therefore, we can reject the null hypothesis that the population correlation coefficient is zero.

Table 9.7 The distance walked, in metres, on a 6 minutes walking test (6MWT) in 13 patients with multiple myeloma awaiting stem cell transplantation before and after a 6-week duration pre-transplant exercise programme.

Subject	Before	After					
i	x_i	y_i	$x_i - \bar{x}$	$y_i - \bar{y}$	$(x_i - x)(y_i - \bar{y})$	$(y_i - \bar{y})^2$	$(x_i - \bar{x})^2$
1	90	285	−256.8	−166.8	42 834.0	27 811.98	65 969.95
2	240	405	−106.8	−46.8	4997.1	2187.36	11 416.10
3	285	420	−61.8	−31.8	1964.8	1009.28	3824.95
4	320	465	−26.8	13.2	−355.2	175.05	720.72
5	330	465	−16.8	13.2	−222.9	175.05	283.79
6	345	405	−1.8	−46.8	86.3	2187.36	3.41
7	380	620	33.2	168.2	5577.5	28 301.59	1099.18
8	390	415	43.2	−36.8	−1586.7	1351.98	1862.25
9	390	405	43.2	−46.8	−2018.3	2187.36	1862.25
10	390	443	43.2	−8.8	−378.4	76.90	1862.25
11	427	525	80.2	73.2	5869.7	5362.75	6424.64
12	442	525	95.2	73.2	6968.2	5362.75	9054.25
13	480	495	133.2	43.2	5756.3	1868.90	17 729.95
Mean	$\bar{x} = 346.8$	$\bar{y} = 451.8$ Sum	0.0	0.0	69 492.5	78 058.3	122 113.7

Source: data from Keen et al. (2018).

Table 9.8 The distance walked, in metres, and ranks of the distance walked in 13 patients with multiple myeloma awaiting stem cell transplantation before and after a six-week duration pre-transplant exercise programme.

Subject	Follow-up		Baseline		Difference in ranks	Difference in ranks^2
i	y_i	Rank y_is	x_i	Rank x_is		
1	285	1	90	1	0	0
2	405	3	240	2	1	1
3	420	6	285	3	3	9
4	465	8.5	320	4	4.5	20.25
5	465	8.5	330	5	3.5	12.25
6	405	3	345	6	−3	9
7	620	13	380	7	6	36
8	415	5	390	9	−4	16
9	405	3	390	9	−6	36
10	443	7	390	9	−2	4
11	525	11.5	427	11	0.5	0.25
12	525	11.5	442	12	−0.5	0.25
13	495	10	480	13	−3	9
				Sum	0.0	153.0

Source: data from Keen et al. (2018).

Spearman's Rank Correlation

In the above example (Table 9.8), the estimated

$$r_{Spearman} = 1 - \frac{6\sum d_i^2}{n^3 - n} = 1 - \frac{6 \times 153}{13^3 - 13} = \frac{918}{2188} = 0.58.$$

Linear Regression

Given a set of pairs of observations $(x_1, y_1), (x_2, y_2), ..., (x_n, y_n)$ the regression coefficient of y given x is

$$b = \frac{\sum_{i=1}^{n}(x_i - \bar{x})(y_i - \bar{y})}{\sum_{i=1}^{n}(x_i - \bar{x})^2}.$$

The intercept is estimated by $a = \bar{y} - b\bar{x}$.

To test whether b is significantly different from zero, calculate

$$E_{xy} = \sum (y - \bar{y})^2 - b^2 \sum (x - \bar{x})^2, E_{xx} = (n - 2) \sum (x - \bar{x})^2,$$

and hence

$$SE(b) = \sqrt{E_{xy}/E_{xx}}.$$

Then compare $t = b/SE(b)$ with the t-distribution of Table T2 with $df = n - 2$.

A 95% CI for the slope is given by

$$b - t_{n-2, 0.05} \times SE(b) \text{ to } b + t_{n-2, 0.05} \times SE(b).$$

Worked Example – Linear Regression

Using the data of Table 9.7 for a linear regression of distance walked (Distance$_{after}$) after a six-week duration pre-transplant exercise programme on distance walked before (Distance$_{before}$) transplant exercise programme, $b = 69\,492.5/122113.7 = 0.569$ and $a = \bar{y} - b\bar{x} = 451.8 - (0.569 \times 346.8) = 254.4$. Thus the regression line is estimated by Distance$_{after} = 254.4 + 0.569 \times$ Distance$_{before}$.

The formal test of significance of the regression coefficient requires $E_{xy} = 78\,058.3 - (0.569^2 \times 121\,113.7) = 38\,511.5$, $E_{xx} = (13-2) \times 122\,113.7 = 1\,343\,250.6$ and hence $SE(b) = (38\,511.5/1343250.6)^{1/2} = 0.169$. From which $t = 0.0569/0.169 = 3.36$. We compare this with a t distribution with $df = 13-2 = 11$. Use of Table T2 gives the P-value between 0.01 and 0.001 (more exactly 0.006) as we had in the correlation coefficient example above.

The 95% CI for the slope is given by $0.569 - (2.201 \times 0.169)$ to $0.569 + (2.201 \times 0.169)$. Finally, that is, 0.196 to 0.942 m.

Worked Example – Calculation of Residuals

The residuals from linear regression of distance walked (Distance$_{after}$) after a six-week duration pre-transplant exercise programme on distance walked before (Distance$_{before}$) the exercise programme of Table 9.7; that is the predicted Distance$_{after} = 254.4 + 0.569 \times$ Distance$_{before}$ are given in Table 9.9.

Table 9.9 Residuals for the linear regression of distance walked (Distance$_{after}$) after a six-week duration pre-transplant exercise programme on distance walked before (Distance$_{before}$) transplant exercise programme in 13 patients with multiple myeloma awaiting autologous haematopoietic stem cell transplantation.

Subject i	Observed y_{obs} Distance$_{after}$	Baseline x_i Distance$_{before}$	Predicted Y_{pred} Distance$_{after}$	Residual $y_{obs} - Y_{pred}$
1	285	90	305.6	−20.6
2	405	240	390.9	14.1
3	420	285	416.6	3.4
4	465	320	436.5	28.5
5	465	330	442.2	22.8
6	405	345	450.7	−45.7
7	620	380	470.6	149.4
8	415	390	476.3	−61.3
9	405	390	476.3	−71.3
10	443	390	476.3	−33.3
11	525	427	497.3	27.7
12	525	442	505.9	19.1
13	495	480	527.5	−32.5
Mean	451.8	346.8	451.7	0.0

Source: data from Keen et al. (2018).

Technical Details: Checking the Assumptions for a Linear Regression Analysis

We defined the model or population linear regression line for the ith subject with a continuous outcome, y_i, as:

$$y_i = \alpha + \beta x_i + \varepsilon_i.$$

Where x_i is an continuous or binary explanatory variable; ε_i is a Normally distributed random error term with mean 0 and variance σ^2_ε often denoted $\varepsilon_i \sim N(0, \sigma^2_\varepsilon)$ and the correlation between the residuals, for any two individual subjects, i and k, is $\text{Corr}(\varepsilon_i, \varepsilon_k) = 0$; α is the expected mean outcome when the explanatory variable x_i is zero and β is the effect on the outcome for a one unit increase in the explanatory variable x_i. For each observed value of x, the observed residual (e_i) is the observed y minus the corresponding fitted or predicted y, i.e. $e_i = y_{\text{obs}} - Y_{\text{pred}}$. Each residual may be positive or negative. As previously indicated, residuals should be Normally distributed with a mean value of zero, and a variance of, σ_ε^2. We can use the residuals to check the following assumptions underlying the linear regression model.

1) *The relationship between the two variables should be linear.*
   Either plot y against x (the data should approximate a straight line) or plot the residuals against x (we should observe a random scatter of points rather than any systematic pattern). Figure 9.5 shows a scatter plot of the relationship between birthweight and gestation. The relationship between the two variables appears to be linear. Figure 9.8 shows a scatter plot of the relationship

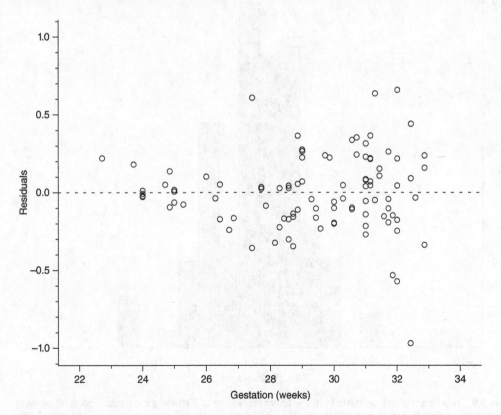

Figure 9.8 Scatter plot of residuals versus gestation from the linear regression of birthweight on gestation in 98 preterm infants. (*Source:* data from Simpson 2004).

between the residuals from the linear regression of birthweight on gestation. The relationship between the two variables appears to be random and does not follow any systematic pattern.

2) *The values of the response variable y should have a Normal distribution for each value of the explanatory variable x.*

This assumption means that the residuals are Normally distributed and should have a mean of zero. We can check this assumption by drawing a histogram, dot plot or box-and-whisker plot of the residuals and look at the results. Figure 9.9 shows a histogram of the residuals from the linear regression of birthweight on gestation for the 98 pre-term infants. The distribution of the residuals is approximately Normal.

3) *The variance (or standard deviation) of y should be the same at each value of x, i.e. there should be no evidence that as the value of y changes, the spread of the x values changes.*

This assumption means that the residuals have the same variability or constant variance for all the fitted values of y. We can check this assumption by a scatter plot of the residuals against the fitted or predicted Y values from the model. We should observe a random scatter of data points. Figure 9.10 shows a scatter plot of the relationship between the residuals from the linear regression of birthweight on gestation and the fitted birthweight values. Note that the graph is essentially the same as Figure 9.8 because fitted birthweight is linearly predicted by gestation. There does appear to be a slight tendency for the variability to increase as the fitted values

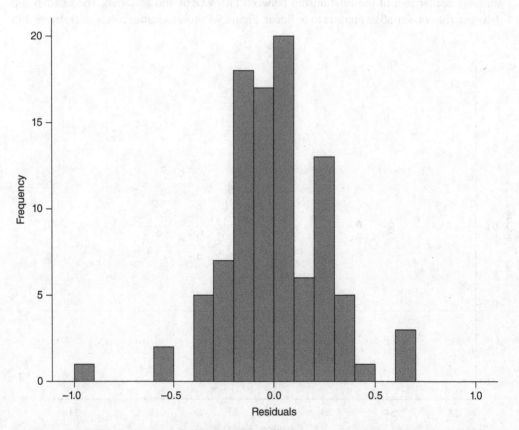

Figure 9.9 Histogram of the residuals from the linear regression of birthweight on gestation in 98 preterm infants. (*Source:* data from Simpson 2004).

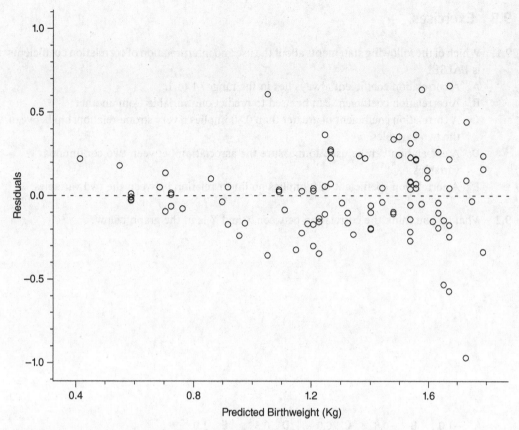

Figure 9.10 Scatter plot of residuals vs. fitted or predicted birthweight from the linear regression of birthweight on gestation in 98 preterm infants. (*Source:* data from Simpson 2004).

increase. This could be investigated further, for example by seeing if taking logs of birthweight, or using more advanced methods to allow for unequal variances. Fortunately, the inferences are quite robust to minor departures such as these.

4) *The observations in the sample are independent.*

The observations in the sample are independent if there is no more than one pair of observations on each subject. In the case where we have single measurements on separate individuals, then there is no problem with independence as there is no reason to suppose that measurements made on one individual are likely to affect a different individual. There are two situations in which the assumption of independence might be violated: (i) if the observations are ordered in time, or (ii) if different numbers of observations are made on some individuals, but all the observations are treated equally. In this latter case the study size is regarded (incorrectly) as the number of data pairs within the regression rather than the number of individuals providing data.

5) *The variable x can be measured without error.*

This is a difficult and almost impossible assumption to check and satisfy! The *x* variable is rarely measured without any error. We have to assume this error is small. Providing this is the case, then this is likely to have little effect on the model and the conclusions from the model.

9.9 Exercises

9.1. Which of the following statements about the use and interpretation of correlation coefficients is FALSE?

A A correlation coefficient always lies in the range –1 to 1.

B A correlation coefficient can be used to predict one variable from another.

C A correlation coefficient of greater than 0.80 implies a very strong relationship between the two variables.

D A correlation can be used to measure the association between two continuous variables.

E A correlation coefficient of 0 implies no linear relation between the two variables

9.2 What do you think the correlation between X and Y is in the graph below?

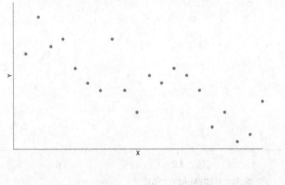

A –1.0   **B** –0.8   **C** 0.0   **D** 0.5   **E** 1.0

9.3 What do you think the correlation between X and Y is in the graph below

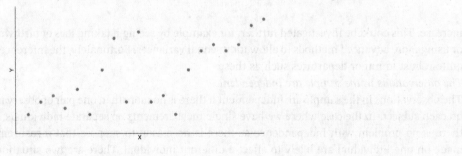

A –1.0   **B** –0.5   **C** 0.0   **D** 0.7   **E** 1.0

9.4 Figure 9.11 shows a scatterplot and regression line of the relationship between the between distance walked, in metres on an endurance shuttle walk test before (pre) and after (post) a physiotherapy rehabilitation programme in 100 patients with Chronic Obstructive Pulmonary (COPD) disease.

From Figure 9.11, what do you think is the approximate correlation between pre and post rehabilitation distance walked?

A −1.0 **B** −0.5 **C** 0.0 **D** 0.4 **E** 0.8

9.5 From Figure 9.11 what do you think is the approximate intercept of the regression line for the relationship between pre and post rehabilitation distance walked?

A 0 **B** 100 **C** 200 **D** 300 **E** 400

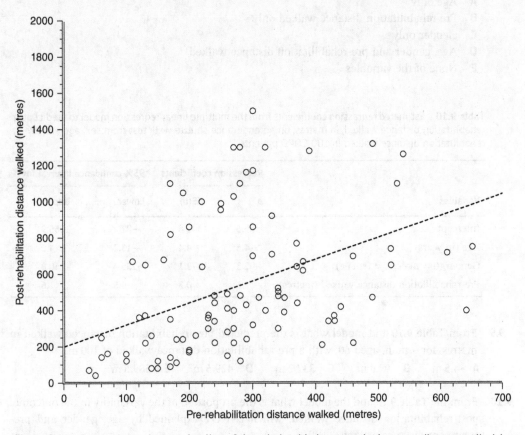

Figure 9.11 Scatterplot and regression line of the relationship between the between distance walked, in metres on an endurance shuttle walk test before (pre) and after (post) a physiotherapy rehabilitation programme in 100 patients with Chronic Obstructive Pulmonary (COPD) disease.

9.6 From Figure 9.11, what do you think is the approximate slope of the regression line for the relationship between pre and post rehabilitation distance walked?

A 0 **B** −1.2 **C** −10 **D** 1.2 **E** 100

9.7 Using the regression line, in Figure 9.11, what is the predicted post-rehabilitation distance walked given a pre-rehabilitation distance walked of 300 m?

A 0 **B** 100 **C** 200 **D** 550 **E** 800

9.8 Table 9.10 below shows the estimated regression coefficients from the multiple linear regression model to predict post-rehabilitation distance walked, in metres, on an endurance shuttle walk test from sex, age and pre-rehabilitation distance walked in 100 COPD patients.

Y or dependent variable: Post-rehabilitation distance walked (metres)

$R^2 = 0.20$, residual SD = 349.2

Which variables are statistically significantly associated with post-rehabilitation distance walked?

A   Age only
B   Pre-rehabilitation distance walked only
C   Gender only
D   Age, gender and pre-rehabilitation distance walked
E   None of the variables

Table 9.10   Estimated regression coefficients from the multiple linear regression model to predict post-rehabilitation distance walked, in metres, on an endurance shuttle walk test from sex, age and pre-rehabilitation distance walked in 100 COPD patients.

	Regression coefficients		95% confidence interval for *b*	
Variables	*b*	SE(*b*)	Lower	Upper
Intercept	589.5	340.8	−87	1265.9
Age (in years)	−4.5	4.4	−13.2	4.2
Gender (0 = male, 1 = female)	−92.3	72.1	−235.4	50.8
Pre-rehabilitation distance walked (metres)	1.1	0.3	0.5	1.6

9.9 From Table 9.10 and model what is the predicted post-rehabilitation distanced walked in metres, for a man, aged 60, with a pre-rehabilitation distance walked of 100 m?

A 4.5 m   **B** 92.3 m   **C** 337.2 m   **D** 429.5 m   **E** 589.5 m

9.10 From the Table 9.10 and the model what is the proportion of the variability in the outcome, post-rehabilitation distance walked, which is NOT explained by age, gender and pre-treatment distance walked?

A 0.10   **B** 0.20   **C** 0.40   **D** 0.60   **E** 0.80

10 Logistic Regression

Medical Statistics: A Textbook for the Health Sciences, Fifth Edition. Stephen J. Walters, Michael J. Campbell, and David Machin.
© 2021 John Wiley & Sons Ltd. Published 2021 by John Wiley & Sons Ltd.
Companion website: www.wiley.com/go/walters/medicalstatistics

Summary

The chi-squared test is used for testing the association between two binary variables. However, it is better to try and model an association rather than simply test whether or not it exists. A logistic regression model is one which suggests a plausible relationship between a binary outcome or dependent variable (such as survive yes/no; diseased yes/no; symptom yes/no) with one or more independent or predictor variables that can be binary, categorical (with more than two categories) or continuous. It enables the investigation of the effect of several predictor variables on this binary outcome. It uses a modification of the outcome data (the logistic transform) to allow a linear relationship to be modelled and gives a set of regression coefficients that represent the relationship between each predictor variable and the binary outcome. When the predictor is a single binary variable then the test of the coefficient associated with this predictor in a logistic regression is equivalent to a chi-squared test. Logistic regression is also useful for analysing case–control studies in general while matched case–control studies require a particular analysis known as *conditional logistic regression*.

10.1 Introduction

Logistic regression is very similar to linear regression but now there is a binary, rather than continuous, outcome of interest and a number of possible predictor or explanatory variables. It enables the investigation of the effect of several predictor variables on this binary outcome. Logistic regression analysis can be used to do one or more of the following:

1) As a substitute for multiple regression, when the outcome variable is binary in cross-sectional and cohort studies and in randomised controlled trials (RCTs). We would use logistic regression to investigate the relationship between a causal variable and binary output variable, allowing for confounding variables which can be categorical or continuous.
2) As a discriminant analysis, to try to find factors that discriminate between two groups. Here the outcome would be a binary variable indicating group membership. For example, one might want to discriminate between men and women on the basis of their psychological test results.
3) To develop prognostic indicators, such as the risk of complications from surgery.
4) To analyse case–control studies and matched case–control studies.

10.2 Binary Outcome Variable

In logistic regression (sometimes known as binary logistic regression), the dependent variable is binary; that is, it can only take a value of one of two categories and these are usually coded 0 and 1. Logistic regression is used to predict binary outcomes such as whether a patient has (code 1) or does not have (code 0) a disease in the presence of a particular diagnostic feature. Another application is to examine whether the chance of cure (success) in patients with, for example, a particular type of cancer depends on the stage of their disease (risk factor).

The model needs to be described with care. It is written in terms of the expected value of a positive result (success) for the outcome variable for an individual, which is assumed to be π. Note that this is not the *observed* outcome, which is just 0 or 1, but the *expected* outcome, which lies between 0 and 1. The logistic model is then

$$\log\left(\frac{\pi}{1-\pi}\right) = \alpha + \beta x.$$

The values of the regression coefficients α and β are chosen as the ones that give expected proportions that are closest (in a particular mathematical sense) to the observed proportions, usually using a technique known as maximum likelihood. The model is described further in the technical details of this chapter.

The above equation may be compared with that for linear regression in Chapter 9. The right-hand side of the logistic equation has the same form, but y on the left-hand side is replaced not by π, but by the so-called logit of π. The essential reason for this is that π itself can take only values between 0 and 1, whereas the logit that is $\log[\pi/(1-\pi)]$ may range from $-\infty$ to $+\infty$ as in theory can the right-hand side of the equation. Essentially this transformation ensures that the probabilities, which we want to estimate, lie between 0 and 1.

The logit transform has the useful property that if an independent variable, x, in the model is binary with values 0 or 1, and has associated regression coefficient β, then $\exp(\beta)$ is the odds ratio, *OR*, of someone with $x = 1$ having a positive result.

Example – Logistic Regression – Foot Corn RCT

The foot corn randomised controlled trial conducted by Farndon et al. (2013) has been described in earlier chapters. If we code the binary outcome corn healed as $y = 1$ (yes) and $y = 0$ (no) and further define the treatment given by $x = 1$ if a patient is randomised to the corn plaster, and 0 if randomised to scalpel, then Table 10.1 shows the data.

A logistic regression with 'corn healed' as the outcome variable gives the output summarised in Table 10.2, from which the OR is estimated by $\exp(0.631) = 1.88$. We can relate this to the 2×2 table of Table 10.1 from which the OR $= (32 \times 74)/(63 \times 20) = 1.88$. The odds of corn healing at three months in the corn plaster group is 1.88 times that of the odds of the corn healing in the scalpel group.

The term 'Wald' in Table 10.2 refers to a statistical test based on the ratio of the estimate (for example, b the estimate of β) to its standard error (SE). The Wald test statistic, z, follows the standard Normal distribution; and its square, z^2, approximates to the chi-squared distribution with 1 df. The P-values obtained are then approximately equal to those from the conventional χ^2 test for 2×2 tables, especially when the numbers in the table are large. A 95% 'Wald' confidence interval (CI) for b, which is the log odds ratio, is given by

$$b \pm \{1.96 \times SE(b)\}.$$

Consequently, an estimated 95% CI for the OR is:

$$\exp\{b - 1.96 \times SE(b)\} \text{ to } \exp\{b + 1.96 \times SE(b)\}.$$

Table 10.1 Relationship between corn healed status and randomised group in 189 patients with foot corns and valid outcome data at post-randomisation.

Treatment Group	x	Index corn healed			Proportion Healed (p_i)
		Yes (1)	No (0)	Total	
Corn plaster (intervention)	1	32	63	95	0.34
Scalpel (control)	0	20	74	94	0.21
Total		52	137	189	

Source: from Table 3.4.

Table 10.2 Output obtained from a logistic regression analysis with outcome variable corned healed (yes or no) and a binary independent variable randomised group.

	Population Regression Coefficient	Sample Estimate	SE	Wald	P-value	Odds Ratio exp(b_Group)	95% CI Lower	Upper
Constant	α	−1.308	0.252					
Group	β_{Group}	0.631	0.333	1.89	0.058	1.88	0.98	3.61

The Wald statistic, which is the ratio of the estimate b to its SE, that is, z = b/SE(b) = 0.631/0.333 = 1.89 with P-value = 0.058.	b_{Group} is the estimate of β_{Group}, and exp(b_{Group}) is the estimated OR associated with x. The coefficient for Group is 0.631, and the OR is exp(0.631) = 1.88 (95% CI: 0.98 to 3.61)

Source: data of Table 10.1.

For the data in Table 10.2 the estimated 95% CI for the OR is:

$$\exp\{0.631 - (1.96 \times 0.333)\} \text{ to } \exp\{0.631 + (1.96 \times 0.333)\}$$

or 0.98 to 3.61.

Note that the 95% CI just includes one, which is to be expected since the Wald test is not statistically significant with a *P*-value greater than 0.05. The CI around the odds ratio is asymmetric, which contrasts with the symmetric CIs of linear regression. This CI is wide, reflecting the uncertainty in the effect of the corn plaster treatment.

10.3 The Multiple Logistic Regression Equation

In the same way that multiple regression is an extension of linear regression, we can extend logistic regression to multiple logistic regression with more than one independent/predictor/explanatory variable. We can also extend it to the case where some independent variables are categorical and some are continuous. Usually for multiple logistic regression we denote the intercept by β_0 rather than by α. Thus if there are p predictor variables $x_1, x_2,...,x_p$, then the model is:

$$\log\left(\frac{\pi}{1-\pi}\right) = \beta_0 + \beta_1 x_1 + \cdots + \beta_p x_p,$$

where x_1 is the first independent variable, x_2 is the second, and so on up to the pth independent variable x_p.

If all the independent variables are categorical then we can tabulate the outcome data by all levels of the covariates. The model then implies that all patients in a particular cell of the table will have the same probability of their corn healing at three-months, say π_i, and this probability may differ from cell to cell. The π_i can be estimated by p_i which is the proportion of patients whose corn healed in that cell. Table 10.1 shows that the estimated proportions healed in the corn plaster and scalpel cells are 0.34 and 0.21 respectively.

If any of the independent variables are continuous, such as baseline corn size, then a table giving the outcome by every combination of independent variables cannot be sensibly constructed. Many cells would be likely to be empty and many contain only a single individual. Thus, the resulting proportions responding in each cell, would almost all be zero or one or missing.

Nevertheless, it is perfectly possible to get valid estimates of the parameters of a logistic model in this extreme (the continuous variable) case using maximum likelihood. In the model, if an independent variable x is continuous and β is the associated regression coefficient, then $\exp(\beta)$ is the change in odds associated with a unit increase in x.

Example – Multiple Logistic Regression – Corn Healed and Baseline Corn Size

For example, if we use multiple logistic regression with two predictors: one continuous baseline corn size (measured in mm); and one binary (randomised group) we obtain Table 10.3. The logistic regression model is

$$\log \left(\frac{\pi}{1-\pi} \right) = \beta_0 + \beta_{1Group} x_{Group} + \beta_{2Size} x_{Size}.$$

Table 10.3 shows some evidence of an effect of corn plasters after adjusting for baseline corn size. The odds ratio for the group term suggests that the odds of the corn healing in the corn plaster groups after adjusting for baseline corn size is 2.01 times the odds of the corn healing in the scalpel group (95% CI: 1.03–3.89). Note that the CI for the treatment group variable now just excludes one after other factors are taken into account. The effect of the continuous variable, baseline corn size, can be interpreted as follows; after taking into account treatment group the odds ratio estimate is the change in the odds of the outcome (corn healing) for a unit (or 1 mm) change in the continuous predictor variable (corn size). Thus, for a patient in the scalpel group with a baseline corn size of 4 mm the odds of a healed corn are $\exp(-0.536 - 0.214 \times 4) = 0.249$. If the baseline corn size was 5 mm the odds of healed corn are $\exp(-0.536 - 0.214 \times 5) = 0.200$. Thus, the odds ratio for corn healing for a 5 mm corn compared to a 4 mm corn are $0.200 / 0.249 = 0.81$ that is, reduced odds of the corn healing. A change of two units (say from 4.0 to 6.0 mm) has an associated OR that is $OR \times OR = OR^2$ (not $2 \times OR$), i.e. $0.81^2 = 0.66$, and a change of three units is shown by OR^3, etc.

Calculating the Probability of an Event
We can rearrange the logistic regression equation to estimate the probability that an individual has the outcome of interest. If we rewrite the fitted multiple logistic regression equation as:

$$p_i = \frac{\exp \left(b_0 + b_1 x_1 + \cdots + b_p x_p \right)}{1 + \exp \left(b_0 + b_1 x_1 + \cdots + b_p x_p \right)}.$$

Table 10.3 Output obtained from a multiple logistic regression analysis with outcome variable corned healed and two independent variables: baseline corn size and group ($N = 188$).

Variable	Population regression coefficient	Sample estimate (b)	SE (b)	Wald z	P-value	OR Exp (b)	95% CI for OR Lower	Upper
Constant	β_0	−0.536	0.452					
Group (0 = scalpel, 1 = plaster	β_{1Group}	0.696	0.338	4.229	0.04	2.01	1.03	3.89
Baseline corn size (mm)	β_{2Size}	−0.214	0.109	3.844	0.05	0.81	0.65	1.00

Here p_i is the estimated probability of the outcome of interest for subject i, with covariates or risk factors $x_1, ..., x_p$; and $b_0, b_1, ..., b_p$ are the estimates of $\beta_0, \beta_1, ..., \beta_p$.

Example – Estimating the Probability that an Individual Has the Outcome of Interest – Corning Healing

If we use multiple logistic regression with two explanatory or predictor variables: one continuous baseline corn size; and one binary (randomised group) we obtain Table 10.3. From this model the estimated probability that an individual patient's corn will have healed by three months, is

$$p_{\text{Healed}} = \frac{\exp(-0.536 + 0.696 \times \text{Group} - 0.214 \times \text{Size})}{[1 + \exp(-0.536 + 0.696 \times \text{Group} - 0.214 \times \text{Size})]}.$$

For example, a patient in the corn plaster (group = 1) with baseline corn size of 4.0 mm has an estimated probability $p_{\text{Healed}} = \exp(-0.536 + 0.696 \times 1 - 0.214 \times 4.0)/[1 + \exp(0.536 + 0.696 \times 1 - 0.214 \times 4.0)] = 0.33$ of their corn healing. A patient in the scalpel group (Group = 0) with the same baseline corn size has an estimated probability $p_{\text{Healed}} = \exp(-0.536 + 0.696 \times 0 - 0.214 \times 4.0)/[1 + \exp(0.536 + 0.696 \times 0 - 0.214 \times 4.0)] = 0.20$ of their corn healing.

Example of Multiple Logistic Regression – Foot Corn RCT

We can analyse the trial conducted by Farndon et al. (2013) by a multiple logistic regression model for the binary outcome healed/not healed, adjusting for centre and size of the index corn at baseline. In the trial, there were seven treatment centres. If we have a nominal categorical explanatory variable, such as centre, that has more than two categories or levels, we have to create a number of *dummy* or *indicator* variables. In general, for a nominal variable with k categories, we create $k - 1$ binary dummy variables. We choose one of the categories to represent the *reference* category. Each dummy variable allows a comparison of one of the remaining $k - 1$ categories with the reference category.

In order to fit a logistic regression model with a categorical variable with seven centres, one centre is chosen as the reference category and a further six dummy variables (each coded 0 and 1) are created (see column 1 of Table 10.4). Thus, if the Central centre is chosen as the reference category,

Table 10.4 Output obtained from a multiple logistic regression model with outcome variable corned healed and independent variables; baseline corn size, centre, and group ($N = 188$).

Variable	b	SE(b)	Wald z	P-value	Odds Ratio	95% CI for OR Lower	Upper
Group (0 = scalpel, 1 = corn plaster)	0.694	0.345	2.01	0.044	2.00	1.02	3.93
Baseline corn size (mm)	−0.204	0.113	−1.81	0.071	0.82	0.65	1.02
Central (0) vs Manor (1)	0.078	0.476	−0.16	0.870	0.93	0.36	2.35
Central (0) vs Jordanthorpe (1)	0.191	0.518	0.37	0.713	1.21	0.44	3.34
Central (0) vs Limbrick (1)	−1.04	1.103	−0.94	0.345	0.35	0.04	3.07
Central (0) vs Firth Park (1)	0.281	0.684	0.41	0.681	1.32	0.35	5.06
Central (0) vs Huddersfield (1)	−0.096	0.879	−0.11	0.913	0.91	0.16	5.09
Central (0) vs Darnall (1)	−0.404	1.169	−0.35	0.730	0.67	0.07	6.60
Constant	−0.550	0.489	−1.13	0.260	0.58	0.22	1.50

then Table 10.4 shows the multiple logistic regression model with outcome variable corned healed and predictor variables: group, baseline corn size and centre. At three-months post-randomisation, 34% (32/94) of participants had a resolved corn with corn plaster compared with 21% (20/94) with scalpel, an odds ratio of 1.91. Adjusting for baseline corn size and centre increases this to 2.00, (95% CI: 1.02 to 3.93, $P = 0.044$) indicating that the odds of a completely healed index corn with corn plaster was twice that with scalpel after adjustment for baseline corn size and centre.

Use of Logistic Regression in Case–Control Studies

Logistic regression is particularly useful in the analysis of case–control studies (see also Chapter 14). It can be shown that if the case (1) or control status (0) is made the dependent variable in a logistic regression then the model will provide valid estimates of the odds ratios associated with risk factors. These odds ratios will give estimates of relative risks (RR) provided the incidence of the disease is reasonably low, say below 20%.

Example from the Literature – Caffeinated Substances and Risk of Crashes in Long Distance Drivers: Case–Control Study

A case–control study to investigate whether there is an association between the use of substances that contain caffeine (coffee, tea, caffeinated soft drinks, caffeine tablets, energy drinks) and the risk of a crash in long distance commercial vehicle drivers was carried out in two areas in Australia (Sharwood et al. 2013). The study participants were 530 drivers of commercial vehicles who had recently been involved in a crash attended by police (cases) and 517 control drivers who had not had a crash (control) whilst driving a commercial vehicle in the past 12 months. The main outcome measure was the risk of a crash associated with the use of substances containing caffeine.

The authors used multiple logistic regression to calculate the risk of a crash, with adjustment for potential confounding factors of: age, distance driven, hours of sleep, night driving, breaks taken and area. Table 10.5 shows that after adjustment for potential confounders, drivers who consumed caffeinated substances had an odds ratio of crashing of 0.37 (95% CI 0.27 to 0.50) compared with drivers who did not take caffeinated substances.

Table 10.5 Associations between use of stimulant substances and crashes in long distance commercial vehicle drivers who were recently involved in crash (cases) and control drivers who had not had crashed in previous 12 months. Figures are numbers (percentage) of participants.

	Cases (n = 530)	Controls (n = 517)	Adjusted[a] OR (95% CI)
Uses caffeinated stimulant:			
No[b]	368 (69.4)	227 (43.9)	1
Yes	162 (30.6)	290 (56.1)	0.37 (0.27 to 0.50)
Uses illegal stimulants[c]:			
Never[b]	520 (98.1)	497 (96.1)	1
Often/sometimes	10 (1.89)	20 (3.87)	0.68 (0.27 to 1.67)
Previous crash[d]	119 (22.5)	75 (14.5)	1.81 (1.26 to 2.62)

[a] Adjusted for age, distance driven, hours of sleep, night driving, and breaks taken and area of crash/recruitment.
[b] Reference category.
[c] Including speed, ecstasy, and cocaine.
[d] Police attended previous crash, in the past five years, not including current crash for cases.
Source: data from Sharwood et al. (2013).

The authors concluded that caffeinated substances are associated with a reduced risk of crashing; and that the use of caffeinated substances could be a useful add-on strategy in the maintenance of alertness while driving.

10.4   Conditional Logistic Regression

Conditional logistic regression is an extension of McNemar's paired test of two proportions described in Chapter 8. The analysis gives adjusted odd ratios for paired binary data, such as may be found in a matched case–control study. In a matched case–control study each case is matched directly with one or more controls. For a valid analysis the matching should be taken into account and for this we use a method known as conditional logistic regression.

Example of Conditional Logistic Regression

Pedersen et al. (2018) identified patients (cases) with non-melanoma skin cancer (NMSC) during 2004–2012 from the Danish Cancer Registry. For each case they chose 20 controls who did not have this disease, matched for age, sex, and calendar time. Cumulative hydrochlorothiazide (HCT) use in 1995–2012 was assessed from the Danish Prescription Registry. Using conditional logistic regression, they calculated odds ratios (ORs) for basal cell carcinoma (BCC) and squamous cell carcinoma (SCC) associated with HCT use.

They found that high use of HCT (>50 000 mg) was associated with ORs of 1.29 (95% CI, 1.23 to 1.35) for BCC and 3.98 (95% CI 3.68 to 4.31) for SCC. Use of other diuretics and anti-hypertensives was not associated with NMSC. They concluded that HCT use is associated with a substantially increased risk of NMSC, especially SCC.

Consequences of the Logistic Model
A question that remains is: is there any interaction between the input variables? For example, corns are often caused by people wearing shoes that fit poorly and certain shoe designs that place excessive pressure on an area of the foot. Ideally, the foot corn trial would have recorded these explanatory variables but unfortunately, it did not. However, in general, females are more likely to wear shoes with high heels so we may regard the sex of the patient as an important risk factor for developing corns and corn healing.

Since the logistic model is described in terms of logarithms, what is additive on a logarithmic scale is multiplicative on the linear scale. To quantify the potential interaction between two binary predictor variables, say x_1 and x_2, (such as treatment group and sex) the multiple logistic regression model is extended by adding a third covariate $x_3 = x_1 \times x_2$. The magnitude of the associated regression coefficient β_3 then indicates whether the two factors interact together in a synergistic (either more or less than multiplicative) way if β_3 is strongly positive or negative or are essentially independent of each other, in which case β_3 will be close to zero.

Example – Foot Corn RCT Group by Sex Interaction

For the foot corn RCT of Farndon et al. (2013), group is coded as 0 = scalpel and 1 = corn plaster and 'sex' takes the value 1 for females and 0 for males; then to investigate interaction between these variables, a new variable 'group × sex' interaction, equal to 'group' multiplied by 'sex', must be included in the logistic model. Table 10.6 shows the output obtained from a multiple logistic

Table 10.6 Output obtained from a multiple logistic regression model with outcome variable corned healed and predictor variables group, sex, and group × sex interaction term (*N* = 188).

Variables	*b*	SE(*b*)	Wald Z	*P*-value	Odds ratio	95% CI for OR Lower	95% CI for OR Upper
Group (0 = scalpel, 1 = plaster)	0.278	0.485	0.328	0.567	1.32	0.51	3.414
Sex (0 = male, 1 = female)	−0.697	0.509	1.873	0.171	0.498	0.184	1.352
Group × sex interaction	0.689	0.672	1.05	0.306	1.992	0.533	7.439
Constant	−0.934	0.356	6.894	0.009			

regression model with outcome variable corned healed and predictor variables group, sex, and group × sex interaction term from the foot corn RCT. From this model, there is no reliable evidence of a group × sex interaction as the associated confidence is wide and includes one.

Model Checking

An important question is whether the logistic model describes the data well. If the logistic model is obtained from grouped data, then there is no problem comparing the observed proportions in the groups and those predicted by the model.

There are a number of ways the model may fail to describe the data well and these include:

i) Lack of an important covariate, a variable which is predictive of the outcome
ii) Outlying observations
iii) 'Extra-Binomial' variation.

The first problem can be investigated by trying all available covariates, and the possible interactions between them. If we believe an unrecorded covariate is predictor of outcome, so provided it is a confounder, then inference about any other covariates is usually not affected.

The influence of covariates with outlying observations can be difficult to check. However, some statistical packages do provide standardised residuals; that is, residuals divided by their estimated SEs. These values can be plotted against values of the predictor variables to examine patterns in the data. It is important also to look for influential observations, perhaps a subgroup of subjects that if deleted from the analysis would result in a substantial change to the values of regression coefficient estimates.

Extra-Binomial variation can occur when the data are not strictly independent; for example, if the data comprise repeated outcome measures from the same individuals rather than a single outcome from each individual, or if patients are grouped for treatment, which may be the case in an intervention trial randomised by clusters rather than for individual patient randomisation. In such cases, although the estimates of the regression coefficients are not unduly affected, the corresponding SEs are usually underestimated. Further details on model checking are described in the technical details section at the end of the chapter.

10.5 Reporting the Results of a Logistic Regression

1) Confirm that the assumptions for the logistic regression were met:
   • The events are independent
   • The relationship is plausibly log-linear

- If the design is matched ensure that the analysis uses an appropriate method such as conditional logistic regression.

2) Summarise the logistic regression to include the number of observations in the analysis, the coefficient of the explanatory variable with its SE and/or the OR and the 95% CI for the OR and the *P*-value.
3) If the predictor variable is continuous, then it is often helpful to scale it for easy interpretation. For example it is easier to think of the increased risk of death every 10 years than the increased risk per year.
4) Report any sensitivity analyses (e.g. model checking) carried out. Is there evidence of over dispersion?
5) Specify whether the explanatory variables were tested for interaction.
6) Name the statistical package used in the analysis.

10.6 Additional Points When Reading the Literature When Logistic Regression Has Been Used

1) Is a logistic regression appropriate? Is the outcome a simple binary variable? If there is a time attached to the outcome then survival analysis (see Chapter 11) might be better.
2) The outcome is often described as 'relative risks'. Whilst this is often approximately true, they are better described as 'approximate relative risks', or better still as odds ratios. Note for an OR, a non-significant result is associated with a 95% CI that includes 1 (not 0 as in multiple linear regression).
3) Has a continuous variable been divided into two to create a binary variable for the analysis? How was the splitting point chosen? If it was chosen after the data have been collected, be very suspicious!
4) If the design is a matched case–control study has conditional logistic regression been carried out?

10.7 Technical Details

The Logistic Regression Model

The dependent/outcome variable can be described as an *event* that is present or absent (sometimes termed '*success*' or '*failure*'). An event might be the presence of disease in a survey or cure from disease in a clinical trial. We wish to examine factors associated with the event. We can rarely predict exactly whether an event will happen or not. What we look for are factors associated with the *probability* of an event happening.

When all the independent variables are categorical, one can form tables in which each cell has individuals with the same values of the independent variables. Consequently, one can calculate the proportion of subjects for whom an event happens. For example, one might wish to examine the presence or absence of disease by gender (two categories) and social class (five categories). Thus, one could form a table with the 10 social class by gender categories and examine the proportion of

Table 10.7 Contingency table of outcome values in which each cell has individuals with the same values of the independent categorical predictor variables.

Outcome	Subgroups		
	1	2	i
Successes	y_1	y_2	y_i
Failures	$n_1 - y_1$	$n_2 - y_2$	$n_i - y_i$
Total	n_1	n_2	n_i

$$p_i = y_i/n_i$$

> p_i is the **sample estimate** of π_i **the population probability** of success for subgroup **i**.

subjects with the disease in each category. With continuous independent variables, such as age, the data table may contain as many cells as there are individuals and the observed proportions of subjects with the outcome in each cell must be 0 out of 1 or 1 out of 1.

If we denote a binary response variable y and its two possible outcomes by 1 'success' and 0 'failure'. The distribution of y is specified by probabilities $P(y = 1) = \pi$ of success and $P(y = 0) = (1 - \pi)$ of failure. The expected proportion or probability of success in the population is $E(y) = \pi$. Table 10.7 shows a $2 \times i$ column contingency table of outcome values in which each cell has individuals with the same values of the independent categorical predictor variables.

As we have said before, the purpose of statistical analysis is to take *samples* to estimate *population* parameters. In logistic regression, the population parameters are the βs. Consider the categorical-grouped case first, the population probability of an event for a cell/subgroup i is π_i. This is also called the 'expected' value. For example, with an unbiased coin the population or expected probability for a 'head' is 0.5. If an event has probability π_i then the *odds* for that event are $\pi_i/(1 - \pi_i)$ to 1. For example the odds of a head to tail are 1 to 1.

The dependent variable, y_i, is the observed number of events in the cell (say, the number of the heads in a set of n_i tosses). We write $E(y_i) = n_i\pi_i$ where E denotes the 'expected value'. We want to describe the proportion of successes $p_i = y_i/n_i$ in each subgroup in terms of factor levels and explanatory variables that characterise each subgroup. As $E(y_i) = n_i\pi_i$ and so $E(p_i) = \pi_i$ we model the probabilities using the logistic regression equation. The model is

$$\log \frac{\pi_i}{1 - \pi_i} = \text{logit}(\pi_i) = \beta_0 + \beta_1 x_{i1} + \ldots + \beta_p x_{ip}$$

where the predictor variables are $x_{i1},\ldots,x_{ip}$ and π_i is the expected probability of an event for cell/subject i. The term on the left-hand side of equation is the log odds of success and is called the *logistic* or *logit* transform.

The exponential of a particular coefficient e^{b1} is an estimate of the odds ratio. For a particular value of x_1 it is the estimated odds of disease for $(x_1 + 1)$ relative to the estimated odds of disease for x_1, while adjusting for all the other xs is in the equation. It is therefore often referred to as an adjusted odds ratio. If the odds ratio is equal to one (unity) then these two odds are the same. A value of the odds ratio above 1 indicates increased odds of having the outcome as x_1 increases by 1 unit. A value below 1 indicates decreased odds of having the outcome as x_1 increases by 1 unit. When the outcome is rare, the odds ratio can be interpreted as a relative risk.

At this stage, the *observed* values of the outcome variable are not in the equation. They are linked to the model by the Binomial distribution. If in cell i we observe y_i successes in n_i subjects, we assume that the y_i are distributed Binomially with probability π_i. Each binary observation is Binomial $\sim(1, \pi_i)$. The parameters in the model are estimated by *maximum likelihood*. Of course, we do not know the population values π_i, and in the modelling process we substitute into the model the estimated or fitted values.

The logistic regression model is often described in the literature with the observed proportion, $p_i = y_i/n_i$ replacing π_i. This misses out the second part of the model, the error distribution that links the two. When the outcome variable is 0 or 1, the logit of the outcome variable does not exist. This may lead some people to believe logistic regression is impossible in these circumstances. However, the model uses the logit of the expected value, not the observed value. The model ensures that the expected value is >0 and <1.

Unlike linear regression models there is no longer an error term in the model and the variance of the outcome is a function of the expected value of the outcome. Since we have no error term in the model, unlike with linear regression we cannot expect an error term to cope with the lack of fit of the model, and the definition of residuals is less obvious.

We can rearrange the logistic regression equation to estimate the probability that an individual has the outcome: $\hat{\pi}_i$.

The estimated linear predictor (LP) for subject i is:

$$LP_i = b_0 + b_1 x_{i1} + \cdots + b_p x_{ip}$$

$$\hat{\pi}_i = \frac{\exp(LP_i)}{1 + \exp(LP_i)}$$

where $\hat{\pi}_i$ is an estimate of π_i and estimates the probability of an event from the model. These are the predicted or fitted values for y_i. A good model will give predictions $\hat{\pi}_i$ close to the observed proportions y_i/n_i.

10.8 The Wald Test

The Wald test statistic, which follows the standard Normal distribution, is equal to the estimated logistic regression coefficient b divided by its SE, i.e. $z = b/SE$. Its square, z^2, approximates the chi-squared distribution with 1 df. The likelihood ratio test and the Wald test give similar results if the sample size is large. The Wald statistic, for the group term in Table 10.2 is the ratio of the estimate b to its SE, i.e. $z = b/SE(b) = (0.631/0.333) = 1.897$ with a P-value $= 0.058$.

10.9 Evaluating the Model and its Fit: The Hosmer–Lemeshow Test

The Hosmer–Lemeshow test assesses the agreement between the observed event probabilities and those predicted by the model. Individuals in the sample are stratified into g groups. We usually take $g = 10$ and base the groups on the deciles of the distribution of predicted probabilities from the model. The expected frequency of the event in each group is the sum of the predicted probabilities of the event for individuals in that group. This is compared with the observed frequency of those

Table 10.8 Output from the Hosmer–Lemeshow test from the logistic regression model using the corn plaster RCT data with binary outcome corn healed and predictor variables group, baseline corn size and centre.

	Hosmer and Lemeshow test		
Step	**Chi-square**	**df**	**Significance**
1	4.399	8	0.819

		Contingency table for Hosmer and Lemeshow test				
		Index corn resolved at three-month post-randomisation (primary outcome) = no		**Index corn resolved at three-month post-randomisation (primary outcome) = yes**		
		Observed	**Expected**	**Observed**	**Expected**	**Total**
Step 1	1	16	16.156	2	1.844	18
	2	15	14.862	3	3.138	18
	3	17	15.104	2	3.896	19
	4	16	17.595	7	5.405	23
	5	10	11.085	5	3.915	15
	6	13	12.258	4	4.742	17
	7	12	13.157	7	5.843	19
	8	14	11.840	4	6.160	18
	9	13	12.383	7	7.617	20
	10	10	11.560	11	9.440	21

with the event in the corresponding group by calculating a test statistic which follows a chi-squared distribution with $(g - 2)$ df. A significant chi-squared value indicates that the model is a poor description of the data. The results from a computer are shown in Table 10.8.

The chi-squared value of 4.399 on 8 df gives $P = 0.819$, which is non-significant and indicates that we have no reliable evidence to suggest that the model is a poor fit or description of the data. However, the power of this test is poor and a non-significant test does not necessarily mean the model is a good one!

10.10 Assessing Predictive Efficiency (1): 2 × 2 Classification Table

Table 10.9 illustrates the ability of the model to correctly discriminate between those who do and do not have the outcome of interest (e.g. corn healed or not). The columns often represent the predicted outcomes from the model. Where an individual is predicted to have or not have the outcome according to whether their predicted probability is greater or less than the (usual) cut-off of 0.5. The rows represent the observed outcomes. If the logistic model is able to classify patients perfectly, the only cells of the table that contain non-zero entries are those lying on the diagonal and the overall percent correct is 100%. Table 10.9 shows that for the logistic regression model using the corn plaster RCT data with binary outcome corn healed and predictor variables group, baseline corn size and centre only 73% (137/188) of the patients correctly had their outcome predicted from the model (using a cut-off of 0.5).

Table 10.9 Classification table from logistic regression model using the corn plaster RCT data with binary outcome corn healed and predictor variables group, baseline corn size and centre.

			Predicted		
			Corn healed		Percentage correct
			No	Yes	
Observed	Corn healed	No	135	1	99.3
		Yes	50	2	3.8
	Overall percentage				72.9

The cut value is 0.500.

10.11 Assessing Predictive Efficiency (2): The ROC Curve

A *receiver operating characteristic (ROC)* curve plots the sensitivity of the model against one minus the specificity for different cut-offs of the predicted probability, $\hat{\pi}_i$. Lowering the cut-off increases the sensitivity. Raising the cut-off increases the specificity. The closer of the curve is to the upper left corner of the diagram, the better the predictive ability of the model. The greater the area under the curve (AUC), upper limit $= 1$, the better the model is discriminating between outcomes. An AUC < 0.5 indicates the model has no predictive efficiency better than chance alone.

Figure 10.1 show the ROC curve from the logistic regression model with multiple covariates (group, centre and baseline corn size) using the corn plaster RCT data. The area under the ROC curve is 0.64, indicating the model with multiple covariates (group, centre and baseline corn size) has some ability to discriminate between outcomes.

10.12 Investigating Linearity

When a predictor variable, x, is continuous, the model assumes the log odds are linearly associated with the covariate. We can check the linearity assumption by categorising individuals into a small number (5–10) of equally sized subgroups according to their values of x. We calculate the log odds for each subgroup and plot this against the mid-point of x from the subgroup. If the assumption of linearity is reasonable, we should expect to see a similarly sized stepwise change in the log odds when moving between adjacent categories of x. If non-linearity is detected, then there a number of approaches to take to deal with it. One approach is to replace x by a set of dummy variables created by categorising the individuals into three or four sub groups according to the magnitude of x (often defined using the *tertiles* or *quartiles* of the distribution). This set of dummy variables can be incorporated into the regression model as categorical explanatory variables. Alternatively, one might try transforming the x variable in some way, e.g. by taking a logarithmic or square root transformation of x, or find some algebraic description that approximates the non-linear relationship using higher orders of x, e.g. quadratic or cubic relationship using polynomial regression. For more explanation of logistic regression see Chapter 3 of Campbell (2006).

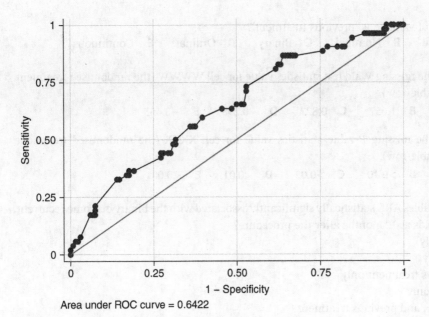

Area under ROC curve = 0.6422

Figure 10.1 ROC curve from the logistic regression model with multiple covariates (group, centre, and baseline corn size) using the corn plaster RCT data.

10.13 Exercises

Table 10.10 shows the computer output from the HubBLE RCT, which aimed to compare of hae-morrhoidal artery ligation (HAL) surgery (intervention) compared with rubber band ligation (RBL) surgery (control) in patients with grade II–III haemorrhoids (Brown et al. 2016). In this trial, 337 patients were randomly allocated to the HAL Intervention surgery (161) or the RBL control surgery (176) group. The primary outcome was the proportion of patients with recurrent haemorrhoids at 12 months after the procedure, derived from the patient's self-reported assessment in combination with resource use from their GP and hospital records.

You may assume a significance level of 0.05 or 5% has been specified for any hypothesis test. Referring to Table 10.10:

Table 10.10 Output obtained from a multiple logistic regression model with outcome variable recurrent haemorrhoids at 12 months after the procedure and predictor variables: age, sex, previous treatment, and group (N = 336).

Variable	b	SE(b)	Wald z	P-value	Odds Ratio	95% CI for OR Lower	Upper
Group (0 = RBL, 1 = HAL)	−0.798	0.231	WWWW	XXXX	YYYY	ZZ	ZZZZ
Age (years)	−0.003	0.009	−0.298	0.766	1.00	0.98	1.02
Sex (0 = female, 1 = male)	0.189	0.23	0.822	0.411	1.21	0.77	1.90
Previous treatment? (0 = no, 1 = yes)	0.425	0.257	1.657	0.098	1.53	0.93	2.53
Constant	−0.128	0.47	−0.271	0.786	0.88		

10.1 What type of variable is 'previous treatment'?

    A Discrete   **B** Nominal   **C** Binary   **D** Ordinal   **E** Continuous

10.2 Calculate the missing Wald test statistics value for cell WWWW (the randomised treatment group variable/row).

    A 3.298   **B** 1.657   **C** 0.822   **D** −0.298   **E** −3.455

10.3 Calculate the missing *P*-value statistics value for cell XXXX (the randomised treatment group variable/row).

    A >0.50   **B** >0.10   **C** >0.05   **D** <0.01   **E** <0.001

10.4 Which variables ARE statistically significantly associated with the binary outcome recurrent haemorrhoids at 12 months after the procedure?

    A Age only

    B Sex only

    C Previous treatment only

    D Group only

    E Age, sex and previous treatment

10.5 Calculate the missing *odds ratio* value for cell YYYY (the randomised treatment group variable/row). The odds ratio for the randomised treatment group variable is:

    A 0.45   **B** 0.88   **C** 1.00   **D** 1.21   **E** 2.22

10.6 Calculate the missing upper and lower limits for the 95% CI estimate for the Odds Ratio (the randomised treatment group variable/row) for cells ZZ and ZZZZ. The 95% CI for the odds ratio for the randomised treatment group variable is:

    A 0.98–1.02   **B** 0.77–1.90   **C** 0.29–0.71   **D** 0.39–0.72   **E** 0.29–1.71

10.7 Table 10.10 reports that the 95% CI for the odds ratio of a recurrent haemorrhoid at 12 months between males and females, after adjustment for age, previous treatment and group is:

0.77 to 1.90.

Which ONE of the following statements is CORRECT?

    A The above 95% CI contains the true population odds ratio for a recurrent haemorrhoid at 12 months between males and females, after adjustment for age, previous treatment and group.

    B The 95% CI, for the odds ratio, is calculated as ±3 SEs away from the odds ratio for a recurrent haemorrhoid at 12 months between males and females.

    C There is a probability of 0.95 that the population odds ratio for a recurrent haemorrhoid at 12 months between males and females, after adjustment for age, previous treatment and group lies between 0.77 and 1.90.

    D The 95% CI for the odds ratio for a recurrent haemorrhoid at 12 months between males and females, after adjustment for age, previous treatment and group is statistically significant and potentially clinically important.

    E The above 95% CI is likely to contain the true population odds ratio for a recurrent haemorrhoid at 12 months between males and females, after adjustment for age, previous treatment.

10.8 Calculate the predicted probability of recurrence of a haemorrhoid at 12 months for a female patient, aged 50, with no previous treatment in the RBL group.

A 0.25   **B** 0.29   **C** 0.34   **D** 0.39   **E** 0.43

10.9 Calculate the predicted probability of recurrence of a haemorrhoid at 12 months for a female patient, aged 50, with no previous treatment in the HAL group.

A 0.25   **B** 0.29   **C** 0.34   **D** 0.39   **E** 0.43

10.10 The sample size calculation for the trial was based on detecting a 15% absolute difference in the proportion of patients who experience a recurrence of a haemorrhoid at 12 months between the RBL and HAL treated groups (i.e. 30% rate in the control treated RBL patients versus a 15% rate in HAL treated patients). Express this difference as an odds ratio effect for recurrence of a haemorrhoid at 12 months between the HAL and RBL groups.

A 0.26   **B** 0.41   **C** 0.85   **D** 2.43   **E** 3.86

10.11 Assume the odds ratio calculated from question 10.10 would be regarded as the smallest effect that was clinically or practically important. Then, using the 95% CI, calculated in 10.6, the odds ratio estimate for participants in the HAL group having a recurrence of a haemorrhoid at 12 months compared to participants in the RBL group, we can say the result of the trial is:

A Statistically significant and potentially clinically important.
B Statistically significant and not clinically important.
C Statistically significant and clinically important.
D Not statistically significant but potentially clinically important.
E Not statistically significant and not clinically important.

11 Survival Analysis

Medical Statistics: A Textbook for the Health Sciences, Fifth Edition. Stephen J. Walters, Michael J. Campbell, and David Machin.
© 2021 John Wiley & Sons Ltd. Published 2021 by John Wiley & Sons Ltd.
Companion website: www.wiley.com/go/walters/medicalstatistics

Summary

The main outcome variable in some clinical studies is the time measured from patient or subject entry into a study until a pre-specified 'critical event' has occurred. These times often have a rather skewed distribution. However, a key feature of 'survival-time' data is the presence of 'censored' observations. Censored observations arise in subjects that are included in the study but for whom the critical event of interest has not yet been observed. We describe the Kaplan–Meier survival curve, the logrank test for comparing two groups, the use of the hazard ratio for data summary and the Cox proportional hazards regression model, which replaces linear regression when the continuous outcome data are survival times with censored observations.

11.1   Time to Event Data

The main outcome variable in some clinical trials is the time from randomisation, and start of treatment, to a specified critical event. The length of time from entry to the study to when the critical event occurs is called the survival time. Examples include patient survival time (time from diagnosis to death), the time a kidney graft remains patent, length of time that an indwelling cannula remains in situ, or the time a serious burn takes to heal. Even when the final outcome is not *actual* survival time, the techniques employed with such data are conventionally termed 'survival' analysis methods.

Example from the Literature – Trial Endpoints – Children with Neuroblastoma

Pearson et al. (2008) describe a randomised clinical trial in children with neuroblastoma in which two chemotherapy regimens are compared. In brief, the object of therapy following diagnosis is first to reduce the tumour burden (to obtain a response); to maintain that response for as long as possible; then following any relapse to prolong survival. Key 'survival type' endpoints are therefore time from start of treatment to: response, progression and death; and duration of response, as shown in Figure 11.1.

However, a key feature of survival time studies is the distinction that needs to be made between calendar time and patient time-on-study, which is illustrated in Figure 11.2. This shows a study including five patients who enter the study at different calendar times. This is typically the situation in any clinical trial in which the potential patients are those presenting at a particular clinic over a period of time and not all on the same date. The progress of patients recruited to the trial are then monitored for a period as

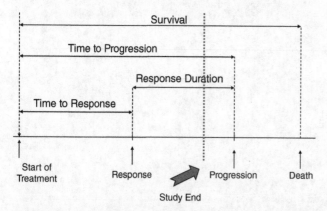

Figure 11.1   Endpoints or critical events relevant to a clinical trial in children with neuroblastoma. (*Source:* Pearson et al. 2008).

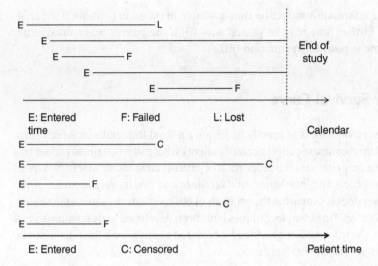

Figure 11.2 'Calendar time' when entering and leaving a study compared to 'patient time' on the study.

is described in the appropriate trial protocol. Also, at some future date (calendar time) the trial will close and an analysis conducted. For a patient recruited late in the trial, this may mean that some of their endpoint observations will not be made. Thus, for such a patient, in the example of Figure 11.1, at the date of analysis only time to response may be observed, in which case time to progression and survival time will both be censored with the same *survival time* value, and response duration will also be censored. The calendar time on which these censorings occur will be the same date.

For the analysis the patients will be viewed as in the lower panel of Figure 11.2, which shows time measured from the start of entry to the study, that is by patient (follow-up) time rather than calendar time.

Although survival time is a continuous variable one often cannot use the standard *t*-test of Chapter 7 for analysis as the distribution of survival times is unlikely to be Normal and it may not be possible to find a transformation that will make it so. However, the major reason for the use of 'survival' methods is not the shape of the distribution but the presence of 'censored' observations. Censored observations arise in patients that are included in a study but for whom the critical event of interest has not yet been observed. For example, although some of the patients recruited to a particular trial may have died and their survival time is calculable, others may still be alive. The time from randomisation to the last date the live patient was examined is known as the censored survival time. Thus, in Figure 11.2, although two patients 'fail', three are 'censored'. Here failure implies that the study endpoint has been reached (perhaps they have died), whilst of those censored, two were censored as the trial analysis was conducted whilst they were still known to be alive (they had therefore not yet died), and one patient had been 'lost'. Essentially 'lost' means known to have lived for the period indicated, and then ceased to be followed by the study team for some reason. Perhaps the patient failed to return for scheduled follow-up visits.

Censored Observations Can Arise in Three Ways

i) The patient is known to be still alive when the trial analysis is carried out.

ii) Was known to be alive at some past follow-up, but the investigator has since lost trace of him or her.

iii) Has died of some cause totally unrelated to the disease in question.

Clearly more survival time information would become available in situation (i) above if the analysis were delayed; possibly further time may be gained with (ii) if the patient was subsequently traced; whilst no further time is possible in situation (iii).

11.2 Kaplan–Meier Survival Curve

One method of analysis of survival data is to specify in advance a fixed time-point at which comparisons are to be made and then compare proportions of patients whose survival times exceed this time period. For example, one may compare the proportion of patients alive at one year in two treatment groups. However, this ignores the individual survival times and can be very wasteful of the available information. Neither does it overcome the problem of observations censored at times less than one year from randomisation. However, techniques have been developed to deal with survival data that can take account of the information provided by censored observations. Such data can be displayed using a Kaplan–Meier (K-M) survival curve.

Example from the Literature – Kaplan–Meier Curves – Aim High Study

Hancock et al. (2004) conducted a randomised controlled trial in 674 patients with malignant melanoma. In this trial, the effect of interferon (Interferon) alfa-2a (3 megaunits 3 times per week for 2 years or until recurrence) on overall survival (OS) and recurrence-free survival (RFS) was compared with that of no further treatment (Control) in radically resected stage IIB and stage III cutaneous malignant melanoma. The corresponding K-M survival curves of time from randomisation to death are shown in Figure 11.3.

If there are no censored observations, then the K-M survival curve for n patients starts at time 0 with a value of 1 (or 100% survival) then continues horizontally until the time the first death occurs, it then drops by $1/n$ at this point. The curve then proceeds horizontally once more until the time of

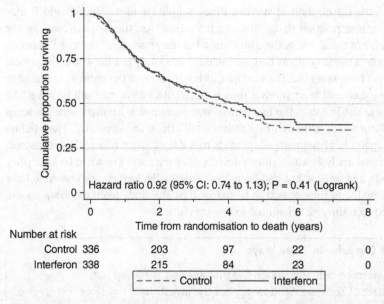

Figure 11.3 Kaplan–Meier survival curves for time from randomisation to death in 674 patients with malignant melanoma randomised to interferon or control. (*Source:* based on Hancock et al. 2004).

the second death when again it drops by $1/n$. This process continues until the time of the last death, when the survival curve drops by the final $1/n$ to take a value of 0 (0%). If two deaths happen to occur at the same time then the step down would be $2/n$.

The K-M estimate of the survival curve when there are censored observations mimics this process. When an observation is censored at a particular time the probability of survival does not change but the number at risk drops by one, so that when another death occurs, if the previous observation was the first censored observation the probability drops by $1/(n-1)$. If there are censored observations which are greater than the longest survival time, the K-M curve does not drop to zero, but should not be plotted beyond the longest observation. The precise method of calculating the K-M survival curve is summarised in the panel below.

Procedure for Calculating a Kaplan–Meier Survival Curve

1) First order (rank) the survival times from smallest to largest. If a censored observation and a time to death are equal, then the censored observation follows the death in the ranking.
2) An event is a death. A censored observation has no associated event.
3) Determine the number at risk, n_i, as the number of patients alive immediately before the event at time t_i.
4) Calculate the probability of survival from t_{i-1} to t_i as $1-d_i/n_i$, where d_i is the number of deaths at t_i. Note the calculation starts at time zero with $t_0 = 0$.
5) The cumulative survival probability, $S(t_i)$, is the probability of surviving from 0 up to t_i. It is calculated as

$$S(t_i) = (1 - d_i/n_i) \times (1 - d_{i-1}/n_{i-1}) \times \ldots \times (1 - d_1/n_1).$$

6) A censored observation at time t_i reduces the number at risk by one but does not change the cumulative survival probability at time t_i since $d_i = 0$.
7) A plot of the cumulative survival probability $S(t_i)$ against t_i, gives the K-M survival curve.

When comparing two or more survival curves, we usually assume that the mechanisms that result in censored observations occurring do not depend on the group concerned, that is, the censoring is 'non-informative' in that it tells us nothing relevant to the comparison of the groups. For example, in a randomised clinical trial, it is assumed that patients are just as likely to be lost to follow-up in one treatment group as in another. If there are imbalances in such losses then this can lead to spurious differences in survival between groups leading to false conclusions being drawn by the analysis. For example, if a trial of rehabilitation for heart disease involved a vigorous run up a steep hill in one arm, there may be more censored observations in this arm, but these are people who died on the way up the hill, and have not been traced since! This would be informative censoring.

Worked Example – K-M Survival Curve

The calculations for the K-M survival curve are easiest to explain by example as in Table 11.1. Here we consider a sample of 20 patients selected at random from the 674 melanoma patients who took part in the AIM High study (Hancock et al. 2004). Some patients are lost to follow-up whilst others have only been observed for short periods of time and so, in both cases, their observations are censored at the time of analysis.

For illustration of the K-M curve, we combine the data from both treatment groups and their ordered (or ranked) survival times, in years from randomisation, are given in Table 11.1, column A. These range from the shortest survival time of 0.909 years to 4.249 years. Patients with censored survival times are denoted with a '*'.

Table 11.1 Illustration of calculations for the Kaplan–Meier survival curve for a random sample of 20 malignant melanoma patients from the AIM High study.

A	B	C	D	E	F
Ordered survival times (years) t_i	Number at risk at start of time interval n_i	Number of deaths d_i	Number censored c_i	Proportion surviving until end of interval $1 - d_i/n_i$	Cumulative proportion surviving $S(t_i)$
0	20			1	1
0.909					
0.909	20	2	0	$1 - 2/20 = 0.900$	0.900
1.112					
1.112	18	2	0	$1 - 2/18 = 0.889$	0.800
1.117	16	1	0	$1 - 1/16 = 0.938$	0.750
1.322	15	1	1	$1 - 1/15 = 0.933$	0.700
1.322*					
1.328	13	1	0	$1 - 1/13 = 0.923$	0.646
1.536					
1.536					
1.536	12	3	0	$1 - 3/12 = 0.750$	0.485
2.713	9	1	0	$1 - 1/9 = 0.889$	0.431
2.741*	8	0	1		
2.743	7	1	0	$1 - 1/7 = 0.857$	0.369
3.524*		0			
3.524*	6	0	2		0.369
4.079*	4	0	1		0.369
4.178*	3	0	1		0.369
4.230*	2	0	1		0.369
4.249	1	1	0	$1 - 1/1 = 0.000$	0.000

* Indicates a censored survival time.

The number of patients who are alive just before 0.909 years is 20 (column B). Since two patients die at 0.909 years (column C), the probability of dying by 0.909 years is 2/20 = 0.10. So, the corresponding probability of surviving up to 0.909 years is 1 minus the probability of dying (column E) or $1 - 2/20 = 0.900$. The cumulative probability of surviving up to 0.909 years is the product of the probability of surviving between 0 and 0.909 years, and surviving throughout the preceding time interval which is, 1 x 0.900 = 0.900 (column F).

The next death(s) occurs at 1.112 when again two patients die (column C), so the probability of dying by 1.112 years is 2/18 = 0.11. So, the corresponding probability of surviving up to 1.112 years is 1 minus the probability of dying (column E) or $1 - 2/18 = 0.889$. The cumulative probability of surviving up to 1.112 years, then, is the probability of surviving at 1.112 years, and surviving throughout the preceding time interval – that is, $0.900 \times 0.889 = 0.800$ (column F). The next death occurs at 1.117 years when 16 subjects are at risk at the start of the interval, so the probability of surviving up to 1.117 years is $1 - 1/16 = 0.938$ and the cumulative proportion surviving is $0.800 \times 0.938 = 0.750$.

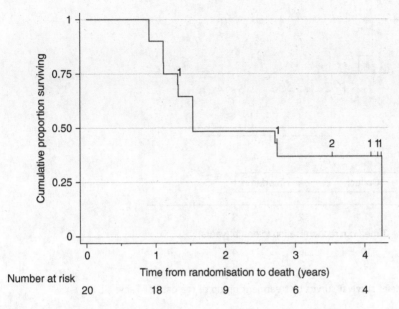

Figure 11.4 Kaplan–Meier survival curve for the 20 patients of Table 11.1.

The fourth time interval (1.322 years) contains a death and a censored observation so the censored observation is denoted 1.322* and is assumed to follow the death in the ranking. The time interval (2.741 years) contains a censored observation so the probability of surviving in this time interval is one or unity, and the cumulative probability of surviving is unchanged from the previous interval. This is the K-M estimate of the survivor function.

The resulting K-M curve is shown in Figure 11.4, from which it can be seen that the step sizes are unequal. In this example the K-M curve does reach the horizontal time-axis as the last (20th) subject died at 4.249 years of follow-up. As occurs in Figure 11.3, if the subject with the longest survival time is censored then the K-M curve will not reach the time-axis as the longest survivors are still alive.

On the K-M survival curve of Figure 11.4, the small spikes correspond to the censored observations. Above each spike, the number of patients censored at that time is given. In this example, all are marked '1' except for the censored observation at 3.5 years where there is a '2' corresponding to two censored observations. When there are a large number of patients and perhaps a large number of censored observations, the 'spikes' may clutter the K-M curve. In which case the numbers at risk, which are a selection of the n_i of Table 11.1, are tabulated at convenient intervals beneath the K-M curves, as illustrated in Figures 11.3 and 11.4.

11.3 The Logrank Test

An important part of survival analysis is to produce a plot of the survival curves for each group of interest. Figure 11.5 shows the K-M survival curves by treatment group for the data of (Tables 11.1 and 11.2).

However, the comparison of the survival curves of two groups should be based on a formal nonparametric statistical test called the *logrank* or log-rank test, and not upon visual impressions. The logrank test is used to test the null hypothesis that there is no difference between the populations in the probability of an event (here a death) at any time point.

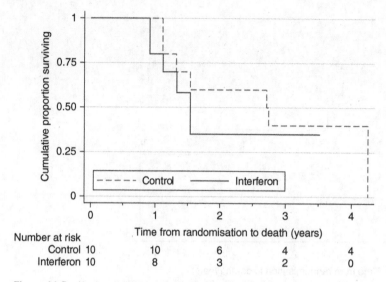

Figure 11.5 Kaplan–Meier survival curves by treatment group of the data of Table 11.1

The appropriate calculations are summarised in the box below. The curious name, logrank, for the test arises because it is related to another statistical test that uses the logarithms of the ranks of the data. Figure 11.3 shows the survival of patients treated for malignant melanoma: the survival of 338 patients on interferon was compared with that of 336 patients in the control. The two groups of patients appear to have similar survival and the logrank test supports this conclusion.

Procedure for Calculating the Logrank Test Comparing Two Groups *A* and *B*

The null hypothesis, H_0, is that the two groups have identical survival curves (or equivalently hazard rates) in the population. The alternative hypothesis (H_A) is that the population survival curves are different.

Using the notation summarised in Table 11.1.

1) The total number of events observed in Groups *A* and *B* are O_A and O_B.
2) Under the null hypothesis, the expected number of events in the group receiving treatment *A* at time t_i is $e_{Ai} = (d_i \, n_{Ai})/n_A$.
3) The expected number of events should not be calculated beyond the last event (at time 4.249 years in this example).
4) The total number of events expected on *A*, assuming the null hypothesis of no difference between treatments is true, is $E_A = \Sigma e_{Ai}$.
    The number expected on *B* is $E_B = \Sigma d_i - E_A$.
5) Calculate

$$\chi^2_{\text{Logrank}} = \frac{(O_A - E_A)^2}{E_A} + \frac{(O_B - E_B)^2}{E_B}.$$

6) This has a χ^2 distribution with $df = 1$ as two groups are being compared.
    If more than two groups are being compared then the test statistic follows a chi-squared distribution on $g - 1 \, df$, where g is the number of groups being compared.

Table 11.2 Illustration of calculations for the logrank test for a random sample of 20 malignant melanoma patients from the Aim High study.

i	Ordered survival time (years) t_i	Status	Total number at risk n_i	Number of deaths at time t_i d_i	Number censored c_i	Kaplan–Meier: Probability of survival in t_{i-1}, t_i $1 - d_i/n_i$	Kaplan–Meier: Cumulative Survival probability $S(t_i)$	Treatment	Logrank test: Number at risk in Interferon Group A (n_{Ai})	Expected number of events in A (E_{Ai})
0	0		20			1	1.000			
1	0.909	Died	20	2	0	0.900	0.900	Interferon	10	1.00
2	0.909	Died						Interferon		
3	1.112	Died	18	2	0	0.889	0.800	Control	8	0.89
4	1.112	Died						Control		
5	1.117	Died	16	1	0	0.938	0.750	Interferon	8	0.50
6	1.322	Died	15	1	1	0.933	0.700	Control	7	0.47
7	1.322	Censored						Interferon	7	
8	1.328	Died	13	1	0	0.923	0.646	Interferon	6	0.46
9	1.536	Died	12	3	0	0.750	0.485	Interferon	5	1.25
10	1.536	Died						Interferon	5	
11	1.536	Died						Control	5	
12	2.713	Died	9	1	0	0.889	0.431	Control	3	0.33
13	2.741	Censored	8	0	1	1.000	0.431	Interferon	3	
14	2.743	Died	7	1	0	0.857	0.369	Control	2	0.29
15	3.524	Censored	6	0	1	1.000	0.369	Interferon	2	
16	3.524	Censored		0	1	1.000	0.369	Interferon	1	
17	4.079	Censored	4	0	1	1.000	0.369	Control	0	
18	4.178	Censored	3	0	1	1.000	0.369	Control	0	
19	4.23	Censored	2	0	1	1.000	0.369	Control	0	
20	4.249	Died	1	1	0	0.000	0.000	Control	0	0.00
				13	7					5.19

Worked Example – Logrank Test

Table 11.2 illustrates the calculations of the logrank test, for the 20 randomly sampled patients from the Aim High trial, in which Interferon (A) and Control (B) groups are compared. This gives $O_A = 6$, $O_B = 7$, $E_A = 5.19$ and $E_B = 7.81$. From which

$$\chi^2_{logrank} = \frac{(6-5.19)^2}{5.19} + \frac{(7-7.81)^2}{7.81} = 0.24.$$

Using the table of the chi-squared distribution (Table T3 in the appendix) with $df = 1$ gives $P = 0.60$ (more precise calculations give 0.62), which suggests that we do not reject the null hypothesis of equal survival curves.

It should be noted that there are a number of alternative statistical tests to the logrank test to compare the equality of survival curves across groups, such as the Wilcoxon (Breslow–Gehan) test, Tarone–Ware test, Peto–Peto–Prentice test and the Fleming–Harrington test. The main distinction between all of these tests is that they all give a different weight to the outcome, and hence its contribution to the calculation of the test statistic, at each distinct failure time (death) compared to a weight of 1 for the logrank test, which treats all failures equally.

For some outcomes, where the result is a positive or favourable event, such as a wound or burn healing then it is definitely preferable to have the Kaplan–Meier plots rising rather than falling by plotting the proportion healed rather than the proportion not healed. Figure 11.6 gives such a plot using data from a randomised controlled trial to compare two interventions for healing leg ulcers (Morrell et al. 1998). All 233 patients began the study with a leg ulcer that was treated either in a specialist clinic or by a district nurse at home. One of the principal outcomes was the time to complete leg ulcer healing. In this example the vertical axis records the cumulative proportion of patients whose initial leg ulcers healed during the 12-month follow-up period.

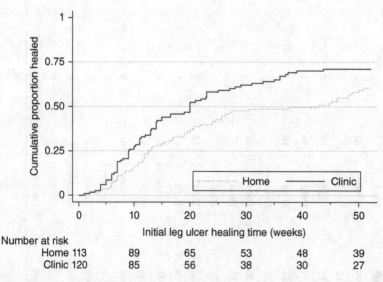

Figure 11.6 Healing times of initial leg ulcers by clinic and home care interventions. (*Source: based* on Morrell et al. 1998).

11.4 The Hazard Ratio

The median survival time may be a suitable summary for survival data as survival times often have rather skew distributions. However, there is a problem if censored data are present. For example, if we were to ignore the censoring in the 20 survival times of Table 11.1, we could calculate the median time, for the 20 patients as the average of the 10th and 11th ordered survival times which is $M = (1.536 + 1.536)/2 = 1.536$ years. However, there are censored values below this 'median' at 1.322^* years, and such observations have the potential to increase and may eventually exceed the current median estimate of 1.536 years. Because of censored observations, we estimate the median in a different way. We first calculate the K-M survival curve, then from the mid-point of the survival axis (survival of 50%) move horizontally until the curve is met, then drop vertically to the time axis to read the median survival time.

Worked Example – Median 'Survival' Time – AIM High

Following the above process for the Interferon group of Figure 11.5 gives a median time to death of approximately 1.5 years and median time to death of approximately 2.75 years in the Control group.

The hazard ratio (HR) has been specifically developed for survival data, and is used as a measure of the relative survival experience of two groups.

Procedure for Calculating the HR when Comparing Two Groups

1) Accumulate the observed number of events in each group, O_A and O_B.
2) Under the hypothesis of no survival difference between the groups, calculate the expected number of events in each group, E_A and E_B, using the logrank test.
3) The ratio O_A/E_A is the relative event rate in group A. Similarly, O_B/E_B is the relative event rate in group B.
4) The HR is the ratio of these relative event rates, that is

$$HR = \frac{O_A/E_A}{O_B/E_B}.$$

When there is no difference between two groups, that is the null hypothesis is true, the value of HR = 1. It is important to note that for the HR the 'expected' deaths in each group are calculated using the logrank method as described previously which allows for censoring. It has parallels with the relative risk, RR, of Chapter 3 and has a similar interpretation. As a consequence, the term RR is often used rather than HR in a survival context also. In general, this is not good practice and we recommend the use of the term HR in survival analysis.

Worked Example – Hazard Ratio – 20 Randomly Sampled Patients from the AIM High Trial

From the calculations summarised in Table 11.2, $O_{A \text{ (Interferon)}} = 6$, $O_{B \text{ (Control)}} = 7$, $E_A = 5.19$ and $E_B = 7.81$. From which $HR = \dfrac{O_A/E_A}{O_B/E_B} = \dfrac{6/5.19}{7/7.81} = 1.29$. Thus, the risk of death with Interferon is

1.3 times that with Control. The corresponding survival curves for the 20 patients are shown in Figure 11.5.

The HR gives an estimate of the overall difference between the survival curves. However, summarising the difference between two survival curves into one statistic can also have its problems. One particularly important consideration for its use is that the ratio of the relative event rates in the two groups should not vary greatly over time.

It also turns out that if M_A and M_B are the respective median survival times of two groups, then the inverse of their ratio, that is $1/(M_A/M_B)$ or M_B/M_A, is approximately the HR.

Confidence Interval for HR

Whenever an estimate of a difference between groups is given, it is useful to calculate a confidence interval (CI) for the estimate. Thus, for the HR obtained from any study, we would like to know a range of values that are not inconsistent with this estimate. In calculating CIs, it is convenient if the statistic under consideration can be assumed to follow an approximately Normal distribution. However, the estimate of the HR is not Normally distributed. In particular it has a possible range of values from 0 to ∞, with the null hypothesis value of unity not located at the centre of this interval. To make the scale symmetric and to enable us to calculate CIs, we transform the estimate to make it approximately Normally distributed. We do this by using the log HR, rather than HR itself, as the basis for our calculation.

95% Confidence Interval (CI) for an HR

1) Calculate the logarithm of the HR estimate: log HR

2) Calculate: $SE(\log HR) = \sqrt{\left(\dfrac{1}{E_A} + \dfrac{1}{E_B}\right)}$, although this should strictly only be used if the number of events $E_A + E_B = O_A + O_B$ is relatively large.

3) Calculate the 95% CI for log HR as

   $\log HR - 1.96 \times SE(\log HR)$ to $\log HR + 1.96 \times SE(\log HR)$.

4) The 95% CI for HR is

   $\exp[\log HR - 1.96 \times SE(\log HR)]$ to $\exp[\log HR + 1.96 \times SE(\log HR)]$.

Worked Example – Confidence Interval for the HR – AIM High Trial

Applying the calculation method to the data of Table 11.2 gives $O_A = 6$, $O_B = 7$, $E_A = 5.19$ and $E_B = 7.81$. From which HR = 1.29 and log(1.29) = 0.111 and

$$SE(\log HR) = \sqrt{\left(\frac{1}{5.19} + \frac{1}{7.81}\right)} = 0.566.$$

A 95% CI for log(HR) sets $z_{0.975} = 1.96$ and gives a range from $0.111 - (1.96 \times 0.566)$ to $0.111 + (1.96 \times 0.566)$ or -0.998 to 1.220. Finally, for the CI for the HR itself, we have to exponentiate these lower and upper limits to obtain $\exp(-0.998) = 0.37$ to $\exp(1.220) = 3.39$, that is 0.4 to 3.4. The wide 95% CI emphasises that reliable conclusions could not be drawn from such data.

11.5 Modelling Time to Event Data

The logrank test cannot be used to explore (and adjust for) the effects of several variables simultaneously, such as age and disease duration, that are known to affect survival. Adjustment for such variables may improve the precision with which we can estimate the treatment effect. The proportional hazards regression method introduced by Cox is used to investigate several variables at a time. Briefly, the procedure models the survival times (or more specifically, the so-called hazard function) on the explanatory variables.

If we think of our own lives for a moment, we are continually exposed to the possibility of our demise. However, having lived until now, we can think of the chance of our demise (say) in the next day, hour or second as our hazard for the next interval be it, a second, hour or day. This can be thought of as our *instantaneous* death rate or failure rate conditional on living until now. Alternatively, it expresses as our hazard at time (our age), t (or now) which is denoted $h(t)$.

In general, suppose n people of a certain age group were alive at the start of a particular year, and d of these died in the following period of duration D, then the risk of death in that period is $d/(nD)$. If we now imagine the width of the time interval, D, getting narrower and narrower then the number of deaths d will get fewer and fewer but the ratio d/D may stay constant. This gives the instantaneous death rate or the *hazard rate*. Thus, at any particular time (say) t, we think of the hazard rate as applying to what is just about to happen in the next very short time period.

Now our own hazard may fluctuate with time and will certainly increase for all of us as t (our age) increases. Similarly, if we become diseased, perhaps with a life-threatening illness, our hazard rate would unquestionably increase in which case the aim of any therapy would be to restore it to the former (lower) value if possible. Individual hazards will differ, even in those of the precisely the same age, and it may be that particular groups may have (on average) higher values than others. Thus, the hazard of developing dental caries may be greater in those who live in areas where fluoridation has not occurred. This leads us to quantify the benefit of fluoridation through the ratio of hazards (the hazard ratio or HR) in those from fluoridation areas to those from non-fluoridation areas whose value may also be influenced by other factors such as dietary intake and tooth brushing frequency.

In Chapters 9 and 10 we described linear regression techniques for continuous data and logistic regression for binary date and both allowed the dependent variable to be related to one or more independent variables or covariates. Although survival time is also a continuous variable the possibility of censored observations has to be taken account of in the regression modelling process. This leads us to the Cox proportional hazards regression model which models, as the dependent variable, the instantaneous hazard, $h(t)$, as it is the change in this that ultimately determines our survival time.

The multivariable Cox model links the hazard to an individual i at time t, $h_i(t)$, to a baseline hazard $h_0(t)$ by

$$\log\{h_i(t)\} = \log\{h_0(t)\} + \beta_1 x_1 + \beta_2 x_2 + \dots + \beta_k x_k,$$

where $x_1, x_2, \dots, x_k$ are covariates associated with individual i. The baseline log hazard, $\log\{h_0(t)\}$, serves as a reference point, and can be thought of as being equivalent to the intercept, α, of a multiple regression equation of Chapter 9; for convenience often labelled β_0.

The Cox model is called the *proportional hazards* model because if we imagine two individuals i and j, then the equation assumes that the ratio of one hazard to the other, $h_i(t)/h_j(t)$, remains constant at whatever time, t, we consider their ratio. Thus, irrespective of how $h_0(t)$ varies over time, the hazards of the two individuals remain proportional to each other.

The above expression for the Cox model can also be written as

$$h_i(t) = h_0(t) \exp\left(\beta_1 x_1 + \beta_2 x_2 + \dots + \beta_k x_k\right).$$

More strictly $h_i(t)$ should be written $h_i(t; x_1, x_2, \dots, x_k)$ as it depends both on t and the covariates x.

Cox Proportional Hazards Regression Model for Two Groups and No Covariates

1) We wish to compare the survival time in two groups (control and intervention) denoted by $x = 0$ and $x = 1$.
2) The Cox model for the single covariate, x, denoting group is $h(t;x) = h_0(t)\exp(\beta x)$.
3) For the control group, $x = 0$, $h(t;0) = h_0(t)\exp(\beta \times 0) = h_0(t) \times 1 = h_0(t)$.
4) For the intervention group, $x = 1$, $h(t;1) = h_0(t)\exp(\beta \times 1) = h_0(t) \times \exp(\beta)$.
5) The ratio of these is the HR $= h(t;1)/h(t;0) = \exp(\beta)$ and this quantifies the effect of the intervention.
6) The regression coefficient of the model, β ($= \log$ HR) is estimated from the survival time data of both groups.

Technical Example

Assume x is a binary variable taking values 0 and 1 for males and females respectively and the estimate of the regression coefficient, β, calculated from the survival data of both groups using the Cox model gives $b = 1.5$ say. With $x = 0$, $h_{\text{Male}} = \exp(1.5 \times 0) = 1.0$ whilst with $x = 1$, $h_{\text{Female}} = \exp(1.5 \times 1) = \exp(1.5) = 4.5$. The associated $HR = h_{\text{Female}}/h_{\text{Male}} = \exp(1.5 \times 1)/\exp(1.5 \times 0) = 4.5/1.0 = 4.5$. In this case, the females have a greater risk of dying.

The Cox model, once fitted to the survival time data, provides a link to the logrank test and the associated HR. In fact, since $\log$ HR $= \beta$, the regression coefficient itself is often referred to as the log hazard ratio.

Worked Example – Cox Model

Fitting the Cox model to the data of Table 11.2, using a computer package gives HR = 1.32. This is quite close to the value of 1.29 resulting from the logrank test that we gave earlier. Such a small difference can be accounted for by the rounding during the respective calculations.

However, the 95% CI for the HR is given as 0.42 to 4.13 is wider than given by the previous calculations. This disparity is caused by using the expression for the SE($\log$ HR) given earlier, which technically is only valid for large samples. Neither method is entirely reliable in the circumstances of our example.

The Cox analysis gives a P-value = 0.63 which compares with the logrank P-value of 0.62 quoted previously.

When the Cox model includes several covariates the fitting procedure is straightforward using standard statistical packages, but care should be taken to avoid including too many variables in the multivariable model. It has to be recognised that it is the number of events observed, rather than the number of subjects in the study that that determines the power of the study. In very broad terms, for every variable included in a multivariable Cox model a minimum of 10 (better 20) events should have been observed. This is to ensure that the regression coefficients estimated have reasonable precision. Thus, no matter whether the number of subjects in the study are 100, or

$10,000$ if the number of events is only 20, one should take care fitting more than one predictor variable.

Example from the Literature – Cox Multivariable Regression – AIM High Trial

The AIM High trial (Hancock et al. 2004) compared the OS of patients treated with interferon (interferon group) with that of no further treatment (control group). Their results are summarised in the K-M plots of Figure 11.3, which seem to suggest broadly similar survival curves.

However, it is known that other factors such as patient age and sex and other features of the disease itself such as its histology (whether the disease was localised or locally metastatic (LM); regionally metastatic at diagnosis (RMD); or regionally metastatic at recurrence (RMR)) may affect prognosis and survival. The trial involved 674 patients and 350 participants were observed to die (the critical event).

If a multivariable Cox regression model is to be used, then with the six independent variables (age, sex, histology [three levels compared to reference level] and treatment group) we have $674/6 \approx 112$ patients per regression coefficient to be estimated and, more importantly, $350/6 \approx 58$ patients per event. This is probably sufficient to obtain reliable estimates of the corresponding coefficients since it is more than 20 events per coefficient. The resulting Cox model is summarised in Table 11.3.

From this analysis, it is clear that even taking account or adjusting for the possible influence of the potentially prognostic variables of age, sex and histology the difference between the groups is not statistically significant (P-value = 0.40) and the group effect is close to one with HR = exp $(-0.0897) = 0.91$ (95% CI 0.74 to 1.13), which suggests we have not got enough evidence to distinguish between the interferon and control groups with regards to survival time.

Although age was thought to be potentially prognostic this did not turn out to be the case as the corresponding 95% CI included the null value of HR = 1. In contrast, the binary predictor variable sex is clearly prognostic with an HR = 0.73 (CI: 0.59 to 0.91) suggesting that female patients have a

Table 11.3 Cox multivariate proportional hazards regression model for 674 patients with malignant melanoma in the Aim High trial of interferon versus no further treatment (control).

Variable	Regression coefficient (*b*)	Standard error SE(*b*)	*Z*	*P*-value	Hazard ratio exp(*b*)	95% CI for HR	
						Lower	Upper
Group (0 = control, 1 = interferon)	−0.0897	0.1076	−0.83	0.40	0.91	0.74	1.13
Age (years)	0.0038	0.0041	0.92	0.36	1.00	1.00	1.01
Sex (0 = male, 1 = female)	−0.3117	0.1103	−2.83	0.005	0.73	0.59	0.91
Histology							
LM (localised = 0, LM = 1)	−0.0331	0.2338	−0.14	0.89	0.97	0.61	1.53
RMD (localised = 0, RMD = 1)	0.4462	0.2039	2.19	0.029	1.56	1.05	2.33
RMR (localised = 0, RMR =1)	0.5688	0.1538	3.70	0.001	1.77	1.31	2.39

Source: based on Hancock et al. 2004.

lower hazard or risk of dying than male patients. The categorical predictor variable histology is also associated with the hazard or risk of dying particularly for the more advanced disease where the cancer has spread to other parts of the body.

The choice of units used in the model and calculations will depend on circumstances but for age, for example, it is very unlikely, even if age does indeed influence survival, that there will be much difference in survival times between individuals of say 69 and 70 years, whereas a marked difference may be seen comparing individuals who are 60 compared to 70 years old. This argues for decades as the unit for analysis rather than years since it is easier to understand. Nevertheless, whichever is chosen, the choice does not affect the *P*-value or the conclusions we draw but just how we express them.

Further details of the Cox model are given by Walters (2010), Campbell (2006), and Tai and Machin (2014).

11.6 Points When Reading Literature

Interpreting the Results of a Survival Analysis

- Is the nature of the censoring specified? As far as possible check that the censoring is non-informative.
- Check that the total number of critical events is reported, as well as subjects and person-time of follow-up, with some measure of variability such as a range for the latter. In trials, are numbers of censored observations given by treatment group?
- Is the estimated survival rate at a conventional time point, by group, with confidence intervals given?
- Are the K-M survival curves displayed by group?
- In the K-M survival curve are the numbers at risk reported at regular time intervals?
- Is the regression model used specified?
- Is the proportional hazards assumption reasonable and has it been validated?
- If a multivariable Cox model is used, are the corresponding HRs and CIs reported for all the variables included in the model?
- Beware when the survival time is time to response to treatment, for example a tumour getting smaller. The problems here include: the results may depend on an arbitrary cut-off (e.g. tumour shrinking by a certain amount and changing the cut-off may change the conclusion; the observation that a patient has responded can be very subjective; time to response is often found not to correlate well with overall survival, which is obviously the most important outcome for patients.
- Are the conclusions drawn critically dependent on the statistical assumptions made?
- Is the computer programme used for the analysis indicated?

Technical Details

The assumption of a constant relationship between the dependent variable and the explanatory variables is termed proportional hazards. This means that the hazard functions for any two individuals at any point in time are proportional. In other words, if an individual has a risk of death at some initial time point that is twice as high as that of another individual, then at all later times the risk of death remains twice as high. This assumption of proportional hazards should be tested.

The testing of the proportional hazards assumption is most straightforward when we compare two groups with no covariates. The simplest check is to plot the Kaplan–Meier survival curves together. If they cross, then the proportional hazards assumption may be violated. For small data sets, where there may be a great deal of error attached to the survival curve, it is possible for curves to cross, even under the proportional hazards assumption. A more sophisticated check is based on what is known as the complementary log–log plot. With this method, a plot of the logarithm of the negative logarithm of the estimated survivor function, that is, $\log(-\log S(t))$, against the logarithm of survival time, $\log(t)$, will yield parallel curves if the hazards are proportional across the groups. An example from the AIM High trial is shown in Figure 11.7. Although there is some visual evidence of a departure from proportional hazards in the early years, these are based on few observations, and later years appear to have very similar risks.

Cox regression is considered a 'semi-parametric' procedure because the baseline hazard function, $h_0(t)$, (and the probability distribution of the survival times) does not have to be specified. Because the hazard function is not restricted to a specific form, the semi-parametric model has considerable flexibility and is widely used. However, if the assumption of a particular probability distribution for the data is valid, inferences based on such an assumption are more precise. That is, estimates of the hazard ratio will have smaller standard errors and hence narrower confidence limits for a valid parametric model.

A fully *parametric proportional hazards model* makes the same assumptions as the Cox regression model but, in addition, also assumes that the baseline hazard function, $h_0(t)$, can be parameterised according to a specific model for the distribution of the survival times. Survival time distributions that can be used for this purpose are usually the *exponential*, *Weibull* and *Gompertz* distributions.

Figure 11.8 shows examples of the hazard functions for the exponential, Weibull and Gompertz distributions. The simplest model for the hazard function is to assume that it is constant over time

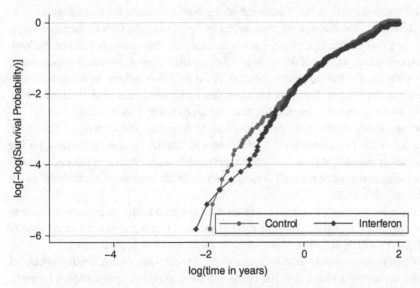

Figure 11.7 Testing the assumption of proportional hazards – a plot of $\log(-\log S(t))$, against $\log(t)$ will yield parallel curves if the hazards are proportional across the groups. (*Source:* based on Hancock et al. 2004).

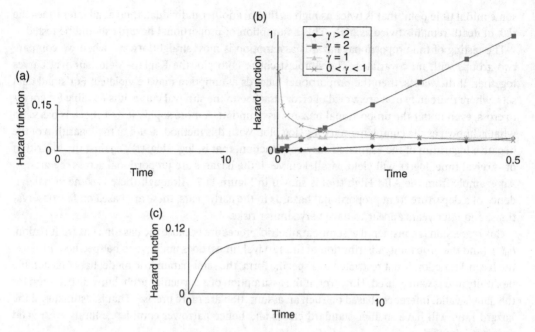

Figure 11.8 Examples of hazard functions over time for (a) exponential, (b) Weibull and (c) Gompertz distributions.

which leads to the exponential model. The hazard of death at any time after the start of the study is then the same, irrespective of the time elapsed, and the hazard function follows an exponential distribution (Figure 11.8a). In practice, the assumption of a constant hazard function (or equivalently exponentially distributed survival times) is rarely tenable. A more general form of hazard function is called the Weibull distribution. The shape of the Weibull hazard function depends critically on the value of the so-called shape parameter, typically denoted by the Greek letter gamma, γ. Figure 11.8b shows the general form of this hazard function for different values of γ. Since the Weibull hazard function can take a variety of forms depending on the value of the shape parameter γ, this distribution is widely used in the parametric analysis of survival data. When the hazard of death is expected to increase or decrease with time in the short term and then to become constant, a hazard function that follows a Gompertz distribution may be appropriate (Figure 11.8c).

Different distributions imply different shapes of the hazard function, and in practice the distribution that best describes the functional form of the observed hazard function is chosen. Fitting three parametric proportional hazard models, assuming exponential, Weibull and Gompertz baseline hazards, to the malignant melanoma trial data produced similar regression coefficients to the standard Cox model in Table 11.3.

One advantage of parametric models is that it enables statistics such as the mean survival time to be estimated. These are useful in health economic models and lead to quantities such as the quality adjusted life year (QALY) which is used to determine cost-effectiveness of treatments,

A family of fully parametric models that accommodate, directly, the multiplicative effects of explanatory variables on survival times, and hence do not have to rely on proportional hazards, are called *accelerated failure time models*. These models are too complex for a discussion here, and a more detailed discussion is given by Collett (2015).

11.7   Exercises

Figure 11.9 and Table 11.4 shows the computer output from the ProGas cohort study that aimed to compare three gastrostomy insertion approaches in terms of safety and clinical outcomes in patients with amyotrophic lateral sclerosis who develop severe dysphagia (ProGas Study Group 2015). A gastrostomy is a feeding tube that is inserted directly into the stomach either surgically under direct vision (open or laproscopic), endoscopically (with a camera), or radiologically (X-ray guidance). A gastrostomy tube allows the delivery of supplemental nutrition and medications directly into the stomach. Survival times from gastrostomy insertion (in days) for 319 patients with amyotrophic lateral sclerosis who underwent percutaneous endoscopic gastrostomy (PEG), radiologically inserted gastrostomy (RIG), or per-oral image-guided gastrostomy (PIG) were recorded.

You may assume a significance level of 0.05 or 5% has been specified for any hypothesis tests.

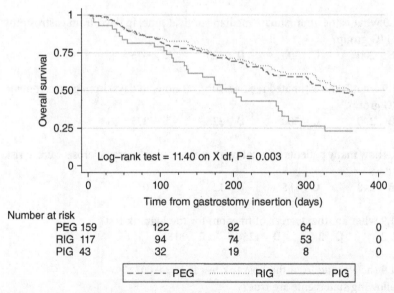

Figure 11.9   Kaplan–Meier survival functions for patients with amyotrophic lateral sclerosis who underwent one of three surgical procedures: PEG (percutaneous endoscopic gastrostomy), RIG (radiologically inserted gastrostomy) or PIG (per-oral image-guided gastrostomy). (*Source:* ProGas Study Group (2015) Gastrostomy in patients with amyotrophic lateral sclerosis (ProGas): a prospective cohort study. *The Lancet Neurology* 14 (7):702–709. Licensed Under CC BY 3.0).

Table 11.4 Output obtained from a multiple Cox proportional hazards regression model with the outcome variable time to death (in days) from gastrostomy insertion and predictor variables: age at onset, site of symptom onset, forced vital capacity, weight loss (% from diagnosis), ALSFRS-R monthly decline rate, and gastrostomy insertion method (*N* = 169).

Variable	*B*	SE(*B*)	*z*	*P*-value	Hazard Ratio	HR 95% CI Lower	Upper
Gastrostomy insertion method							
RIG (vs PEG)	−0.343	0.282	−1.219	0.223	0.71	0.41	1.23
PIG (vs PEG)	0.343	0.329	WWWW	XXXX	YYYY	ZZ	ZZZZ
Age at onset (years)	0.032	0.013	2.491	0.013	1.03	1.01	1.06
Site of symptom onset[1] (1 = limb, 2 = bulbar)	−0.199	0.279	−0.714	0.475	0.82	0.47	1.42
Forced vital capacity (litres)	−0.010	0.005	−1.805	0.071	0.99	0.98	1.00
Weight loss (% from diagnosis)[2]	−0.045	0.014	−3.205	0.001	0.96	0.93	0.98
ALSFRS-R monthly decline rate[3]	0.086	0.061	1.424	0.155	1.09	0.97	1.23

[1]Site of amyotrophic lateral sclerosis symptom onset (limb or bulbar).
[2]Percentage of weight difference at gastrostomy compared with diagnosis weight
[3]Monthly rate of decline of the revised amyotrophic lateral sclerosis functional rating scale (ALSFRS-R).

11.1 From Figure 11.9 what is the approximate median survival time, in days, from gastrostomy to death in the PIG group?
    A 100   **B** 200   **C** 300   **D** 325   **E** 375

11.2 From Figure 11.9 what is the estimated median survival time, in days, from gastrostomy to death in the RIG group?
    A 100   **B** 200   **C** 300   **D** 325   **E** 375

11.3 From Figure 11.9 how many patients (in total) with amyotrophic lateral sclerosis were at risk of dying at 300 days?
    A 319   **B** 248   **C** 185   **D** 125   **E** 0

11.4 From Figure 11.9 what are the degrees of freedom for the logrank test?
    A 1   **B** 2   **C** 3   **D** 125   **E** 318

11.5 From Figure 11.9 the *P*-value from the Logrank test is *P* = 0.003.
Which of the following statements are true?
    A This result is not statistically significant.
    B The probability of getting the value of the Logrank test or more extreme by chance if there had been no difference in the population survival curves between the three groups is 0.850.
    C The probability of getting this difference or more extreme is 0.003.
    D There is sufficient evidence to reject the null hypothesis.
    E The results are unlikely when the null hypothesis is true.

11.6 From Table 11.4, what type of variable is 'site of symptom onset'?

    A Discrete   **B** Nominal   **C** Binary   **D** Ordinal   **E** Continuous

11.7 Using the data in Table 11.4 calculate the missing test statistics value for cell WWWW (the PIG vs PEG variable/row).

    A 1.043   **B** 1.657   **C** 0.822   **D** −0.298   **E** −3.458

11.8 Using the data in Table 11.4 calculate the missing *P*-value for cell XXXX (the PIG vs PEG variable/row)?

    A >0.80   **B** >0.20   **C** <0.05   **D** <0.01   **E** <0.0001

11.9 From Table 11.4 which variables ARE statistically significantly associated with the hazard or risk of dying after the gastrostomy procedure?

    A Age only

    B Weight only

    C Site of symptom onset

    D Gastrostomy insertion method only

    E Age and weight loss

11.10 Using the data in Table 11.4 calculate the missing *hazard ratio* value for cell YYYY (the PIG vs PEG variable/row).

    A 0.45   **B** 0.88   **C** 1.00   **D** 1.41   **E** 2.20

11.11 Using the data in Table 11.4 calculate the missing upper and lower limits for the 95% confidence interval estimate for the Hazard Ratio (the PIG vs PEG variable/row) for cells ZZ and ZZZZ.

    A 0.58 to 1.02

    B 0.74 to 2.69

    C 0.88 to 1.05

    D 0.39 to 0.72

    E 0.29 to 1.71

12   Reliability and Method Comparison Studies

Medical Statistics: A Textbook for the Health Sciences, Fifth Edition. Stephen J. Walters, Michael J. Campbell, and David Machin.
© 2021 John Wiley & Sons Ltd. Published 2021 by John Wiley & Sons Ltd.
Companion website: www.wiley.com/go/walters/medicalstatistics

Summary

In the health sciences, we often make measurements that need to be validated. Physiotherapists may need a reliable method of measuring pain, and an occupational therapist a reliable method of assessing whether someone is lifting a heavy weight correctly. In addition, different observers may come to different conclusions. Radiologists may disagree on the interpretation of an X-ray, physiotherapists on the level of pain actually experienced or pathologists on the histological grade of a tumour. Many projects start with a proposed method of measuring something, and the important question is: 'does this instrument measure what it purports to measure?' In many disciplines new techniques evolve that are simpler or less invasive than earlier procedures and an important question is whether the new procedure can replace of the earlier one. This chapter has a different emphasis to preceding ones in that we are not *testing* whether something is reliable but rather *measuring* how reliable it is.

12.1   Introduction

Many measurements that are taken during any investigation require some degree of subjective judgement, whether this is when taking a temperature with a thermometer, assessing the results of diagnostic procedures or observing the effects of therapies. As a consequence, were the same observer to repeat, or different observers to appraise, the same outcome measure they may not obtain identical results. Observer agreement studies investigate the reproducibility of a single observer, and the level of the consensus between different observers, assessing the same unit, be it a specimen, radiograph or pathology slide.

Typically, in observer agreement studies, several observers make assessments on each of a series of experimental units and these assessments are compared. For example, to examine the variation in measurements of the volume of intracranial gliomas from computed tomography, different observers might evaluate scans from a series of patients. The values of tumour volume so recorded could then be compared. In other circumstances, the assessments may be binary such as a conclusion with respect to the presence or absence of metastases seen on liver scintigraphy. Clearly an ideal situation is one in which all the observers agree *and* the answer is correct. The correct answer can only be known if there is a 'gold' standard means of assessment available. For some diseases this may be only possible at autopsy but this is clearly too late for patient care purposes.

Assessment of *reliability* consists of determining that the process used for measurement yields reproducible and consistent results. Any measurement whether on a numerical scale or by more subjective means, should yield reproducible or similar values if it is used repeatedly on the same patient whilst the patient's condition has not changed materially. In these circumstances, reliability concerns the level of agreement between two or more repeated measures. This is sometimes known as the *test–retest* reliability.

If the measuring instrument is a questionnaire, perhaps to measure patient quality of life (QoL), then during the development stage of the questionnaire itself reliability of the scales is of particular concern. Thus, for scales containing multiple items, all the items should have *internal reliability* and therefore be consistent in the sense that they should all measure the same thing. Just as with any quantitative measurement the final questionnaire should have test–retest reliability also.

12.2   Repeatability

A basic requirement of a measurement is that it is repeatable; if the same measurement is made on a second occasion, and nothing has changed then we would expect it to give the same answer, although some experimental error may be anticipated.

Coefficient of Variation

For a continuous observation that is measured several times a simple measure of repeatability is the *coefficient of variation* (CV) which is the within subject standard deviation divided by the mean and is expressed as a percentage.

Coefficient of Variation

$$CV = \frac{100 \times (\text{Within subject SD})}{\text{Mean}} = \frac{100 s_{\text{Within}}}{\bar{x}},$$

where $\bar{x}$ and s_{Within} are calculated from continuous data obtained from the same subject in a stable situation.

The CV is independent of the units in which the observation is measured. It is often used in, for example, clinical biochemistry where repeated assays are made on a substance with known concentration to test the assay method. Commonly a CV of <5% is deemed acceptable.

Example – CV – Total Steps Per Day
In the example of Figure 2.10 in which total steps per day walked by a subject, assessed by a pedometer was recorded every day for 100 days. The mean of steps per day was $\bar{x} = 14\,107$ and the within-subject standard deviation, $s_{\text{Within}} = 4959$. Thus, the CV $= 100 \times (4959/14\,107) = 35.2\%$. This suggests a high level of variability. To be generally useful, there is an implicit assumption that the mean and within subject standard deviation are proportional, so for example a more sedentary person, with a mean of 3000 steps per day would be expected to have a standard deviation of $3000 \times 35.2/100$ or about 1000 steps. Thus, the CV% is most useful where subjects are expected to have similar mean values, such as in biochemistry.

Intra-class Correlation Coefficient (ICC)

Rather than repeated measures being confined to only a single subject, the more usual situation is to have repeated (often duplicate and by the same rater) measures on a number of subjects. In this case there are two sources of variability that must be taken into account when assessing repeatability. The first source, as with the CV, is the within patient standard deviation and the second, since we are now concerned with several subjects on which the duplicates are taken, is the between subject standard deviation, s_{Between}.

In these circumstances, repeatability can be assessed by the intra-class correlation coefficient (ICC). This measures the strength of agreement between repeated measurements, by assessing the proportion of the between-patient variance (the square of the standard deviation), to the total variance, comprising the sum of both the within and between variances.

Intra-Class Correlation Coefficient

$$ICC = \frac{s_{\text{Between}}^2}{s_{\text{Within}}^2 + s_{\text{Between}}^2},$$

where s_{Within} and s_{Between} are the within and between subject standard deviations.

It is evident that, if we only have only one observation per person, we cannot estimate the within person standard deviation. If we have several observations per person, we can estimate the standard deviation for that person and take the average variance of all the individuals concerned as an estimate of s^2_{within}. As shown in Section 12.5, the estimate of the between person variance can be obtained once the variance of the means for each person is known.

If the ICC is large (close to 1), then the within rater (or random error) variability is low and a high proportion of the variance in the observations is attributable to variation between raters. The measurements are then described as having high reliability. Conversely, if the ICC is low (close to 0), then the random error variability dominates and the measurements have low reliability. If the error variability is regarded as 'noise' and the true value of rater scores as the 'signal', then the ICC measures the signal-to-noise ratio.

The ICC is the most commonly used method for assessing reliability with continuous data. It is also sometimes used for ordered categorical data that have more than five or more response categories. A value of at least 0.90 is often recommended if the measurements of concern are to be used for evaluating future patients for which therapeutic decisions are to be made (Streiner et al. 2015; Koo and Li 2016).

In the context of a questionnaire, say to assess QoL, if a patient is in a stable condition, an instrument should yield repeatable and reproducible results if it is used repeatedly on that patient. This is usually assessed using a test–retest study, with patients who are thought to have stable disease and who are not expected to experience changes due to treatment effects or toxicity. The patients are asked to complete the same QoL questionnaire on several occasions. The level of agreement between the occasions is a measure of the reliability of the instrument. It is important to select patients whose condition is stable, and to choose carefully a between-assessment time-gap that is neither too short nor too long. As would be the case for a pathologist making a diagnosis from slides, too short a period might allow the pathologist to recall his or her earlier responses, and too long a period might allow a deterioration in the quality of the specimens under review. However, problems associated with developing and using QoL and other instruments are often rather specialist in nature and readers are referred to Fayers and Machin (2016) for a more detailed discussion.

Example from the Literature – ICC – Paediatric Asthma Quality of Life Questionnaire
Juniper et al. (1996) evaluated the Paediatric Asthma Quality of Life Questionnaire (PAQLQ) by examining reliability in children aged 7 to 17 who had stable asthma. The corresponding ICC values are shown in Table 12.1, and all are above 0.80. These findings suggest that the PAQLQ has high test–retest reliability in stable patients.

Comparison Between the Intraclass Correlation and Pearson's Correlation

If there are only two measurements per unit, for example a measurement is repeated for each individual, or two raters look at each patient, then an alternative correlation coefficient to consider is Pearson's, as described in Section 9.2. However, Pearson's correlation is a measure of *association* and not *agreement*. For example, suppose one was measuring lung function using two spirometers,

Table 12.1 ICC values for reliability of items in the PAQLQ.

Item	Within-subject SD	Between-subject SD	Intraclass correlation ICC
Overall QoL	0.17	0.73	0.95
Symptoms	0.22	0.84	0.93
Activities	0.42	0.96	0.84
Emotions	0.23	0.64	0.89

Source: after Juniper et al. (1996).

and one spirometer consistently read 10 ml higher than the other. Then the Pearson correlation would be 1, but the ICC would be less than 1, the value depending on the variance of the observations. Clearly one cannot substitute one spirometer blindly for the other, since they don't agree. Another difference between the two statistics is that in the ICC, the data are centred and scaled using a pooled mean and standard deviation, whereas in the Pearson correlation, each variable is centred and scaled by its own mean and standard deviation. This pooled scaling for the ICC makes sense because all measurements are of the same quantity (albeit on units in different groups).

12.3   Agreement

A common problem is measuring how well two observers make a binary (yes/no) diagnostic deci-sion say after examining a patient or perhaps a specimen taken from a patient. A similar problem is how consistently does a single observer make the same decision. To assess the latter, we would require the same assessments to be repeated by the same observer. For example, the same slide would need to be reviewed by the reviewing pathologist on two occasions. The second review would need to be undertaken 'blind' to the results of the first review and clearly sometime later. A 'wash-out' period long enough to ensure that the pathologist does not 'recognise' the slide but not too much later as an extended period may cause deterioration of the specimen or the observer (now more experienced) may change his/her methods in a systematic way.

For a single observer examining the same specimen on two occasions, or two observers examin-ing the same specimen but independently of each other, the degree of reproducibility is quantified by the probability of making a chance error. In the context of making a definitive (and binary) diag-nosis, this is the probability of ascribing either absent (coded 0) to a diagnosis when it should be present (coded 1), or a 1 to a diagnosis that should be 0. For N_{Repeat} specimens this process is described in Table 12.2.

It is important to note that tests of statistical significance are rarely appropriate for reliability studies. Thus Table 12.2 looks like a standard (paired) 2×2 contingency table to be analysed by McNemar's test of Chapter 8, but the test will not tell us whether or not the reviewer(s) is reliable.

One method of measuring whether a reviewer agrees with him or herself, or two reviewers agree, is simply to calculate the percentage of occasions the same response is obtained.

Observer(s) Agreement
The estimated probability the observer(s) agrees is

$$P_{\text{Agree}} = \frac{x_{00} + x_{11}}{N_{\text{Repeat}}}.$$

Observer(s) Disagreement
The estimated probability observer(s) disagree is

$$P_{\text{Disagree}} = \frac{x_{10} + x_{01}}{N_{\text{Repeat}}}.$$

Cohen's Kappa (κ)

If the diagnostic choice is binary, then there are only two options for each patient or specimen so that if observers made their repeated choices at random, rather than by careful examination, these will agree by chance alone some of the time. Jacob Cohen developed the kappa (κ) statistic to allow

Table 12.2   The possible outcomes for a single observer reviewing the same material on two occasions, or two observers reviewing the same material independently of each other.

Second	First review(er)		
Review(er)	Absent	Present	Total
Absent	x_{00}	x_{01}	n_0
Present	x_{10}	x_{11}	n_1
Total	m_0	m_1	N_{Repeat}

for chance agreements of this kind. It is essentially the proportion of cases that the raters agree minus the proportion of cases they are likely to agree by chance, scaled so that if the observers agree all the time, then κ is one. Thus, if κ is equal to 1, there is perfect agreement, and when $\kappa = 0$ the agreement is no better than chance. Negative values indicate an agreement that is even less than what would be expected by chance.

Cohen's κ

$$\kappa = \frac{P_{\text{Agree}} - P_{\text{Chance}}}{1 - P_{\text{Chance}}},$$

where P_{Chance} is the proportion expected to show agreement by chance alone. The method of calculating P_{Chance} is given in Section 12.5.

Interpretation of κ is subjective, but Fayers and Machin (2015) suggest using the guideline values in Table 12.3.

Example from the Literature – Cohen's κ – Arteriovenous Malformations (AVM)
Al-Shahi et al. (2014) used two observers to review angiograms of 38 patients with AVM of the brain to determine inter-observer agreement. Consequently 13 binary features of each angiogram were reviewed with κ ranging from 0.14 to 0.62 (median 0.36). The investigators concluded that inter-observer agreement was slight to moderate and that there was a need for more robust definitions of AVM.

The concept of a binary diagnostic division may be extended to that of an ordered categorical variable where, for example, a pathologist may grade patient material into different grades perhaps indicative of increasing severity of the disease. In which case the results may be summarised in a square $R \times R$ contingency table where R is the number of possible grades that can be allocated to the specimen.

Table 12.3   Guideline values of κ to indicate the strength of agreement.

κ	Agreement
<0.20	Poor
0.20 to <0.40	Slight
0.40 to <0.60	Moderate
0.60 to <0.80	Good
0.80 to 1.00	Very High

Source: Fayers and Machin (2015).

Table 12.4 Pathologist agreement resulting from independent reviews of the same biopsy specimens from patients with lesions of the uterine cervix.

	Grade	Pathologist 2				
		I	II	III	IV	Total
Pathologist 1	I	**22**	2	2	0	26
	II	5	**7**	14	0	26
	III	0	2	**36**	0	38
	IV	0	1	14	**7**	22
Total		27	12	66	7	112

Worked Example – Cohen's κ – Pathology Review

Table 12.4 shows a comparison of two pathologists reviewing biopsy material from 112 patients with lesions of the uterine cervix. The grade categories were I = negative, II = squamous hyperplasia, III = carcinoma in situ and IV = squamous carcinoma.

The **bold** observed values in the diagonal are $O_{11} = 22$, $O_{22} = 7$, $O_{33} = 36$ and $O_{44} = 7$. The corresponding expected values are $E_{11} = 26 \times 27/112 = 6.27$, $E_{22} = 2.79$, $E_{33} = 22.39$ and $E_{44} = 1.38$. Hence $p_{\text{Observed}} = (22 + 7 + 36 + 7)/112 = 0.64$, $p_{\text{Expected}} = (6.27 + 2.79 + 22.39 + 1.38)/112 = 0.29$ and $\kappa = (0.64 - 0.29)/(1 - 0.29) = 0.493$.

This is only 'moderate' agreement and such a low value may then stimulate the pathologists concerned to review their classification methods in detail.

Kappa was developed for categorical classifications, where disagreement is assumed equally likely between categories. However, when the categories are ordered, disagreement between more extreme categories is less likely than amongst the intermediate ones. Consequently, the concept of κ can be extended to give more weight to the more extreme disagreements. One set of weights (that weight the disagreement by the square of the distance between categories), leads to the equivalent of the *ICC*. For example, for these data we find weighted κ is 0.777, showing that the few disparities of misclassification by two categories have had a large effect on κ. The intraclass correlation is 0.779, which is very close to the weighted kappa.

Kappa (κ) has a number of limitations:

(i) The maximum value of $\kappa = 1$ is only obtainable when observers agree completely with each other.

(ii) For a given level of agreement, κ increases when the number of categories decreases. Thus, comparisons between κ from different studies should only be made when the number of categories in each study are the same.

(iii) κ depends on the marginal distributions, (the values of n_0, n_1, m_0, and m_1 in Table 12.2). Thus, one can obtain a particular value of κ, even though the two assessors have different agreement patterns. For example, one observer may have a bias with a systematic direction whilst the other may make more random decisions.

(iv) Some computer programmes give a p-value associated with κ. These should be ignored since the null hypothesis they are testing has no meaning.

12.4 Validity

Cronbach's Alpha (α_{Cronbach})

Some questionnaires, such as those used to assess concepts such as anxiety and depression in patients, often comprise a series of questions. Each question is then scored, and the scores combined in some way to give a single numerical value. Often this is done by merely summing the scores for each answer to give an overall scale score. The internal validity of each of the component questions of the scale is indicated if they are all positively correlated with each other; a lack of correlation of two such items would indicate that at least one of them was not measuring the concept in question. Alternatively, one might frame a question in two different ways, and if the answers are always similar, then the questions are internally consistent.

A measure of internal consistency is Cronbach's (sometimes spelled Chronbach) alpha, $\alpha_{Cronbach}$. It is essentially a form of correlation coefficient; a value of 0 would indicate that there was no correlation between the items that make up a scale, and a value of 1 would indicate perfect correlation.

Cronbach's Alpha, $\alpha_{Cronbach}$

If a questionnaire has k items, and this has been administered to a group of subjects, then the standard deviation, s_i, of the ith item and s_T the standard deviation of the sum score T of all the items is required. From which

$$\alpha_{Cronbach} = \frac{k}{k-1}\left(1 - \frac{\sum s_i^2}{s_T^2}\right).$$

A worked example is given in Section 12.5. For comparing groups, $\alpha_{Cronbach}$ values of 0.7 to 0.8 are regarded as satisfactory, although for clinical applications higher values are necessary. However, a value of 1 would indicate that most of the questions could in fact be discarded, since all the information is contained in just one of them. Clearly one would like items that all refer so a single concept such as pain to be related to each other. However, if they are too closely related then some of the questions are redundant. When constructing a questionnaire, one might omit items which have a weak or very strong correlation with other items in the domain of interest.

Example from the Literature – $\alpha_{Cronbach}$ – Patients with Pressure Ulcers (PU)
Gorecki et al. (2013) developed the PU-QOL instrument for assessing patient-reported outcomes for patients with pressure ulcers. A validation of the scales developed was carried out on 229 patients The scales included, for example, pain, sleep, and emotional well-being. They found values of $\alpha_{Cronbach}$ for each of the 10 scales ranging from 0.89 to 0.95 (median 0.925) and concluded that the instrument had satisfactory internal validity.

12.5 Method Comparison Studies

A feature of laboratory work, and of many aspects of clinical work, is the evaluation of new instruments. It is usual in such studies to compare results obtained from the new with that obtained from some standard. Alternatively, two devices may be proposed for measuring the same quantity and one may wish to determine which is the better. Essentially one is assessing the same subject or specimen in two ways each determining the same outcome using the same units of measurement.

Example – Method Comparisons – Two Spirometers

Forced expiratory volume (FEV_1), which is the volume of air expelled in the first second of maximal forced expiration from a position of full inspiration, is measured using a spirometer. Figure 12.1 presents the results of a study in which 56 subjects had their FEV_1 measured by both a Respiradyne and a Vitalograph spirometer. The purpose of the study was to see if the Respiradyne spirometer could be used in place of the Vitalograph.

As previously indicated, a common but inappropriate method of analysis is first to calculate the correlation coefficient between the two sets of readings and then calculate a significance level on the null hypothesis of no association.

Why Calculating the Correlation Coefficient is Inappropriate

1) The correlation coefficient is a measure of *association*. What is required here is a measure of agreement. We will have perfect association if the observations lie on any straight line, but there is only perfect agreement if the points lie on the line of equality $y = x$.
2) The correlation coefficient observed depends on the range of measurements used. So, one can increase the correlation coefficient by choosing widely spaced observations. Since investigators usually compare two methods over the whole range of likely values (as they should), a good correlation is almost guaranteed.
3) Because of (2), data that have an apparently high correlation can, for individual subjects, show very poor agreement between the methods of measurement.
4) The test of significance is not relevant since it would be very surprising if two methods designed to measure the same thing were not related.

Bland and Altman (1986) give these arguments and recommend an alternative approach. As an initial step one should plot the data as in Figure 12.1, but omit the calculation of the corresponding correlation coefficient and the associated test of significance. They then argue that a plot of the paired difference, d, between the two observations on each subject against their mean value is more likely to reveal features of these data, in particular any systematic differences between methods. Common features would be that one method consistently gives a higher reading than the other, or that the differences relate to the mean, for example the scatter plot fans out suggesting that the differences are larger with bigger measurements.

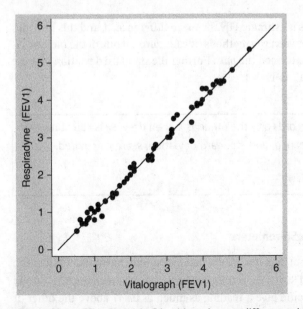

Figure 12.1 FEV$_1$ (litres) in 56 subjects by two different spirometers with the line of equality.

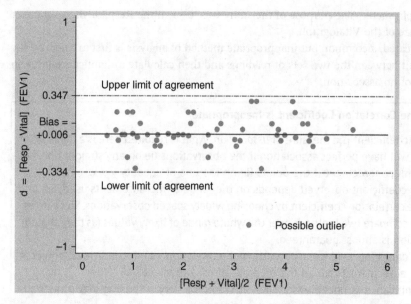

Figure 12.2 Scatter diagram of the difference between methods against the mean of both for the 56 subjects of Figure 12.1.

Example – Bland and Altman Plots – Comparing Respiradyne and Vitalograph Spirometers

Figure 12.2 displays the scatter plot of the difference in FEV_1, as assessed by the two spirometers in each patient, against their mean value. From this plot it can be seen that the size of the difference calculated remains essentially the same as their joint mean increases in value. The bias = +0.006 indicates that Respiradyne readings are very marginally higher than those of the Vitalograph although the possible outlier (with $d = -0.8$) is in the reverse direction and appears more prominent than in Figure 12.1.

The lack of agreement between methods is estimated by the mean difference, $\bar{d}$, and this provides an estimate of the systematic difference between the methods (ideally zero). If one of the methods is a gold standard then the mean difference is termed the *bias*. Further the standard deviation of these differences allows the 'limits of agreement' to be set.

> **Method Comparisons** If one method records as y the other as x, then $d = y - x$ is calculated for each subject, and the corresponding mean, $\bar{d}$, and standard deviation, s, are calculated.
> Systematic difference or bias: $\bar{d}$,
> 95% 'limits of agreement' $\bar{d} - 2s$ to $\bar{d} + 2s$.

Example – Limits of Agreement – Two Spirometers

For the FEV_1 data comparing the two spirometers $n = 56$, the mean Respiradyne minus Vitalograph difference in assessments of $\bar{d} = 0.0064$ and $SD(d) = s = 0.1703$. The 'limits of agreement' are -0.334 to $+0.347$ implying that one spirometer could give a reading as much as 0.347 above the other or

0.334 below it. In this case, the bias observed is negligible but whether the limits of agreement are acceptable needs to be judged from a clinical viewpoint.

If an outlier is present it is good practice to check the results for this subject. Perhaps there has been a mistake entering the data, and if necessary that subject could be excluded from the calculations for the limits of agreement.

Example from the Literature – Limits of Agreement – Positron Emission Tomography (PET) and Endoscopic Ultrasound (EUS)

Foley (2017) compared the length of disease, defined as the total extent of the primary tumour and the involved regional lymph nodes, in 160 patients with oesophageal cancer as assessed by both PET and EUS. They used the Bland–Altman methodology and concluded that on average the tumour as measured by PET measured 2.2 cm shorter than that by EUS and the 95% levels of agreement of −9.6 and +5.2 cm. The authors concluded that these results highlight the continued benefit of EUS in the oesophageal cancer staging and treatment pathway.

12.6   Points When Reading the Literature

1) When a new instrument has been used, has it been tested for reliability and validity?
2) When two methods of measurement have been compared, has correlation been used to assess whether one instrument can be used instead of another? If so, are there systematic biases?
3) When Cohen's kappa is compared, are the marginal distributions similar? If not, then be careful about making comparisons.

12.7   Technical Details

Suppose we measured FEV_1 on four patients with the results given in Table 12.5.

Table 12.5 FEV_1 (litres) for four patients measured on two occasions.

Subject (i)	First occasion (x_{i1})	Second occasion (x_{i2})	Difference ($x_{i1} - x_{i2}$)	Mean $\bar{x}_i = \dfrac{(x_{i1} + x_{i2})}{2}$
1	2.1	2.2	−0.1	2.15
2	2.3	2.5	−0.2	2.40
3	2.6	2.6	+0.0	2.60
4	2.8	2.7	+0.1	2.75
Mean	2.45	2.50	−0.050	2.475
SD	0.31	0.22	0.129	0.260

The corresponding model is $y_{ij} = \mu + \tau_i + \varepsilon_{ij}$ where μ is the overall mean, τ_i is the additional effect of subject i and ε_{ij} is the random error from one measurement, j, to another. We assume τ and ε are random independent variables. The variance of τ is the *between subject variance* and the variance of ε is the *within subject variance*. It is important to note that we are not assuming an 'occasion' effect here. The calculations will give the same result if some of the observations on the two occasions are swapped. This is known as an *exchangeable error*.

With n pairs of observations (x_{i1}, x_{i2}), $i = 1,...,n$, the within subject variance is estimated by $s^2_{\text{Within}} = \sum_{i=1}^{n} (x_{i1} - x_{i2})^2/2n$. Also, if $\overline{x}_i = (x_{i1} + x_{i2})/2$ then $\text{Var}(\overline{x}_i) = s^2_{\text{Between}} + \dfrac{s^2_{\text{Within}}}{2}$. From the data of Table 12.5, $s^2_{\text{Within}} = \{(-0.1)^2 + (-0.2)^2 + 0^2 + 0.1^2\}/8 = 0.0075$ and $\text{Var}(\overline{x}_i) = 0.260^2 = 0.0675$. Hence, $s^2_{\text{Between}} = 0.0675 - 0.0075/2 = 0.06375$ and $\text{ICC} = 0.06375/(0.0075 + 0.06375) = 0.895$. The ICC is close to unity which suggests the measurement of FEV_1 may be regarded as repeatable.

Agreement by Chance (P_{Chance})

From Table 12.2, $p_{\text{Agree}} = (x_{00} + x_{11})/N_{\text{Repeat}}$. To get the expected agreement we use the row and column totals to estimate the expected numbers agreeing for each category.

For negative agreement (absent, absent) the expected proportion is the product of $(x_{01} + x_{00})/N_{\text{Repeat}}$ and $(x_{10} + x_{00})/N_{\text{Repeat}}$, giving $(x_{00} + x_{01})(x_{00} + x_{10})/N^2_{\text{Repeat}}$. Likewise, for positive agreement the expected proportion is $(x_{10} + x_{11})(x_{01} + x_{11})/N^2_{\text{Repeat}}$. The expected proportion of agreements for the whole table is the sum of these two terms, that is

$$P_{\text{Chance}} = \frac{(x_{00} + x_{01})(x_{00} + x_{10})}{N^2_{\text{Repeat}}} + \frac{(x_{10} + x_{11})(x_{01} + x_{11})}{N^2_{\text{Repeat}}}.$$

Suppose we have an $R \times R$ contingency table, where $R > 2$, and the rows contain the categories observed by one rater and the columns the categories observed by the other rater. By analogy with Table 12.2, then the numbers in the diagonals of the table, that is x_{ii}, are the numbers observed when the two raters agree. The corresponding numbers expected by chance in category i are labelled e_{ii}.

If N is the number of specimens classified and we denote $P_{\text{Agree}} = \Sigma x_{ii}/N$ and $P_{\text{Chance}} = \Sigma e_{ii}/N$, then

$$\kappa = \frac{P_{\text{Agree}} - P_{\text{Chance}}}{1 - P_{\text{Chance}}}.$$

Calculation of Cronbach's Alpha

Suppose a section of a questionnaire has three items, which measure pain say, each of which can have a score between 1 (no pain) and 5 (severe pain). The total of the three items make up the total pain score for a particular dimension of the questionnaire.

If a questionnaire has k items, and this has been administered to a group of subjects, then if s_i is the SD of the ith item, T is the sum score of all the items, and s_T is the SD of T, then Cronbach's alpha is $\alpha_{\text{Cronbach}} = \dfrac{k}{k-1}\left(1 - \dfrac{\sum s_i^2}{s_T^2}\right)$. Thus, for the data of Table 12.6, $k = 3$, and $\sum s_i^2 = 1.63^2 + 1.71^2 + 0.95^2 = 6.4835$, $s_T^2 = 16.9744$ and so $\alpha_{\text{Cronbach}} = \dfrac{3}{(3-1)}\left(1 - \dfrac{6.4835}{16.8744}\right) = 0.924$.

Table 12.6 Responses to three questions and total score for four subjects.

Subject	Q1	Q2	Q3	Total score
1	1	1	2	4
2	3	3	2	8
3	5	5	4	14
4	3	2	3	8
SD	1.63	1.71	0.95	4.12

The reason that α_{Cronbach} is a measure of correlation is as follows. If $X_1, \ldots, X_k$ are independent random variables, then $T = X_1 + \ldots + X_k$ and $\text{Var}(T) = \text{Var}(X_1) + \ldots + \text{Var}(X_k)$. Thus $s_T^2 = \sum s_i^2$ so that the numerator and denominator in the braces in the equation for Cronbach's alpha are the same and so $\alpha_{\text{Cronbach}} = 0$. In contrast, if $X_1, \ldots, X_k$ are perfectly correlated so that $X_1 = X_2 = \ldots = X_k$ (all equal to X say) then $T = kX$ and $s_T^2 = k^2\text{Var}(X)$, whereas $\sum s_i^2 = k\text{Var}(X)$. Thus, the ratio in the braces is now $1/k$ and so $\alpha_{\text{Cronbach}} = 1$. Clearly between these two extreme situations, when there is likely to be some association between the X_i, α_{Cronbach} will be between 0 and 1.

12.8 Exercises

Two radiologists reviewed 50 dual energy X-ray absorptiometry (DXA) spine radiographs for the detection of vertebral fractures in children aged 5–15 years. The results are shown in Table 12.7.

Table 12.7 Radiologist agreement resulting from independent reviews of the same DXA spine radiographs for the detection of vertebral fractures in 50 children aged 5–15 years.

	Any fracture from DXA scan	Observer 2		Total
		No	Yes	
Observer 1	No	23	6	29
	Yes	1	20	21
Total		24	26	50

12.1 From the data in Table 12.7 calculate the estimated probability that the two radiographers will agree on the diagnosis of a vertebral fracture.

- **A** 0.09
- **B** 0.14
- **C** 0.50
- **D** 0.72
- **E** 0.86

12.2 From the data in Table 12.7 calculate the Kappa statistic.
  A 0.09
  B 0.14
  C 0.50
  D 0.72
  E 0.86

12.3 The Kappa value from 12.2 indicates which of the following strengths of agreement:
  A Poor
  B Slight
  C Moderate
  D Good
  E Very High

Table 12.8 shows the responses of 10 children with osteogenesis imperfecta (OI) to six questions asked about being safe and careful measured on a five-point Likert scale (1 = always, 2 = most of the time, 3 = sometimes, 4 = not much, 5 = never). The children were part of a study to develop a diseases specific QoL measure for children with OI. The six items and total score are scaled so that a higher score indicates a better health state (Hill et al. 2014; Hill 2015).

Table 12.8 Responses to six questions on being safe careful and total score for 10 subjects with OI.

Subject	Q1	Q2	Q3	Q4	Q5	Q6	Total score
1	4	2	2	2	1	1	12
2	3	3	4	3	2	3	18
3	4	5	5	5	5	5	29
4	3	1	1	1	3	1	10
5	5	5	5	4	4	3	26
6	3	2	2	2	3	1	13
7	4	4	4	3	5	2	22
8	2	1	1	1	3	5	13
9	4	2	3	4	3	3	19
10	3	3	3	3	4	5	21
Mean	3.50	2.80	3.00	2.80	3.30	2.90	18.30
SD	0.85	1.48	1.49	1.32	1.25	1.66	6.33

Q1 Does someone give you extra help to keep you safe?
Q2 Do you keep away from busy areas to keep safe?
Q3 Do you keep away from crowds to keep safe?
Q4 Do you try to keep safe to stop you breaking a bone?
Q5 Do you keep away from some activities to stop you having a broken bone?
Q6 Do you think before playing sports to avoid having a broken bone?

12.4 Calculate Cronbach's alpha for the data in Table 12.8.
    A 0.09
    B 0.14
    C 0.50
    D 0.72
    E 0.86

12.5 Which of the following are TRUE?
    A If items of a scale are all essentially measuring the same thing then Cronbach's α is expected to be close to 1.
    B Cronbach's α can be used with nominal categorical scales
    C Cohen's kappa can be negative.
    D Cohen's weighted kappa can be used with ordered categorical scales
    E The ICC can be negative.

12.6 Which of the following are TRUE?
    A A measurement with a CV of 50% is repeatable
    B The Bland–Altman method can be used to compare instruments with different scales.
    C The limits of agreement will get narrower as the number of measurements increases.
    D If the output from one instrument has a high correlation with the output from a different instrument, they can be used interchangeably.
    E Reliability means the instrument measures what it is intended to measure.

12.7 Table 12.9 shows the central lung distance (CLD) in mm measured on two occasions by a single radiographer in 10 women undergoing radiotherapy treatment for breast cancer.

Table 12.9 Central lung distance (CLD), in mm, measured on two occasions by a single radiographer in 10 women undergoing radiotherapy treatment for breast cancer.

	CLD (mm)			
Subject	First occasion	Second occasion	Difference	Mean
1	18	15	−3	16.5
2	14	13	−1	13.5
3	18	10	−8	14
4	15	13	−2	14
5	12	10	−2	11
6	16	16	0	16
7	10	8	−2	9
8	14	13	−1	13.5
9	12	12	0	12
10	14	18	4	16
Mean			−1.500	13.550
SD			2.991	2.374
Variance			8.944	5.636

12.8 Calculate the ICC for the data in Table 12.9.

    A 0.09

    B 0.14

    C 0.37

    D 0.72

    E 0.86

13   Evaluation of Diagnostic Tests

Medical Statistics: A Textbook for the Health Sciences, Fifth Edition. Stephen J. Walters, Michael J. Campbell, and David Machin.
© 2021 John Wiley & Sons Ltd. Published 2021 by John Wiley & Sons Ltd.
Companion website: www.wiley.com/go/walters/medicalstatistics

Summary

Diagnosis is an essential part of clinical practice. A diagnostic test may be used together with a clinical examination to diagnose or exclude a particular disorder in a patient or as a screening test to ascertain which individuals in an apparently healthy population are likely to have (or not) the disease of interest. Individuals flagged in these ways will then usually be subjected to more rigorous investigations in order to have their initial diagnosis confirmed or otherwise. The two major elements associated with the clinical value of diagnostic tests are their sensitivity and their specificity. When the result of a diagnostic test is a continuous variable, there may be difficulty in deciding an appropriate cut-point to categorise those with and without the condition of interest. In this case, a receiver operating characteristic (ROC) curve may be used to help with cut-point determination.

13.1   Introduction

Many different diagnostic tests can be used to diagnose disease and such tests are usually used as an alternative to a definitive or 'gold standard' test when the gold standard is not practical for use in routine clinical practice. Thus, the reason for not giving angiographs to all patients with suspected heart disease is that it is a difficult and expensive procedure, and carries a non-negligible risk to the patient. An alternative test such as an exercise test might be tried, and only if it is positive would angiography then be carried out. If the exercise test is negative then the next stage would be to carry out biochemical tests, and if these turned out positive, once again angiography could be performed. An extreme example is the diagnosis of Alzheimer's dementia which can only be confirmed after death by a post mortem examination of the brain under a microscope.

A diagnostic test is used to classify individuals into one of two categories such as: diseased or not diseased; positive or negative; high or low risk. Diagnostic tests do not always give the 'correct' diagnosis and so it is important to be able to quantify how accurate a particular test is. There is no single statistical summary measure of a diagnostic test's accuracy and several measures are commonly used to summarise a test's performance. The statistical analysis of diagnostic tests is fairly straightforward, but causes difficulty because of unfamiliar and confusing terminology.

13.2   Diagnostic Tests

In making a diagnosis, a clinician first establishes a possible set of diagnostic alternatives and then attempts to reduce these by progressively ruling out specific diseases or conditions. Alternatively, the clinician may have a strong hunch that the patient has one particular disease and they then set about confirming its presence. Given a particular diagnosis, a good diagnostic test should indicate either that the disease is very unlikely or that it is very probable. In a practical sense it is important to realise that a diagnostic test is useful only if the result influences patient management since, if the management is the same for two different conditions, there is little point in trying strenuously to distinguish between them.

The simplest case to consider is that where patients can be classified into two groups according to the results of an investigation, perhaps an X-ray or MRI scan. Table 13.1 shows the relationship between the results of an MRI scan and the diagnosis of prostate cancer based on a biopsy from 576 men with suspected prostate cancer (Ahmed et al. 2017). In this example the gold or reference

Table 13.1 Notation and results of the multi-parametric magnetic resonance imaging (MP-MRI) test to diagnose prostate cancer compared to the gold standard test of template prostate mapping (TPM) biopsy in 576 men with suspected prostate cancer.

Test result	TRUE disease status: confirmed diagnosis of prostate cancer by TPM-biopsy		
Diagnostic test MP-MRI	Present $(D+)$	Absent $(D-)$	Total
Positive $(T+)$	213 (a)	205 (b)	418 $(a+b)$
Negative $(T-)$	17 (c)	141 (d)	158 $(c+d)$
Total	230 $(a+c)$	346 $(b+d)$	576 (N)

Source: based on Ahmed et al. (2017).

standard diagnosis is the template prostate mapping (TPM)-biopsy result. The reference test was done using core biopsies taken every 5 mm and the result reported by one of two expert uropathologists blinded to all MR images. The question of interest here is how good is the MRI scan at diagnosing prostate cancer?

Assuming that the diagnostic test can be positive or negative, indicating the present or absence of disease, then the different test results can be represented as a basic 2×2 contingency table with the notation of Table 13.1.

13.3 Prevalence, Overall Accuracy, Sensitivity, and Specificity

In Table 13.1 the proportion of subjects with the disease (prostate cancer) is termed the *prevalence* of the disease, or condition. Using the general notation this is calculated as $(a+c)/N$. The overall agreement between the test result and true diagnosis is the sum of the numbers in the top left and bottom right cells of Table 13.1 where the two classifications agree; from which the *overall accuracy* of the test and is calculated as $(a+d)/N$.

The problem with calculating the overall agreement between the two classifications, is that it assumes that the positive and negative diagnoses of disease have the same importance or weight and there is a symmetric relationship between the two classifications. That is having a positive test result and true diagnosis of prostate cancer is of equal importance as having a negative test result and a true diagnosis of no prostate cancer. However, these two options may not always be equally desirable.

Another approach is to calculate the proportion of patients with positive (correct diagnosis) and negative (incorrect diagnosis) test results within each of the gold standard diagnostic groups. These two proportions summarise the accuracy of a diagnostic test and are termed the *sensitivity* (or true positive rate) and *specificity* (or true negative rate.).

The *sensitivity* is the proportion of subjects who have the disease who are correctly identified by the test as positive and, in the notation of Table 13.1, it is estimated by $a/(a+c)$ and often expressed as a percentage. Note that 'c' is the number of false negatives (test is negative when disease is truly present) so that sensitivity is also one minus the proportion of false negatives. Now as sensitivity is the probability of a positive test result (event $T+$) given that the disease is present (event $D+$) it can be written as $P(T+|D+)$, where the '|' is read as 'given'.

The *specificity* of the test is the proportion of those without disease who give a negative test result and is estimated $d/(b + d)$ and also often expressed as a percentage. Note that '*b*' is the number of false positives (test is positive when although the disease absent) so that specificity is also one minus the proportion of false positives. Thus, specificity is the probability of a negative test result (event *T*-) given that the disease is absent (event *D*-) and can be written as $P(T\text{-}|D\text{-})$.

Sensitivity measures how good the test is at correctly identifying 'diseased' individuals and specificity measures how good the test is at correctly identifying 'non-diseased' individuals. Ideally good and accurate tests should have both sensitivity and specificity close to 1 (or 100%); although it is often difficult in reality to have both high sensitivity and specificity. The consequences of a false positive or false negative test result will depend on the setting. For example, a false positive X-ray or mammogram result on screening for breast cancer would be overturned on further testing, although the anxiety associated with a positive test result that turns out to be false is also an important factor in evaluating a test's performance. Conversely, a false negative mammogram test result may lead to a delayed diagnosis of breast cancer, causing a worse prognosis. In pregnant women, a false positive test for Down's syndrome may result in an unnecessary abortion.

Example of Calculations for Sensitivity and Specificity – Diagnosis of Prostate Cancer (Ahmed et al. 2017)

Consider the results of the MP-MRI and TPM-biopsy tests in men with suspected prostate cancer summarised in Table 13.1. The prevalence of prostate cancer in these subjects is $(a + c)/N = 230/576 = 0.3993$ or approximately 40%. Thus, the probability of a subject chosen at random from the combined group having the disease is estimated to be $P(D+) = 0.40$. The corresponding sensitivity of the test is $a/(a + c) = 213/230 = 0.9261$ or 93% whilst the specificity is $d/(b + d) = 141/346 = 0.4075$ or 41%.

Since sensitivity is *conditional* on the disease being present, and specificity on the disease being absent, in theory, they are unaffected by disease prevalence. For example, if we doubled the number of subjects with prostate cancer from 230 to 460 in Table 13.1, so that the prevalence was now $460/576 = 80\%$, then we could expect twice as many subjects to give a positive test result. Thus $2 \times 213 = 426$ would have a positive result. In this case the sensitivity would be $426/460 = 0.93$, which is unchanged from the previous value. A similar result is obtained for specificity.

Sensitivity and specificity are useful statistics because they yield consistent results for the diagnostic test in a variety of patient groups with different disease prevalence. This is an important point: sensitivity and specificity are characteristics of the test, not the population to which the test is applied. Although indeed they are independent of disease prevalence, in practice if the disease is very rare, the accuracy with which one can estimate the sensitivity will be limited.

13.4 Positive and Negative Predictive Values

At first sight, the calculations of the sensitivity and specificity of the new diagnostic test appear to have answered the question posed, namely: how good is the MRI scan at diagnosing prostate cancer? However, we have answered the question from one perspective only. The whole point of a diagnostic test, such as an MRI scan, is that it is used to make a diagnosis. In clinical practice the test result is all that is known; not the true disease status. So, we want to know how good the test is in giving the correct diagnosis, whether the outcome is a positive or negative diagnosis.

The *positive predictive value (PPV)* is the probability that someone has the disease when the test is positive; alternatively expressed as the proportion of individuals with the disease when the test is positive. Using the notation of Table 13.1, PPV = $a/(a + b)$. The PPV is what most people need to know. However, its value depends on the prevalence of the disease in question, that is, the frequency of affected individuals in the type of population being tested.

The *negative predictive value (NPV)* is the probability that someone is without disease when the test is negative, or the proportion of individuals without disease when the test is negative, which is estimated by NPV = $d/(c + d)$. This too depends on the prevalence of the disease.

Since sensitivity = 1 – probability(false negative) and specificity = 1 – probability(false positive), a possibly useful mnemonic to recall this is that 'se*n*sitivity' and '*n*egative' have *n*s in them and 's*p*ecificity' and '*p*ositive' have '*p*'s in them'.

Example of Calculations for PPV and NPV – Diagnosis of Prostate Cancer (Ahmed et al. 2017)

The PPV is the proportion of individuals with disease when the test is positive. Using the notation and data of Table 13.1, PPV = $a/(a + b) = 213/418 = 0.5096$ or 51%.

The NPV is the proportion of individuals without disease when the test is negative. Hence, NPV = $d/(c + d) = 141/158 = 0.8924$ or 89%.

Table 13.2 provides an overview of the four measures used to summarise the performance of a diagnostic test as well as some alternative nomenclature for the cells of the 2×2 contingency table of Table 13.1.

13.5 The Effect of Prevalence

Since sensitivity and specificity are conditional on having or not having the disease, they are properties of the test, not the disease. Therefore, they should not change when the test is applied to a population with low or high prevalence of disease. As we have indicated, the disadvantage of sensitivity and specificity is that they do not assess the accuracy of the test in a clinically useful way. However, since PPV is the proportion of patients with positive test results who are correctly diagnosed and NPV is the proportion of patients with negative test results who are correctly diagnosed, they give a direct assessment of the usefulness of the test in practice. However,

Table 13.2 Four measures used to summarise the performance of a diagnostic test.

| Test result | True diagnosis of disease | | Total | |
	Present	Absent		
Positive	a True positive (TP)	b False positive (FP)	$(a + b)$	*Positive predictive value* $a/(a + b)$ or TP/(TP + FN)
Negative	c False negative (FN)	d True negative (TN)	$(c + d)$	*Negative predictive value* $d/(c + d)$ or TN/(FN + TN)
Total	$(a + c)$	$(b + d)$	N	
	Sensitivity $a/(a + c)$ or TP/(TP + FN)	*Specificity* $d/(b + d)$ or TN/(FP + TN)		

Table 13.3 Predicted effect on MRI scan results for a prevalence of abnormality of 80%.

Test result	TRUE disease status: confirmed diagnosis of prostate cancer by TPM-biopsy		
Diagnostic test	Present	Absent	
MP-MRI	$(D+)$	$(D-)$	Total
Positive $(T+)$	429 (a)	68 (b)	497 $(a+b)$
Negative $(T-)$	32 (c)	47 (d)	79 $(c+d)$
Total	461 $(a+c)$	115 $(b+d)$	576 (N)

Table 13.4 Comparison of diagnostic test summary measures of the accuracy of the MRI scan for diagnosing prostate cancer when the prevalence of disease is 10, 40 and 80% respectively.

Diagnostic test	Prevalence (%)		
Summary statistic	10	40	80
Sensitivity	0.93	0.93	0.93
Specificity	0.41	0.41	0.41
Positive predictive value (PPV)	0.15	0.51	0.86
Negative predictive value (NPV)	0.98	0.89	0.59
Total correct predictions	0.46	0.61	0.83

their values depend very strongly on the prevalence of the disease, condition or abnormality in question.

In different clinical settings the prevalence of the abnormality will vary greatly. In the MRI scan study of Table 13.1 the prevalence of prostate was approximately 40%; implying 4 out of 10 patients who had an MRI scan will have prostate cancer. Suppose we double the prevalence from 40 to 80%, or 8 out of 10 then, using the data of Tables 13.1, then Table 13.3 shows the MRI scan results we would expect in such a group of patients. In this table (Table 13.3), the entries in the $D+$ column are twice those of the earlier table (Table 13.1) whilst those in the $D-$ column are smaller.

The corresponding diagnostic test summary statistics for three prevalence values are given in Table 13.4. This shows the PPV increasing as the prevalence of disease increases and conversely the NPV decreasing as the prevalence increases. Thus, the predictive values of a test depend on the prevalence of abnormality in the patients being tested, which may not be known. We should not take the predictive values observed in the sample as applying universally.

13.6   Confidence Intervals

Sensitivity, Specificity, PPV, NPV and prevalence are proportions, so we can calculate confidence intervals for them using standard methods (as described in Chapter 5). Confidence intervals (CIs) present a range of values, on the basis of the sample data, in which the population value for such a proportion is likely to lie. Confidence intervals convey only the effects of sampling variation on the estimated proportions and cannot control for other non-sampling errors such as biases in study design, conduct, or analysis. Table 13.5 shows the 95% CIs for the diagnostic test summary statistics obtained for the prostate cancer example of Table 13.1.

Table 13.5 Ninety-five percent confidence intervals for the MRI scan data.

Diagnostic test summary statistic	Estimate	Standard error	95% CI Lower	Upper
Prevalence	0.40	0.02	0.36	0.44
Overall accuracy	0.61	0.02	0.57	0.65
Sensitivity	0.93	0.02	0.89	0.96
Specificity	0.41	0.03	0.36	0.46
PPV	0.51	0.02	0.46	0.56
NPV	0.89	0.02	0.84	0.94

13.7 Functions of a Screening and Diagnostic Test

Diagnostic tests are rarely performed on their own but usually as part of a battery of clinical investigations during which the function of any test might change at different stages from screening to diagnosis. With a screening test, such as a mammogram for breast cancer on (apparently) healthy women; we need the test to have high *sensitivity* to rule out those without disease (SnNout).

A test with 100% sensitivity will recognise all patients with the disease by testing positive; as by definition there will be no false negative test results (cell $c = 0$ in Table 13.6a). A negative test result would definitely rule out the presence of the disease in the patient. Note the n in false *n*egative and in se*n*sitivity. When a result is negative, tests with high sensitivity are useful for ruling out a diagnosis.

For a diagnostic test on people with a high suspicion of disease, a test with high specificity to include those with disease (SpPin) is required. Suppose a test is 100% specific and we get a positive result which can only be in cell a of Table 13.6b. A test with 100% specificity will read negative, and

Table 13.6 Example of acreening tests with (a) 100% sensitivity and (b) with 100% specificity.

(a) 100% sensitivity				(b) 100% specificity			
	True diagnosis (gold standard) Disease				True diagnosis (gold standard) Disease		
Test result	Present Positive	Absent Negative	Total	Test result	Present Positive	Absent Negative	Total
Positive	a	b	$a + b$	Positive	a	$b = 0$	a
Negative	$c = 0$	d	d	Negative	c	d	$c + d$
Total	a	$b + d$	N	Total	$a + c$	d	N

accurately exclude disease from all healthy patients. The subject definitely has disease. Note 'p' in false *p*ositive and in s*p*ecificity. When a result is positive, tests with high specificity are useful for ruling in a diagnosis (SpPin).

13.8   Likelihood Ratio, Pre-test Odds and Post-test Odds

For any test result we can compare the probability of getting that result, if the patient truly had the condition of interest, with the corresponding probability if they were healthy. The ratio of these probabilities is called the likelihood ratio (LR). The LR is a measure combining sensitivity and specificity. The LR for a positive test result (LR^+) is calculated, using the notation of Table 13.1, as

$$LR^+ = \frac{\text{Prob}(T + \mid D +)}{\text{Prob}(T + \mid D -)} = \frac{\text{Sensitivity}}{1 - \text{Specificity}}.$$

An LR^+ greater than 1 indicates that the test is more likely to give a positive result if the individual had the disease than if they did not. The greater the value of LR^+, the more discriminating the test. A large LR^+, such as 10 or more, suggests the diagnostic test may be useful in ruling in a diagnosis. Conversely, the LR for a negative test results (LR^-) is calculated as:

$$LR^- = \frac{\text{Prob}(T - \mid D +)}{\text{Prob}(T - \mid D -)} = \frac{1 - \text{Sensitivity}}{\text{Specificity}}$$

An LR^- for a negative result of 0.5 means that a negative test is half as likely to occur in patients with the disease in question than patients without the disease.

Example – Likelihood Ratio – MRI Scan for Diagnosing Prostate Cancer

From the MRI scan data, in Table 13.1, for diagnosing prostate cancer the LR for a positive (abnormal) MRI scan result is:

$$LR^+ = 0.93/(1 - 0.41) = 1.58.$$

Thus, a positive MRI scan result is 1.58 times more likely in a patient with prostate cancer than in a patient without prostate cancer.

In contrast, for a negative MRI scan result:

$$LR^- = (1 - 0.93)/0.41 = 0.17.$$

Thus, a negative or normal MRI scan result is 0.17 times likely in a patient with prostate cancer than in a patient without prostate cancer. An LR for a negative result of 0.17 means that a negative test is 0.17 times as likely to occur in patients with prostate cancer than patients without.

The LR can be combined with the odds of having the condition, to quantify the information given by the test that an individual with a positive test result actually has the disease. The prevalence is the probability of disease before the test is performed. The *pre-test odds* of having the disease are:

Pre-odds = prevalence/(1 − prevalence).

Following a positive test result the *post-test odds* is given by:

Post-odds = Pre-odds × LR^+.

The post-test odds are another way of quantifying the information that a positive test result provides about whether an individual truly has the disease.

From Table 13.1, the prevalence of prostate cancer in these subjects is $= 230/576 = 0.3993$, so the pre-test odds of disease are $0.3993/(1–0.3993) = 0.66$. Further $LR^+ = 1.58$, and so the post-odds of the disease after the test are $0.66 \times 1.56 = 1.04$. This can be verified from the post-test probability, or PPV, of $P(D + |T+) = 0.51$ calculated earlier, so that the post-test odds are $0.51/(1–0.51) = 1.04$.

13.9   Receiver Operating Characteristic (ROC) Curve

Sometimes diagnosis is made using a continuous measurement such as an assay or a person reported outcome measure. When a diagnostic test produces a continuous measurement, then a convenient diagnostic cut-off must be selected to calculate the sensitivity and specificity of the test.

For example, can we use a self-reported 10-item Edinburgh Postnatal Depression Scale (EPDS) at six weeks postnatally to satisfactorily diagnose postnatal depression (PND)? Each item within the questionnaire is scored 0, 1, 2, or 3 and these responses are then summed generating a score from 0 to 30 with higher scores indicating greater risk of PND. Table 13.7 shows the results of completing the EPDS amongst a sample of new mothers known to experience PND or not. For example, in those 24 new mothers with an EPDS $= 0$ there are none who were subsequently diagnosed with PND whereas 23 of the 37 whose score is 17 have PND. If we wish to use the EPDS prospectively to diagnose PND then we need to choose an appropriate cut-point score. For each possible cut-off we can calculate the sensitivity and specificity, of the test and from these determine the optimal cut-point for the EPDS for diagnosing PND. Note that with a continuous outcome, sensitivity and specificity are complementary; one can always get a test with a high sensitivity by reducing the specificity and vice versa.

Example of Calculations – Diagnosis of PND Using the EPDS

Table 13.7 shows that 859 new mothers completed and returned the EPDS questionnaire by post at six weeks postnatally. The 'gold standard' diagnosis of depression was determined from Schedules for Clinical Assessment in Neuropsychiatry (SCAN) diagnostic interview with all 859 mothers. Overall, 132/859 new mothers had a diagnosis of PND based on the SCAN interviews whilst 727/859 were classified as not depressed. Convention suggested that an EPDS score of more than 10 indicates minor or major depression may be present and that further evaluation is recommended. Table 13.8 shows the results using this cut-off value and gives a sensitivity of 122/132 or 92%, and a specificity of 338/727 or 46%.

In this example, we need not have chosen an EPDS score of 10 or more as the cut-off value; we could choose any value between 0 and 27 as this is the EPDS score range. The corresponding sensitivity and specificity for each possible cut-point are given in Table 13.7. Thus, a cut-off of 5 or more would detect all those with post-natal depression, at a cost of stating that 84% of women who in fact do not have post-natal depression are depressed.

We can display these calculations by graphing the sensitivity on the *y*-axis (vertical) and the false positive rate (1 – specificity) on the *x*-axis (horizontal) for all possible cut-off values of the diagnostic test. The resulting curve is known as the *relative (or receiver) operating characteristic* (ROC) curve.

Table 13.7 Results of completing the Edinburgh Postnatal Depression Scale amongst a sample of 859 new mothers with and without postnatal depression (PND).

EPDS Score	Postnatal depression Yes	No	Total	Potential EPDS score Cut-off	Sensitivity	Specificity	1 – Specificity
0	0	24	24	0 or more	1.00	0.00	1.00
1	0	19	19	1 or more	1.00	0.03	0.97
2	0	25	25	2 or more	1.00	0.06	0.94
3	0	19	19	3 or more	1.00	0.09	0.91
4	0	29	29	4 or more	1.00	0.12	0.88
5	1	37	38	5 or more	1.00	0.16	0.84
6	0	32	32	6 or more	0.99	0.21	0.79
7	5	30	35	7 or more	0.99	0.25	0.75
8	0	37	37	8 or more	0.95	0.30	0.70
9	4	86	90	9 or more	0.95	0.35	0.65
10	*4*	*82*	*86*	*10 or more*	*0.92*	*0.46*	*0.54*
11	3	67	70	11 or more	0.89	0.58	0.42
12	10	61	71	12 or more	0.87	0.67	0.33
13	8	51	59	13 or more	0.80	0.75	0.25
14	10	35	45	14 or more	0.73	0.82	0.18
15	10	24	34	15 or more	0.66	0.87	0.13
16	8	19	27	16 or more	0.58	0.91	0.09
17	14	23	37	17 or more	0.52	0.93	0.07
18	11	9	20	18 or more	0.42	0.96	0.04
19	13	4	17	19 or more	0.33	0.98	0.02
20	8	7	15	20 or more	0.23	0.98	0.02
21	8	4	12	21 or more	0.17	0.99	0.01
22	1	1	2	22 or more	0.11	1.00	0.00
23	5	2	7	23 or more	0.11	1.00	0.00
24	4	0	4	24 or more	0.07	1.00	0.00
25	3	0	3	25 or more	0.04	1.00	0.00
26	1	0	1	26 or more	0.02	1.00	0.00
27	1	0	1	27 or more	0.01	1.00	0.00
Total	132	727	859				

Source: data from Morrell et al. (2009).

Example from the Literature – ROC – Diagnosis of Postnatal Depression Using the EPDS

The ROC curve when using the EPDS to diagnose PND is shown in Figure 13.1.

A perfect diagnostic test would be one with no false positive (that is specificity = 1) or false negative (sensitivity = 1) results and would be represented by a line that started at the origin and went up the *y*-axis to a sensitivity = 1, and then across to a false positive rate of 0 (1 – specificity = 1).

Table 13.8 Number of subjects above and below 10 on the EPDS by true diagnosis of postnatal depression from the SCAN interview.

EPDS score	True diagnosis from SCAN interview		Total
	Depressed	Not depressed	
Positive ≥ 10	122	389	511
Negative <10	10	338	348
Total	132	727	859

Source: data from Morrell et al. (2009).

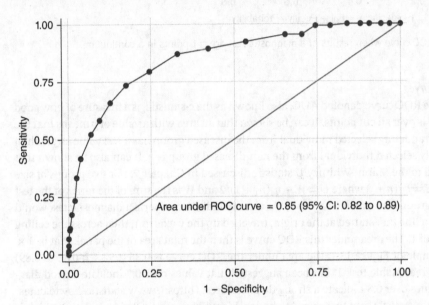

Figure 13.1 Receiver operating characteristic (ROC) curve for diagnosing PND using the EPDS (Edinburgh Postnatal Depression Scale) in new mothers (*n* = 859). (*Source:* data from Morrell et al. 2009).

A test that produces false positive results at the same rate as true positive results would produce an ROC on the diagonal line $y = x$. Any reasonable diagnostic test will display an ROC curve in the upper left triangle of Figure 13.1.

When more than one laboratory test is available for the same clinical problem one can compare ROC curves, by plotting both on the same (schematic) diagram as in Figure 13.2.

An ROC curve for a useless test will approximately lie along 45° line. The better test is the one whereby the sensitivity is always greater for a given 1 − specificity as shown in Figure 13.2. When comparing two curves overall the one with the largest area under the ROC is considered more accurate.

The selection of an optimal combination of sensitivity and specificity for a particular test requires an analysis of the relative medical consequences and costs of false positive and false negative interpretations.

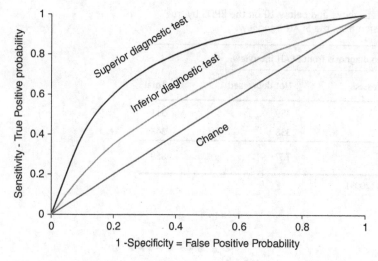

Figure 13.2 The ROC curve when results of a diagnostic test are cut-points in a continuum.

Analysis of ROC Curves

The area under the ROC curve denoted AUC, also known as the c-statistic, is a measure of how good the diagnostic test is over all cut points. It can be shown that an area with a value of p means that the probability that a randomly selected individual from the diseased group has a test value larger than that for a randomly selected individual from the non-diseased group is p. It can also be shown that the AUC is related to the Mann–Whitney U statistic discussed in Chapter 7. For two groups of size n_1 and n_2 the AUC $= U/(n_1 n_2)$ where $U = W - n_1(n_1 + 1)/2$ and W is the sum of the ranks of the test scores in the first group (Box 7.4 in Chapter 7). As already indicated, a perfect diagnostic test would be represented by a line that started at the origin, travelled up the y-axis to 1, then across the ceiling to an x-axis value of 1. The area under this ROC curve is then the total area of the panel; that is, $1 \times 1 = 1$. In the example of Figure 13.1, the area under the ROC curve is 0.85 (95% CI: 0.82 to 0.89) which indicates a reasonable test. It has been suggested that values over 0.7 indicate a good diagnostic test and values over 0.8 indicate a strong diagnostic test (https://www.statisticshowto.datasciencecentral.com/c-statistic) but these need to be considered in context. Obviously, a test which is perfect at discriminating between the disease outcomes has an AUC of 1; and a non-discriminating test, with performance no better than chance has an AUC of 0.5.

Discussion

Leeflang et al. (2013) showed in 416 studies that the assumption that sensitivity and specificity are independent of prevalence is not found in practice. They found that specificity tended to be lower with higher disease prevalence but found no such systematic effect for sensitivity. They suggest that the distribution of symptoms and severity in different populations may change with varying prevalence and this may influence sensitivity and specificity. They also suggest that the patient care pathway by which patients are referred may be influenced by the spectrum of disease in the population which again may influence sensitivity and specificity. Because it may be difficult to identify such mechanisms, they suggest clinicians should use prevalence as a guide when selecting studies that most closely match their situation to obtain the sensitivity and specificity of the test they are using.

13.10 Points When Reading the Literature About a Diagnostic Test

1) To whom has the diagnostic test been applied? It is possible that characteristics of the patients or stage and severity of the disease can influence the sensitivity of the test. For example, it is likely that a test for cancer will have greater sensitivity for advanced rather than early disease. Have the authors given enough information to enable us to be sure of the disease status?

2) How has the group of patients used in the analysis been selected, and in particular how has the decision to verify the test by the gold standard been made? A common error is to select patients in some manner for verification of a previous diagnosis; this usually leads to positive tests being over-represented in the verified sample and the sensitivity being inflated. It is also common for an investigation to assume that unverified cases are disease-free, which can lead to inflated specificity estimates. The best way to avoid such bias is to construct a prospective study in which all patients receive definite verification of disease status.

3) How have the investigators coped with specimens they were not able to interpret? If the reason for failure to interpret is essentially random, and is unrelated to disease status, then the test characteristics can be estimated. If it is related to disease status, then these results cannot be ignored when interpreting the results. In either case, the proportion of non-interpretable results should be reported in any diagnostic test efficacy study, since it is an important consideration in the cost-effectiveness of the test.

4) Did the investigator who provided the diagnostic test result know other clinical results concerning the patients? Diagnostic tests are usually carried out during or, in conjunction with, the clinical examination. Where there is an element of subjectivity in a test, such as an ECG stress test, a remarkable improvement in sensitivity can be shown when the investigator is aware of other symptoms of the patient!

5) Was the reproducibility of the test result determined? This could be done by repeating the test with different operators, or at different times, or with different machines, depending on the circumstances.

6) Did the patients who had the test actually benefit as a consequence of the test?

7) How good is the gold standard? An ideal gold standard either may not exist or be very expensive or invasive and therefore not carried out. In this case, the test used as the gold standard may be subject to error, which in turn will make the estimates of sensitivity and specificity problematical.

8) Does the report of the study follow the STAndards for the Reporting of Diagnostic accuracy studies (STARD) statement?
   http://www.stard-statement.org
   http://www.equator-network.org/reporting-guidelines/stard

Technical Details

Bayes' Theorem

A conditional probability is a probability of one event happening given that another event has also happened. For example, we may wish to know the probability that a patient has a particular disease given that they have a positive result on a diagnostic test. This conditional probability can be calculated using a result called Bayes' theorem.

For any two events A and B, the probability of A happening given that B has already happened is denoted by $P(A|B)$. This leads to what is known as *Bayes' theorem* or

$$P(A \mid B) = \frac{P(B \mid A) \times P(A)}{P(B)}.$$

This formula is not appropriate if $P(B) = 0$, that is if B is an event which cannot happen. Also, the probability of A given B, $P(A|B)$, is not the same as probability of B given A, $P(B|A)$, unless P $(A) = P(B)$.

Example: Conditional Probabilities and Diagnostic Testing

Bayes' theorem can be used to calculate the conditional probability that a patient with a positive test results on a diagnostic test really has the disease. Using the data of Table 13.1 one can use Bayes' theorem to calculate $P(D + |T+)$, probability of the patient having prostate cancer, given a positive test result. In terms of Bayes' theorem, the diagnostic process is summarised by

$$P(D + \mid T +) = \frac{P(T + \mid D +)P(D +)}{P(T +)}.$$

Here the prevalence $P(D+)$ is termed the a priori probability of disease, $P(T+)$ the probability of a positive test result, $P(D + |T+)$ the a posteriori probability, and $P(T + |D+)$ the sensitivity of the test. From Table 13.1, $P(T+) = 418/576 = 0.73$, $P(D+) = 230/576 = 0.40$ and $P(T+|D+) = 213/230 = 0.93$.

The probability of patient having the disease (prostate cancer), given a positive test result (MRI scan) is also known as the PPV of the test and for the data in Table 13.1

$$P(D + \mid T +) = \frac{\text{Sensitivity} \times \text{Prevalence}}{\text{Probability of a positive result}} = \frac{0.93 \times 0.40}{0.73} = 0.51.$$

13.11 Exercises

A new blood test is being developed to diagnose bowel cancer. Table 13.9 below shows the results of using the new test on a sample of 250 individuals with suspected bowel cancer. The new test results are compared to the gold standard test of a biopsy which provides a definitive diagnosis of the condition.

Table 13.9 Results of new blood test for diagnosis of bowel cancer in a sample of 250 individuals with suspected disease.

Test results	True diagnosis		
	Disease	No disease	Total
Positive	40	5	45
Negative	10	195	205
Total	50	200	250

13.1 What is the *prevalence* of disease (bowel cancer) in this sample?
   A 5%
   B 10%
   C 15%
   D 20%
   E 25%

13.2 What is the *sensitivity* of the new test?
   A 80%
   B 89%
   C 94%
   D 95%
   E 98%

13.3 What is the *specificity* of the new test?
   A 80%
   B 89%
   C 94%
   D 95%
   E 98%

13.4 What is the *PPV* of the new test?
   A 80%
   B 89%
   C 94%
   D 95%
   E 98%

13.5 What is the *NPV* of the new test?
   A 80%
   B 89%
   C 94%
   D 95%
   E 98%

13.6 What proportion of individuals in the sample were correctly diagnosed by the new test?
   A 80%
   B 89%
   C 94%
   D 95%
   E 98%

13.7 Which ONE of the following statements about the sensitivity of a diagnostic test is INCORRECT?
   A Given the patient has the disease, sensitivity is the proportion of times the test is positive.
   B Sensitivity is the proportion of positives (patients with a true positive diagnosis of disease) that are correctly identified by the new test.
   C Sensitivity is the probability that someone with disease has a positive test result.

D Sensitivity is one minus the proportion of false negatives (test is negative when patient has the disease).

E Sensitivity is the probability that someone has the disease when the test is positive.

13.8 Which ONE of the following statements about the specificity of a diagnostic test is INCORRECT?

A Given the subject is free of disease, specificity is the proportion of times the test will be negative.

B Specificity is the proportion of negatives (subjects with a true negative diagnosis of disease) that are correctly identified by the new test.

C Specificity is one minus the proportion of false positives (test is positive when person does not have the disease).

D Specificity is the probability that a person without disease has a negative test result.

E Specificity is the probability that someone is without disease when the test is negative.

13.9 Which ONE of the following statements about diagnostic tests is INCORRECT?

A The PPV is the proportion of patients with positive test results who are correctly diagnosed.

B The NPV is the proportion of patients with negative test results who are correctly diagnosed.

C Positive (and negative) predictive values depend on the prevalence of disease.

D Both sensitivity and specificity are conditional on having or not having the disease. They are properties of the test, not the disease.

E Both PPV and NPV are conditional on having or not having the disease.

13.10 Which ONE of the following statements about the ROC curve (when the results of a diagnostic test are cut-points in a continuum) is INCORRECT?

A The ROC curve is obtained by plotting sensitivity vs specificity for every distinct cut-off value.

B A ROC curve that is no better than chance will lie along a 45° line.

C The area under the ROC would be 1 for a perfect test.

D When comparing two ROC curves, for two different tests on the same sample, the one with the higher ROC is considered more accurate.

E The best cut-point for the diagnostic test is the one nearest the upper left-hand corner

14 Observational Studies

Medical Statistics: A Textbook for the Health Sciences, Fifth Edition. Stephen J. Walters, Michael J. Campbell, and David Machin.
© 2021 John Wiley & Sons Ltd. Published 2021 by John Wiley & Sons Ltd.
Companion website: www.wiley.com/go/walters/medicalstatistics

Summary

This chapter considers the design of observational studies: cross-sectional surveys, case–control studies and cohort studies together with the problems of inferring causality from such studies. A vital tool for eliciting information from subjects is the questionnaire and we discuss how these may be constructed and also how samples may be chosen.

14.1 Introduction

In an observational study one cannot decide which subjects get exposed to a risk, or given a new treatment. This is in contrast to the randomised controlled trial, to be described in Chapter 15. In many situations where an investigator is looking for an association between exposure to a risk factor and subsequent disease, it is not possible to randomly allocate exposure to subjects; you cannot insist that some people smoke and others do not, or randomly expose some industrial workers to radiation and protect others. Thus studies relating exposure to outcome are often observational; the investigator simply observes what happens and does not intervene. The options under the control of the investigator are restricted to the choice of subjects, whether to follow them retrospectively or prospectively, and the size of the sample.

The major problem in the interpretation of observational studies is that although an association between exposure and disease can be observed, this does not necessarily imply a causal relationship. For example, many studies have shown that smoking is associated with subsequent lung cancer. Those who refuse to believe causation argue, however, that some people are genetically susceptible to lung cancer, and this same gene predisposes them to smoke! Factors that are related to both the exposure of a risk factor and the outcome are called confounding factors (see Figure 1.1 in Chapter 1). In observational studies it is always possible to think of potential confounding factors that might explain away an argument for causality. However, some methods for strengthening the causality argument are given later in the chapter.

14.2 Risk and Rates

Although methods of summarising binary data were introduced in Chapter 3 we now provide more detail of these and some others.

Risk is Defined as:

$$\text{Risk} = \frac{\text{Number of events observed}}{\text{Number in the group}}.$$

Thus if 100 people sat down to a meal and 10 suffered food poisoning, we would say the *risk* of food poisoning was 0.1 or 10%.

Often, however, we are interested in the number of events over a period of time. This leads to the definition of a *rate*, which is the number of events, for example deaths or cases of a disease, per unit of population, in a particular time span. For example, Figure 4.2, shows that the crude United Kingdom probability of dying, or mortality rate per person per year, is about 0.010. Since this is a small number, it is usually multiplied by a larger number such as 100 000, and expressed as a mortality rate of 1000 deaths per 100 000 of the population per year.

To Calculate a Rate the Following Are Needed

1) A defined period of time (for example, a calendar year).
2) A defined population, with an accurate estimate of the size of the population during the defined period (for example the population of a city, estimated by a census).
3) The number of events occurring over the period (for example the number of deaths occurring in the city over a calendar year).

The event could be a permanent one (like death) or a temporary one (like a cold). After a permanent event the person is no longer at risk of the event, and is removed from the 'at risk' population. Strictly we should measure the amount of time that each member of the population is at risk. For people who have a permanent event this would be the time from the start of the period to the time of the event. For people who do not have an event it is the length of the period, such as one year. Usually, incidence and rates are expressed per 100,000 people.

Incidence is Defined as:

$$\text{Incidence} = \frac{\text{Number of events in a defined period}}{\text{Total person-time at risk}} \times 100000.$$

When the number of events is relatively small compared with the population at risk, then the total person-time at risk can be approximated by the mid-period population multiplied by the length of the period.

Crude Mortality Rate

When the length of the period is one year, an example of a rate is the crude mortality rate (CMR) for a particular year which is given by

$$\text{CMR} = \frac{\text{Number of deaths occuring in year}}{\text{Mid-year population}} \times 100000.$$

It is important to remember that rates must refer to a specific period of time.

Example of Crude Mortality Rates

Table 14.1 and Figure 14.1 show the number of deaths from breast cancer in females and prostate cancer in males in 19 five-year age bands; the age-specific rates (ASRs) of deaths from cancer (per 100 000) as well as the mid-year population estimates for England in 2016.

Table 14.1 shows there were 9852 male deaths from prostate cancer in England in 2016 and a mid-year population estimate of 27 300 920. The CMR for male prostate cancer is:

$$\text{CMR}_{\text{Prostate}} = \frac{9852}{27\ 300\ 920} \times 100\ 000 = 36.1 \text{ per } 100\ 000 \text{ population per year.}$$

The corresponding CMR for female breast cancer is 34.4 deaths/100 000 population per year. Thus males and females appear to have similar CMRs for prostate and breast cancer respectively.

Age-Specific Rates (ASRs)

ASRs may be calculated for each age group and these are defined as the number of deaths per 100 000 population in the same age group.

Table 14.1 Number of deaths from prostate cancer in males and breast cancer in females in England in 2016, the mid-year population estimates for England and the age-specific rates of deaths from cancer (per 100 000), and the 2013 European Standard population.

Age group k	Prostate cancer deaths 2016 d_k	Population estimates England mid-2016 Males p_k	Age-specific Prostate cancer mortality Rate/100 000 ASR_k	Breast cancer deaths 2016 d_k	Population estimates England mid-2016 Females p_k	Age-specific Breast cancer mortality Rate/100 000 ASR_k	European standard population 2013 ESP_k	Prostate $ASR_k \times ESP_k$	Breast $ASR_k \times ESP_k$
0–4	1	1 757 639	0.1	0	1 671 407	0.0	5000	284.5	0.0
5–9	0	1 755 683	0.0	0	1 672 583	0.0	5500	0.0	0.0
10–14	0	1 572 421	0.0	0	1 497 833	0.0	5500	0.0	0.0
15–19	0	1 631 799	0.0	0	1 547 611	0.0	5500	0.0	0.0
20–24	0	1 824 091	0.0	3	1 735 865	0.2	6000	0.0	1036.9
25–29	0	1 924 216	0.0	17	1 887 371	0.9	6000	0.0	5404.3
30–34	0	1 874 897	0.0	58	1 874 726	3.1	6500	0.0	20 109.6
35–39	1	1 773 846	0.1	140	1 783 165	7.9	7000	394.6	54 958.5
40–44	0	1 756 427	0.0	230	1 778 839	12.9	7000	0.0	90 508.5
45–49	12	1 919 824	0.6	463	1 963 255	23.6	7000	4375.4	165 083.0
50–54	48	1 911 583	2.5	699	1 961 512	35.6	7000	17 577.1	249 450.4
55–59	151	1 670 419	9.0	699	1 707 241	40.9	6500	58 757.7	266 131.1
60–64	325	1 436 605	22.6	725	1 494 368	48.5	6000	135 736.7	291 093.0
65–69	748	1 470 578	50.9	1012	1 561 477	64.8	5500	279 753.9	356 457.4
70–74	1152	1 137 445	101.3	1000	1 243 844	80.4	5000	506 398.1	401 979.7
75–79	1625	827 832	196.3	1053	968 214	108.8	4000	785 183.5	435 027.8
80–84	2032	584 219	347.8	1226	761 140	161.1	2500	869 536.9	402 685.4
85–89	2130	324 015	657.4	1085	516 231	210.2	1500	986 065.5	315 265.8
90 and over	1627	147 381	1103.9	1203	340 465	353.3	1000	1 103 941.5	353 340.3
	9852	27 300 920	36.1	9613	27 967 147	34.4	$\sum_k ESP_k = 100\,000$	47.5	34.1

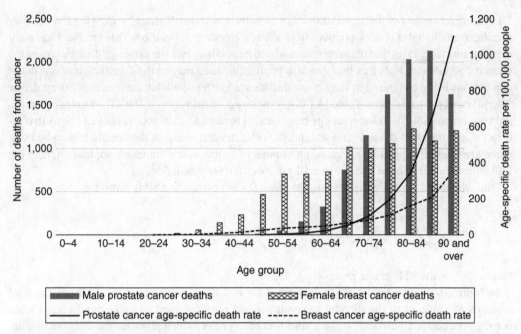

Figure 14.1 Number of deaths from breast cancer in females and prostate cancer in males and age-specific rates of deaths from cancer (per 100 000) in England, 2016. (*Source:* National Cancer Registration and Analysis Service within Public Health England; Office for National Statistics).

Age-Specific Rate

If a particular age group is specified, the age-specific mortality rate (ASR) for age group k is obtained as

$$\mathrm{ASR}_k = \frac{\text{Number of deaths occurring in specified age group } (d_k)}{\text{Mid} - \text{year number in that age group } (p_k)} \times 100\ 000.$$

Where ASR_k = age-specific rate for age group k; d_k = deaths in age group k; p_k = population in age group k = 0–4, 5–9, …, 85–89, and 90 and over years.

ASRs may be calculated separately for males and females (as in Table 14.1), or for both sexes combined. The ASRs shown in Table 14.1 and Figure 14.1 are derived from the deaths from breast and prostate cancer in England in 2016 for a particular age group and the corresponding mid-year resident population in that age-group.

Direct and Indirect Age-Standardised Rates

The incidence and mortality from cancer varies greatly with age. Thus, if we wish to compare countries for mortality, we need to allow for different age structures. For example, it would give misleading results if we compared the incidence of cancer in countries with a young population, such as those in South America, with those with an old population such as Japan, without allowing for age. One method is just to look at the age-specific death rates, but it can be helpful to have an overall summary measure and there are two ways of doing this; either using direct or indirect standardisation. These can be used to compare countries, or regions within a country or subgroups of a population such as social class.

In the *direct method* of standardisation, 'age adjusted rates' are obtained by applying the category specific mortality rates of each population to a single standard population. This produces age standardised mortality rates that these countries would have if they had the same age distribution as the standard population. Note that the 'standard population' used may be the distribution of one of the populations being compared or may be an outside standard population such as the 'European' or 'World' standard population. Table 14.1 displays the age-distribution of the 2013 European Standard Population (ESP) in 19 five-year age-bands scaled to add up to 100 000. Table 14.1 shows that in direct standardisation the age- and sex-specific rates in each group in the populations to be compared are multiplied by the corresponding number of people in the 'standard' population, here the ESP, and then summed to give an overall rate per 100 000 population.

Thus, the directly standardised mortality rate (DASR) using the ESP is given by:

$$DASR(ESP) = \frac{\sum_k (ASR_k \times ESP_k)}{\sum_k ESP_k},$$

where ESP_k is the ESP in age group k.

Such directly standardised rates are presented for breast and prostate cancer deaths in the final columns of Table 14.1. The directly age standardised rates are used to make valid comparisons between the breast cancer and prostate cancer mortality rates (which allow for the different population age structures and distributions for males and females). The DASR for prostate cancer is 47.5 per 100 000 population per year compared to 34.1 per 100 000 population per year for breast cancer. Thus, overall, the mortality rate from prostate cancer is higher than the mortality rate from breast cancer, although as can be seen from Figure 14.1 the rate for breast cancer is higher at younger age groups.

The *indirect method* of standardisation is commonly used when ASRs are not available for individual populations or the numbers within a specific population in some age groups are too small to enable accurate rate estimates. In this method, instead of taking one population structure as standard and applying sets of rates to it to estimate expected events, a set of rates from a standard population (or the comparator populations combined) is applied to each of the populations being compared to calculate standardised incidence/mortality ratios.

After lung cancer, prostate cancer is the second most common cause of death from cancer in Scottish men and 894 died from the disease in 2016 (Information Services Division (ISD) 2017). Table 14.2 uses the indirect method of standardisation to calculate how many prostate cancer deaths would be expected in Scotland if it had the same age-specific prostate cancer mortality rates as England. The expected deaths in Scotland are calculated by multiplying the ASR for England by the population of Scotland in the corresponding age group. The sum of the age categories then gives the expected total number of deaths that would be experienced in Scotland.

An overall summary measure can then be calculated, that is, the standardised mortality ratio (SMR), which is the ratio of the observed number of deaths to the expected number of deaths.

Standardised Mortality Ratio (SMR)

$$SMR = \frac{\text{Observed number of deaths } (O)}{\text{Expected number of death } (E)} \times 100.$$

From Table 14.2 the SMR = $(894/925.5) \times 100 = 97$, which means that the number of observed deaths in males from prostate cancer in Scotland in 2016 is 3% lower than the number we would expect if Scotland had the same mortality experience as England.

Table 14.2 Calculation of the indirect age standardised mortality ratio for prostate cancer in Scotland compared to England in 2016 using the mid-year population estimates for England and Scotland and the age-specific rates of deaths from prostate cancer for England.

Age group	England				Scotland	
	Prostate cancer deaths 2016	Population estimates mid-2016 males	Age-specific Prostate cancer mortality rate	Expected deaths ASR$_{Eng\_k}$ × p_{Eng_k}	Population estimates mid-2016 males	Scotland expected deaths ASR$_{Eng\_k}$ × p_{Scot_k}
k	d_{Eng_k}	p_{Eng_k}	ASR$_{Engd\_k}$		pP_{Scot_k}	p_{Scot_k}
0–4	1	1 757 639	0.000001	1	147 527	0.1
5–9	0	1 755 683	0.000000	0	152 292	0.0
10–14	0	1 572 421	0.000000	0	140 381	0.0
15–19	0	1 631 799	0.000000	0	152 614	0.0
20–24	0	1 824 091	0.000000	0	181 688	0.0
25–29	0	1 924 216	0.000000	0	186 149	0.0
30–34	0	1 874 897	0.000000	0	172 305	0.0
35–39	1	1 773 846	0.000001	1	161 268	0.1
40–44	0	1 756 427	0.000000	0	164 929	0.0
45–49	12	1 919 824	0.000006	12	189 422	1.2
50–54	48	1 911 583	0.000025	48	197 429	5.0
55–59	151	1 670 419	0.000090	151	180 737	16.3
60–64	325	1 436 605	0.000226	325	156 406	35.4
65–69	748	1 470 578	0.000509	748	153 467	78.1
70–74	1152	1 137 445	0.001013	1152	111 869	113.3
75–79	1625	827 832	0.001963	1625	82 515	162.0
80–84	2032	584 219	0.003478	2032	56 201	195.5
85–89	2130	324 015	0.006574	2130	28 287	186.0
90 and over	1627	147 381	0.011039	1627	12 017	132.7
	9852	27 300 920		9852	2 627 503	925.5
Total observed deaths (*O*)	9852					894
Total expected deaths (*E*)	9852					925.5
SMR (*O/E*) × 100	100					97

Issues in the Use of Standardisation

Standardised rates represent a weighted average of the group-specific rates taken from a 'standard population' and are not actual rates. They are commonly used for age standardisation, but can be used to compare groups with different burdens of disease (case-mix). The direct method of standardisation requires that the ASRs for all populations being studied are available and that a standard population is defined. The indirect method of standardisation requires the total number of cases. The ratio of two directly standardised rates is called the *comparative incidence ratio* or *comparative mortality ratio*. Indirect standardisation is more appropriate for use in studies with small numbers or when the rates are unstable. One major assumption in using the indirect method is that the group-specific risk is the same for each population. This may seem reasonable for age, but may not be suitable for adjusting for different case-mixes. For example the death rate from a specific disease may vary between countries simply because the diagnosis criteria differs. This assumption (the constant risk) has been shown to fail in some circumstances (Nicholl 2007).

As the choice of a standard population will affect the comparison between populations, it should always be stated clearly which standard population has been applied. Standardisation may be used to adjust for the effects of a variety of confounding factors including age, sex, race, or socio-economic status.

Incidence and Prevalence

The prevalence and incidence of a disease are closely related. If the incidence of a disease is low but the duration of disease (that is until recovery or death) is long, the prevalence will be high relative to the incidence. For example, diseases like leprosy or tuberculosis tend to persist for a longer duration, from months to years, hence the prevalence (old and new cases) would be larger than the incidence. Conversely, if the incidence of a disease is high and the duration of the disease is short, the prevalence will be low relative to the incidence. For example, acute conditions like diarrhoea have a relatively short duration (a few days) and so there will be few cases at any point in time, but the cumulative number of people suffering the disease may be quite high.

A change in the duration of a disease, for example the development of a new treatment that prevents death but does not result in a cure, will lead to the rather paradoxical result that the new treatment, which is beneficial, leads to an increase in prevalence! Fatal diseases or diseases from which a rapid recovery is common have a low prevalence, whereas diseases with a low incidence may have a high prevalence if they are incurable but rarely fatal and have a long duration.

The incidence rate refers to the number of new cases of a particular disease that develop during a specified time interval. The *prevalence* of a disease (which is strictly not a rate since no time period is specified) refers to the number of cases of disease that exist at a specified point in time. For diseases that only last a short time, sometimes the *period prevalence* is used, such as the proportion of cases of influenza over three months. Often the time period is implicit and risk and incidence are used synonymously.

14.3 Taking a Random Sample

For any observational studies, it is necessary to define the subjects chosen for the study in some way. For example, if a survey were to be conducted then a random sample of the population of interest would be required. In this situation, a simple random sample could be obtained first by numbering all the individual members in the target population, and then computer-generating random numbers from that list. Suppose the population totals 600 subjects, which are numbered 001 through to 600. If we use the first line of the random number table in Table T5 and find the random sequence 5345542567. We would take the first three subjects as 534, 554, and 256, for example. These subjects are then identified on the list and sent a questionnaire.

There are other devices which might be appropriate in specific circumstances. For example, suppose a researcher wanted to estimate the prevalence of menstrual flushing in the country. Rather than sampling a national list containing millions of women, one may first randomly choose one county from a list of counties, from within each county a sample of electoral wards, and then obtain only lists for these wards from which to select the women. Such a device is termed *multi-stage random sampling*.

In other circumstances one may wish to ensure that equal numbers of men and women are sampled. Thus the list is divided into strata (men and women) and equal numbers sampled from each stratum, and this is termed *stratified random sampling*.

14.4 Questionnaire and Form Design

Purpose of Questionnaires and Forms

It is important to distinguish between questionnaires and forms. Forms are used largely to record factual information, such as a subject's age, blood pressure or treatment group. They are commonly used in clinical trials to follow a patient's progress and are often completed by the responsible investigator. For forms, the main requirement is that the form be clearly laid out and all investigators are familiar with it. A questionnaire on the other hand, although it too may include basic demographic information, can be regarded as an instrument in its own right. For example, it may try to measure personal attributes such as attitudes, emotional status or levels of pain and is often completed by the individual concerned.

For questionnaires the pragmatic advice is, if possible, do not design your own, use someone else's! There are a number of reasons for this apparently negative advice. First, use of a standardised format means that results should be comparable between studies. Secondly, it is a difficult and time-consuming process to obtain a satisfactory questionnaire. Help with designing health measurement scales is given in Streiner et al. (2015).

Types of Questions

There are two major types of question: open or closed. In an open question respondents are asked to reply in their own words, whereas in a closed question the possible responses are given.

The advantages of open type questions are that more detailed answers are possible. They give the responders the feeling that they can express their own ideas. On the other hand, they take more time and effort to complete and they can be difficult to code and hence analyse since there may be a wide variety of disparate responses from different individuals. Closed questions can be answered by simply circling or ticking responses. When constructing responses to closed questions it is important to provide a suitable range of replies, or the responder may object to being forced into a particular category, and simply not answer the question. A useful strategy is to conduct a pilot study using open questions on a limited but representative sample of people. From their responses one can then devise suitable closed questions.

Another type of closed question is to make a statement and then ask whether the respondent agrees or disagrees. When a closed question has an odd number of responses, it is often called a Likert scale.

Some researchers prefer to omit central categories, such as 'average' or 'don't know' so as to force people to have an opinion. The danger is that if people do not wish to be forced, then they will simply not reply.

An alternative method of recording strength of feeling is by means of a visual analogue score (VAS). The VAS is scored by measuring the distance of the respondent's mark from the left-hand end of the scale.

Examples – Types of Questions

Open question
'Please describe how you feel about the treatment you have just received?'

Closed question
'How would you rate the treatment you have just received?'

(1) Excellent, (2) Good, (3) Average, (4) Poor, (5) Very poor.

Likert rating scales
'Medical statistics is not very interesting'
(a) Strongly agree, (b) Agree, (c) Don't know, (d) Disagree, (e) Strongly disagree.

Visual analogue score
'Please rate your pain by marking a line on the following scale:'

No Pain   Worst
possible
pain

14.5 Cross-sectional Surveys

A cross-sectional study describes a group of subjects at one particular point in time. It may feature the proportion of people with a particular characteristic, which is a prevalence study. It may look at how the prevalence varies by other features such as by age or gender.

Suppose an investigator wishes to determine the prevalence of menstrual flushing in women aged 45–60. Then an appropriate design may be a survey of women in that age group by means of a postal questionnaire. In such a situation, this type of survey may be conducted at, for example, a town, county, or national level. However, a prerequisite before such a survey is conducted is a list of women in the corresponding age groups. Once such a list is obtained it may be possible to send a postal questionnaire to all women on the list. More usually one may wish to draw a sample from the list and the questionnaire be sent to this sample. The sampling proportion will have to be chosen carefully. It is important that those women who are selected are selected by an appropriate random sampling technique.

In some situations a visit by an interviewer to those included in the sample may be more appropriate than a postal survey. However, this may be costly both in time and money and will require the training of personnel. As a consequence, this will usually imply a smaller sample than that possible by means of a postal questionnaire. On the other hand, response rates to postal questionnaires may be low. A low response rate can cause considerable difficulty in interpretation of the results as it can always be argued (whether true or not) that non-responders are atypical with respect to the problem being investigated and therefore estimates of prevalence, necessarily obtained from the responders only, will be inherently biased. Thus in a well-designed survey, every attempt should be made to keep the numbers of non-responders to a minimum, and the potential non-response rate taken into account when estimating sample size.

Volunteers as participants in cross-sectional surveys often present considerable problems. Suppose one is interested in the prevalence of hypertension in a community then one approach might be to ask volunteers to come forward by advertising in the local newspaper. The difficulty here is that people may volunteer simply because they are worried about their blood pressure (this is known as *selection bias*) and also there is no way one can ascertain the response rate, or investigate reasons why people did not volunteer. A better approach would be to take a random sample from the community, either from an electoral roll or a general practitioner, and then invite each one individually to have their blood pressure measured. In that way the response rate is known and the non-responders identified. In contrast, if the object of interest is a relationship within subjects, for example physiological responses to increasing doses of a drug, then one cannot avoid the use of volunteers.

Market research organisations have complex sampling schemes that often contain elements of randomisation. However, in essence they are grab or convenience samples, in that only subjects who are available to the interviewer can be questioned. So-called *quota samples* ensure that the sample is representative of the general population in say, age, gender and social class structure. Problems associated with the interpretation of quota samples are discussed in detail by Machin and Campbell (2005). They are not recommended, in general, for use in medical research.

Other biases are possible in cross-sectional studies. Consider a study that reveals a negative association between height and age. Possible interpretations include: people shrink as they get older, younger generations are getting taller, or tall people have a higher mortality than short people!

One of the differences between a cross-sectional study and other designs discussed in this chapter is that in the latter subjects are included without reference to either their exposure or their disease. Cross-sectional studies usually deal with exposures that do not change, such as blood type or chronic smoking habit. However, in occupational studies a cross-sectional study might contain all workers in a factory, and their exposures determined by a retrospective work-history. Here the problem is the *healthy worker effect* in that people in work tend to be healthier than people not in work, even those in jobs which expose them to health hazards. A cross-sectional study resembles a case–control study (see Section 15.8) except that the numbers of cases are not known in advance, but are simply the prevalent cases at the time of the survey.

Example from the Literature – Prevalence of Asthma in Greece

Gangadi et al. (2016) evaluated the prevalence of asthma in a randomly selected sample representative of the adult general population in Greece. A total of 5137 participants were included using a multi-stage stratified random sampling method, involving localities throughout the country. Information on asthma and asthma-like symptoms (ALS) during the last 12 months was collected through questionnaires administered by trained interviewers. Prevalence of asthma and ALS was determined taking into account the design of the study and additional adjustments for age and sex. The prevalence was found to be 6.3% (CI 95%: 5.6 to 7.0%) and it was higher in women than in men (7.2% vs 5.3% $p = 0.011$).

14.6   Non-randomised Studies

Pre-test/Post-test Studies

A pre-test/post-test study is one in which a group of individuals are measured, then subjected to an intervention, and then measured again. The purpose of the study is to observe the size of the resulting effect. The major problem is ascribing the change in the measurement to the intervention since other factors may also have changed in that interval.

Example from the Literature – Before-and-After Studies
Christie (1979) describes a consecutive series of patients admitted to a hospital with stroke in 1974 who were then followed prospectively until death and their survival time determined. Subsequently

Table 14.3 Survival pre- and post-availability of a CT scan.

Survival	CT scan in 1978	
	Yes	No
1978 better than 1974	9 (31%)	34 (38%)
1978 equal to 1974	18 (62%)	38 (43%)
1978 worse than 1974	2 (7%)	17 (19%)
	29	89

Source: data from Christie (1979).

a CT head scanner was installed in the hospital and so in 1978 the study was repeated so that the scanner could be evaluated.

Successive patients in the 1978 series who had had a CT scan were matched by age, diagnosis, and level of consciousness with patients in the 1974 series. A total of 29 matched pairs were obtained and their survival times compared. The results, given in Table 14.3, column 2, appeared to show a marked improvement in the 1978 patients over those from 1974 with 31% with better survival and only 7% worse. This was presumed to be due to the CT scanner.

However, the study was then extended to an analysis of the 1978 patients who had *not* had a CT scan (Table 14.3, column 3) compared with a matched group of 89 patients from 1974 using the same matching criteria. This second study again found an improvement; with 38% of the 1978 patients were doing better than the 1974 patients, and 19% doing worse. Thus looking at the two components of the study together, then whether or not patients had received a CT scan, the outcome had improved over the years.

In the absence of the control study, the comparison of patients who had had no CT scan, the investigators may well have concluded that the installation of a CT head scanner had improved patient survival time. There are two possible explanations of the apparent anomaly. One is to suppose that other improvements in treatment, unrelated to CT scanning, had taken place between 1974 and 1978. The other is to ask what would a clinician do with a stroke patient even if he knew the outcome of a CT scan? The answer is, usually, very little. It is therefore possible that the patients in 1978 were, in fact, less seriously ill than those in 1974, despite the attempts at matching, and hence would live longer.

However, in certain circumstances before-and-after studies without control groups are unavoidable if the design is not under the direct control of the investigator. Such situations may arise when national policy legislates for a change, for example compulsory seat belt wearing, the value of which may still need to be evaluated.

Example from the Literature – Observational Study – Acute Myocardial Infarction
In June 2002 the town of Helena, Montana, USA imposed a law requiring smoke-free work and public places but in December 2002 opponents won a court order suspending enforcement. Sargent et al. (2004) found that there were 24 admissions to hospital for acute myocardial infarction in the six months of the smoking ban, compared with an average of 40 for the same six months in the years before and after the ban (difference 16 admissions, 95% CI 0.3 to 31.7). They concluded that the smoking ban may reduce morbidity from heart disease, and this result encouraged smoking bans in other areas.

Quasi-experimental Designs

A prospective study that has both a test group and a control group, but in which the treatment is not allocated at random, is known as a quasi-experimental design. It is often used to take advantage of information on the merits of a new treatment that is being implemented in one group of patients, but where randomisation is difficult or impossible to implement.

The main disadvantage of a quasi-experimental study is that, because treatments are not randomised to the subjects, it is impossible to state at the outset that the subjects are comparable in the two groups. Thus, for example, when comparing survival rates in patients undergoing different types of surgery each performed by different surgeons, it is possible that different surgeons will have different selection thresholds of risk for admitting patients to surgery. As a consequence, any difference in mortality observed between types of surgical intervention may be clouded by systematic patient differences, and hence not reflect the relative mortality of the surgical alternatives.

Example from the Literature – Quasi-experimental Study – Cancer in Gulf War Veterans
Macfarlane et al. (2003) compared the incidence rates of cancer in UK service personnel who were deployed in the Gulf War of 1990 to the incidence rate for service personnel not employed in the Gulf War. They followed up 51 721 Gulf War veterans for 11 years, and chose a control group of 50 755 personnel matched for age, gender, rank, service, and level of fitness. There were 270 incident cancers in those who went to the Gulf, compared with 269 in the control, an incidence rate ratio for all cancers of 0.99 (95% CI 0.83 to 1.17). It was concluded that there was no excess risk of cancer in Gulf War veterans.

Clearly it is impossible to randomly choose whether people went to the Gulf or not, but there is no reason to suppose that people selected for Gulf service were at any different risk of cancer at the time than those not selected, when age, gender, and other factors are controlled for.

Interrupted Time Series

Interrupted time series (ITS) analysis is arguably the strongest quasi-experimental research design. The approach usually involves constructing a time series of population-level rates for a particular quality improvement focus and testing for a change in the outcome rate in the time periods before and time periods after implementation of a policy/programme designed to change the outcome. In parallel, investigators often analyse rates of negative outcomes that might be (unintentionally) affected by the policy/programme. The main strengths of ITS is the ability to control for secular trends in the data (unlike a before-and-after study) and it lends itself to easy graphical presentation of results. The limitations of ITS include the need for a number of time periods before and after an intervention to evaluate changes statistically, difficulty in analysing the independent impact of separate components of a programme that are implemented close together in time, and existence of a suitable control population.

Example of an Interrupted Time Series

Pearson et al. (2016) took advantage of a six-day closure of London Heathrow Airport in April 2010 caused by volcanic ash to examine if there was a decrease in emergency cardiovascular hospital admissions during or immediately after the closure period, using an interrupted daily time-series study design. The population living within the 55 dB(A) noise contour was substantial at 0.7 million. The average daily admission count was 13.9 (SD 4.4). After adjustment for covariates, there was no evidence of a decreased risk of hospital admission from cardiovascular disease during the closure period – relative risk 0.97 (95% CI 0.75 to 1.26).

14.7 Cohort Studies

A cohort is a component of a population identified so that its characteristics for example, causes of death or numbers contracting a certain disease can be ascertained as it ages through time.

The term 'cohort' is often used to describe those born during a particular year but can be extended to describe any designated group of persons who are traced over a period of time. Thus, for example, we may refer to a cohort born in 1950, or to a cohort of people who ever worked in a particular factory. A cohort study, which may also be referred to as a follow-up, longitudinal, or prospective study, is one in which subsets of a defined population can be identified who have been exposed (or will be exposed) to a factor which may influence the probability of occurrence of a given disease or other outcome. A study may follow two groups of subjects, one group exposed to a potential toxic hazard, the other not, to see if the exposure influences, for example, the occurrence of certain types of cancers. Cohort studies are usually confined to studies determining and investigating aetiological factors, and do not allocate the equivalent of treatments. They are termed observational studies, since they simply *observe* the progress of individuals over time.

Design

The progress of a cohort study is described in Figure 14.2 and Table 14.4 provides the corresponding notation. Thus members of the 'without' disease group are first identified (clearly those who already have the disease of interest are not of concern here) and their 'exposure' status determined. They are then followed for a pre-specified duration after which time their disease status (present/absent) is determined.

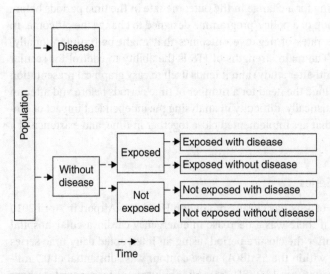

Figure 14.2 Definition and progress of a cohort study.

Table 14.4 Notation for a cohort study.

Develop the disease in the follow-up period	Risk factor Exposed	Risk factor Not exposed	Total
Yes	a	b	$a + b$
No	c	d	$c + d$
Total	$a + c$	$b + d$	N

Relative Risk

From Table 14.4, the risk of developing the disease within the follow-up time is $a/(a + c)$ for the exposed population and $b/(b + d)$ for the unexposed population.

The relative risk (RR) is the ratio of these two, that is

$$\text{RR} = \frac{a/(a + c)}{b/(b + d)} = \frac{a(b + d)}{b(a + c)}.$$

Example from the Literature – Cohort Study – Mortality in Slate Workers

Campbell et al. (2005) studied a cohort of people living in towns in North Wales associated with slate mining. Over a period of 24 years they followed up a group of men who worked or had worked with slate and a control group comprising men who had never been exposed to slate dust. The slate workers and controls were well matched for age and smoking habit. The results are given in Table 14.5.

The risk of death to slate workers is $379/726 = 0.5220$ whilst that for the non-slate workers is $230/529 = 0.4348$, giving RR $= 0.5220/0.4348 = 1.20$ with 95% CI 1.07 to 1.36 (see Section 14.12).

In fact the published report took note of the actual survival times and so analysed this study using the survival techniques of Chapter 11. They found a hazard ratio HR $= 1.24$ (95% CI 1.04 to 1.47, $p = 0.015$) and concluded that exposure to slate increases a man's risk of death at any point in time by about 25%.

It is useful to note that in this study the RR and HR are numerically close.

Table 14.5 Results of a slate workers study.

Outcome:	Exposure or risk factor – occupation Slate worker	Exposure or risk factor – occupation Non-slate worker
Died in follow-up period	379	230
Survived follow-up period	347	299
Total	726	529

Source: data from Campbell et al. (2005).

The Population Attributable Risk

If very few men were exposed to slate dust, the effect of slate exposure on the health of the population is not going to be large, however serious the consequences for the individual. The effect of a risk factor on community health is related to both relative risk and the percentage of the population exposed to the risk factor and this can be measured by the attributable risk (AR).

Attributable Risk

The terminology is not standard, but if $I_{Population}$ is the incidence of a disease in the population and I_E and I_{NE} are the incidence in the exposed and not exposed respectively, then the excess incidence attributable to the risk factor is simply $I_{Population} - I_{NE}$ and the population AR is

$$AR = (I_{Population} - I_{NE})/I_{Population}.$$

That is the proportion of the population risk that can be associated with the risk factor.

Some authors define the *excess risk* (or *absolute risk difference*) as $I_E - I_{NE}$ and the population AR as $(I_E - I_{NE})/I_{NE}$, but the definition given above has the advantage of greater logical consistency.

If we define, from Table 14.4, $\theta_E = (a + b)/N$ to be the proportion of the population exposed to the risk factor, then it can be shown that

$$AR = \frac{\theta_E(RR - 1)}{1 + \theta_E(RR - 1)}.$$

The advantage of this formula is that it enables us to calculate the AR from the relative risk, and the proportion of the population exposed to the risk factor. Both of these can be estimated from cohort studies and also from case–control studies in certain circumstances when the controls are a random sample of the population.

Worked Example – Attributable Risk

The RR of dying for slate workers compared to non-slate workers is RR = 1.20 and RR – 1 = 1.20 – 1 = 0.20. Suppose the slate workers represented 5% of the population in the towns in North Wales where they lived, then the AR = $(0.05 \times 0.20)/(1 + 0.05 \times 0.20) = 0.01$, or about 1%. Thus one might conclude that slate working increased overall mortality by about 1% in those towns.

Why Quote a Relative Risk?

The relative risk provides a convenient summary of the outcome of a cohort study. It is in many cases independent of the incidence of the disease and so is more stable than the individual risks. For example, if we studied the effect of slate exposure on a different population of men, the death rate in the unexposed group may be different, say for illustration half that of the original population. The incidence or death rate in the exposed group is also likely to be half that of the first group, and so the relative risk of slate exposure compared with non-exposure remains unaltered.

Also, it is often the case that if a factor in addition to the principal one under study acts independently on the disease process, then the joint relative risk is just the product of the two relative risks.

Thus if smokers, had a relative risk of 2.0 of dying compared with non-smokers, then the risk of dying amongst smokers who are also exposed to slate is likely to be $2.0 \times 1.2 = 2.4$.

The interpretation of cohort studies is often that much more difficult than that for a randomised trial as bias may influence the measure of interest. For example, to determine in a cohort study if the rate of cardiovascular disease is raised in men sterilised by vasectomy, it is necessary to have a comparison group of non-vasectomised men. However, comparisons between these two groups of men may be biased as it is clearly not possible to randomise men to sterilisation or non-sterilisation groups. Men who are seeking sterilisation would certainly not accept the 'no sterilisation' option. Thus the comparison that will be made here is between those men who opt for sterilisation against those who do not, and there may be inherent biases present when comparisons are made between the two groups. For example, the vasectomised men may be fitter or better educated than the non-vasectomised men and this may influence cardiovascular disease rates.

In the design of a cohort study, careful consideration before commencement of the study must be taken to identify and subsequently measure important prognostic variables that may differ between the exposure groups. Provided they are recorded, differences in these baseline characteristics between groups can be adjusted for in the final analysis.

Size of Study

The required size of a cohort study depends not only on the size of the risk being investigated but also on the incidence of the particular condition under investigation. In the vasectomy example, cardiovascular events are not particularly rare amongst a cohort of men aged 40–50, and this may determine that the cohort of middle-aged men be investigated. On the other hand, if a rare condition were being investigated very few events would be observed amongst many thousands of subjects, whether exposed to the 'insult' of interest or not. This usually prevents the use of cohort studies to investigate aetiological factors in rare diseases.

Problems in Interpretation of Cohort Studies

When the cohort is made up of employed individuals, the risk of dying in the first few years of follow-up is generally less than that of the general population and so we have the 'healthy worker' effect. It is due to the fact that people who are sick are less likely to be employed. It is also known that people who respond to questionnaires are likely to be fitter than those who do not. Both these effects can lead to problems in the interpretation of risks from employed populations. Another problem arises when follow-up is poor, or when it is more complete for the exposed group than for the unexposed group. We are then led to ask: Are the people lost to follow-up different in any way and could a poor follow-up bias the conclusions?

Post-marketing Surveillance

Post-marketing surveillance is a particular type of cohort study carried out on a population of people receiving an established drug. In such an example, a drug that is in routine use nationwide may be monitored; not for its efficacy but for any untoward medical event happening to patients receiving the drug. The incidence of such adverse events with the new drug is then compared with the incidence in patients receiving alternatives to the new medicine.

14.8 Case–Control Studies

Design

A case–control study, also known as a case-referent study or retrospective study, starts with the identification of persons with the disease (or other outcome variable) of interest, and a suitable control (reference) group of persons without the disease. The relationship of a risk factor to the disease is examined by comparing the diseased and non-diseased with regard to how frequently the risk factor is present. If the variable under consideration is quantitative, the average levels of the risk factor in the cases and controls are utilised.

The design and progress of a case–control study is shown in Figure 14.3. Here people with a disease and select a group of controls who do not have the disease are identified. Then whether, in the past, how much exposure to the risk factor of interest each group has had is retrospectively determined.

There are two possible variations in design. The control subjects can be chosen to match individual cases for certain important variables such as age and gender, leading to what is known as a matched design. Alternatively the controls can be a sample from a suitable non-diseased population, leading to an unmatched design. It is a common misconception that there must be matching criteria in all case–control studies, but this is not so. However, it is important that the statistical analysis utilised reflects the chosen design.

Unmatched Study

As just indicated, in an unmatched design the controls can be a sample from a suitable non-diseased population and Table 14.6 gives the notation for this situation.

Example from the Literature – Case-Control Study – Mobile Phone Use and Glioma
Hepworth et al. (2006) describe a case–control study of mobile phone use and glioma (a type of brain tumour). The cases were 966 people with diagnosed with a glioma between certain dates.

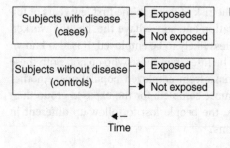

Figure 14.3 Design and progress of a case–control study.

Table 14.6 Notation for an unmatched case–control study.

Risk factor	Cases (with disease)	Controls (without disease)
Exposed	a	b
Not exposed	c	d
Total	a + c	b + d

Table 14.7   Results from a case–control study on glioma and mobile phone use.

Mobile phone use	Cases	Controls
Regular	508	898
Never/non-regular	456	818
Total	964	1716

Source: data from Hepworth et al. (2006).

The controls were randomly selected from general practitioner lists. Telephone use was defined as regular use for at least six months in the period up to one year before diagnosis.

The controls were interviewed in exactly the same way as the cases, using a computer assisted personal interview. The results of the study are summarised in Table 14.7.

The question of interest is the relative risk of glioma in people who regularly use mobile phones. This cannot be estimated directly in a case–control study because, as discussed below, a case–control study is retrospective, and relative risk is measured in a prospective cohort study. Instead the odds ratio for exposure and disease (as defined in Chapter 3) is calculated.

Odds Ratio

From Table 14.6, given that a subject has a disease, the odds of having been exposed are a/c. Given that a subject does not have a disease, the odds of having been exposed are b/d. Then the odds ratio is

$$OR = \frac{a/c}{b/d} = \frac{ad}{bc}.$$

An OR of unity implies that cases are no more likely to be exposed to the risk factor than controls.

Worked Example – Odds Ratio – Mobile Phone Use and Glioma
From Table 14.7 the odds ratio for mobile phone use and glioma is

$$OR = (508 \times 818)/(456 \times 898) = 1.01$$

The corresponding 95% CI is 0.87 to 1.19 (see Section 14.12). This shows that regular phone users are no more at risk of glioma than never or non-regular users. As the confidence interval is narrow we have good evidence that there is little or no effect as the null hypothesis value of OR = 1 is within this narrow interval.

Matched Studies

In some case–control studies each case is matched on an individual basis with a particular control. In this situation the analysis should take matching into account. The notation for a matched case–control study is given in Table 14.8.

In this situation we classify each of the N case–control pairs by exposure of the case and the control. An important point here is that the concordant pairs, that is, situations where the case and control are either both exposed or both not exposed, tell us nothing about the risk of exposure

Table 14.8 Notation for a matched case–control study.

Cases	Controls		Total
	Exposed	**Not exposed**	**Total**
Exposed	e	f	a
Not exposed	g	h	c
Total	b	d	N

separately for cases or controls. Consider a situation where it was required to discriminate between two students in tests which resulted in either a simple pass or fail. If the students are given a variety of tests, in some they will both pass and in some they will both fail. However, it is only by the tests where one student passes and the other fails, that a decision as to who is better can be given.

Odds Ratio for a Matched Case–Control Study

The odds ratio for a matched case–control study is given by

$$OR = f/g.$$

The main purpose of matching is to permit the use of efficient analytical methods to control for confounding variables that might influence the case–control comparison. In addition it can lead to a clear identification of appropriate controls. However, matching can be wasteful and costly if the matching criteria lead to many available controls being discarded because they fail the matching criteria. In fact if controls are too closely matched to their respective cases, the odds ratio may be underestimated. Usually it is worthwhile matching only one, or at most two or three, variables which are presumed or known to influence outcome strongly, common variables being age, gender, and social class.

Example from the Literature – Matched Case Control Study – Adverse Childhood or Adult
Experiences and Risk of Bilateral Oophorectomy
Gazzuola Rocca et al. (2017) matched 128 women who underwent bilateral oophorectomy before age 46 years for a non-cancerous condition (cases) and 128 age-matched (within one year) controls. A bilateral oophorecectomy is surgical removal of both ovaries. One variable of interest was whether or not women who suffered adverse childhood experiences (ACEs) or adult abuse are at increased risk of undergoing bilateral oophorectomy before menopause. ACEs were summarised using the ACE score. The 10-item ACE score has been used to assess long-term effects of childhood adversity on later health and illness. The ACE score was derived from information abstracted from medical records rather than from a patient interview. The results are given in Table 14.9.

The odds ratio for an ACE as a risk for bilateral oophorectomy is given by OR = 42/13 = 3.23, with 95% CI 1.79 to 5.82 (see Section 14.12); suggesting that women who suffered ACEs are at increased risk of undergoing bilateral oophorectomy before menopause.

Analysis by Matching?

In many case–control studies, matching is not used with the control of bias or increase of precision of the odds ratio in mind, but merely as a convenient criterion for choosing controls. Thus for

Table 14.9 Results of matched case control study to investigate the possible association between adverse childhood experience (ACE score ⩾ 1) before age of 19 and the occurrence of bilateral oophorectomy.

Cases (bilateral oophorectomy)	Controls (women without oophorectomy)		
ACE score ⩾ 1	ACE score ⩾ 1		
	Yes	No	Total
Yes	59	42	101
No	13	14	27
Total	72	56	128

Source: from Gazzuola Rocca et al. (2017).

example, a control is often chosen to be of the same sex, of a similar age and with the same physician as the case for convenience. The question then arises whether one should take this matching into account in the analysis. The general rule is that the analysis should reflect the design.

Selection of Controls

The general principle in selecting controls is to select subjects who *might* have been cases in the study, and to select them independently of the exposure variable. Thus if the cases were all treated in one particular hospital the controls should represent people who, had they developed the disease, would also have gone to the same hospital. Note that this is not the same as selecting hospital controls (see the example below). Since a case–control study is designed to estimate relative, and not absolute, risks, it is not essential that the controls be representative of all those subjects without the disease, as has been sometimes suggested. It is also not correct to require that the control group be alike in every respect to the cases, apart from having the disease of interest. As an example of this 'over-matching' consider a study of oestrogens and endometrial cancer. The cases and controls were both drawn from women who had been evaluated by uterine dilatation and curettage. Such a control group is inappropriate because agents that cause one disease in an organ often cause other diseases or symptoms in that organ. In this case it is possible that oestrogens cause other diseases of the endometrium, which requires the women to have dilatation and curettage and so present as possible controls.

The choice of the appropriate control population is crucial to a correct interpretation of the results.

Confounding

Confounding arises when an association between an exposure and an outcome is being investigated, but the exposure and outcome are both strongly associated with a third variable. An extreme example of confounding is 'Simpson's paradox', when the third factor reverses the apparent association between the exposure and outcome.

Table 14.10 A hypothetical illustration of Simpson's paradox.

Vital status	Insulin dependent	
	No	Yes
Alive	326	253
Dead	218	105
Total	544	358
Percentage dead	40%	29%

Vital status	Patients aged ≤ 40 insulin dependent		Patients age > 40 insulin dependent	
	No	Yes	No	Yes
Alive	15	129	311	124
Dead	0	1	218	104
	15	130	529	228
Percentage dead	0%	1%	41%	46%

Source: Julious and Mullee 1994.

Example from the Literature – Simpson's Paradox

As an illustration of Simpson's paradox, Julious and Mullee (1994) give an example describing a cohort study of patients with diabetes; where the exposure was type of diabetes (insulin or non-insulin dependent) and the outcome was mortality.

It would appear from the top panel of Table 14.10 that a higher proportion of patients (40%) with non-insulin dependent diabetes died compared to 29% with insulin dependent diabetes, implying that non-insulin diabetes carried a higher risk of mortality. However, non-insulin diabetes usually develops after the age of 40. Indeed when the patients are split into those aged <40 years and those aged ⧠40, it is found that in both age groups a smaller proportion of patients with non-insulin diabetes died compared with those with insulin diabetes (0% versus 1% and 41% versus 46%). As might be expected, the insulin-dependent patients had the higher mortality.

Thus, a problem arises when the outcome (mortality) and the variable of interest (the exposure – type of diabetes) is expected to be confounded with another factor (age) or when there is an important imbalance of a factor at the different levels of the variable of interest (such as an imbalance in the proportion of the sexes on two treatments). To adjust for this, factors such as age should also be included in a multiple regression or multiple logistic regression model together with the exposure variable of interest.

Limitations of Case–Control Studies

Ascertainment of exposure in case–control studies relies on previously recorded data or on memory, and it is difficult to ensure lack of bias between the cases and the controls. Since they are suffering a disease, cases are likely to be more motivated to recall possible risk factors. One of the major difficulties with case–control studies is in the selection of a suitable control group, and this has often been a major source of criticism of published case–control studies. This has led some investigators to regard them purely as a hypothesis-generating tool, to be corroborated subsequently by a cohort study.

14.9   Association and Causality

Once an association between a risk factor and disease has been identified, a number of questions should be asked to try to strengthen the argument that the relationship is causal. These are known as the *Bradford Hill* criteria.

1) Consistency. Have other investigators and other studies in different populations led to similar conclusions?
2) Plausibility. Are the results biologically plausible? For example, if a risk factor is associated with cancer, are there known carcinogens in the risk factor?
3) Dose–response. Are subjects with a heavy exposure to the risk factor at greater risk of disease than those with only slight exposure?
4) Temporality. Does the disease incidence in a population increase or decrease following increasing or decreasing exposure to a risk factor? For example, lung cancer in women increased some years after the numbers of women taking up smoking increased.
5) Strength of the relationship. A large relative risk may be more convincing than a small one (even if the latter is statistically significant). The difficulty with statistical significance is that it is a function of the sample size as well as the size of any possible effect. In any study where large numbers of groups are compared some statistically significant differences are bound to occur.
6) Reversibility. If the putative cause is removed, the effect should diminish. For example, lung cancer in men is diminished, sometime after the prevalence of smoking in men declined.
7) No other convincing explanations are available. For example, the result is not explained by confounding.

14.10   Modern Causality Methods and Big Data

There are numerous problems in ascribing causality to observational data as attested to by recent debates on, say, the role of dietary fat or the use of hormone replacement therapy (HRT) in heart disease, the role of serum serotonin in the prevention of depression. The Bradford Hill criteria cannot prove causality, they just provide some means of strengthening the causal argument. The basic problem is that all observational studies can only measure correlation and there are many ways in which spurious correlations can arise. In recent years, there have been many advances in epidemiological methods covered by the general topic of *causal inference* (see Hernán and Robins 2017) which are beyond the scope of this book. The proponents of these techniques argue that their methods can strengthen causality arguments, but at a cost of being more opaque. Contemporaneous with this is the rise of disciplines such as *data science* and the availability of large data sets, garnered by routine electronic surveillance, known collectively as *big data*. Time will tell whether these methods will provide greater insight into the relationships between exposures and health. However, it is well to be cautious of analysing data when the reason for collection is somewhat obscure. If there is some bias in the way the data are generated, then increasing the size of the data set will not reduce the bias, and if the factors associated with the bias are not measured, then statistical models will not be able to account for it.

For example, in 2009, a team of researchers from Google announced a remarkable achievement in the journal *Nature*. They were able to track the spread of influenza across the USA more quickly than the Centers for Disease Control and Prevention (CDC). Google's tracking had only a day's delay, compared with the week or more it took for the CDC to assemble a picture based on reports from doctors' surgeries. Google was faster because it was tracking the outbreak by finding a correlation between what people searched for online and whether they had flu symptoms. However four years later Google's model pointed to a severe outbreak of flu but when the data from the CDC arrived, they showed that Google's estimates of the spread of flu-like illnesses were overstated by almost a factor of two. The problem was that Google did not know what linked the search terms with the spread of flu. Google's engineers were not trying to figure out what caused what, they were merely finding statistical patterns in the data. They cared about correlation rather than causation. This is common in big data analysis. Figuring out what causes what is hard. Figuring out what is correlated with what is much cheaper and easier. A theory-free analysis of mere correlations is inevitably fragile. If one has no idea what is behind a correlation, you have no idea what might cause that correlation to break down. One explanation of the flu trends failure is that the news was full of scary stories about flu and that these stories provoked internet searches by people who were healthy. Another possible explanation is that Google's own search algorithm moved the goalposts when it began automatically suggesting diagnoses when people entered medical symptoms.

14.11 Points When Reading the Literature

1) In a cohort study, have a large percentage of the cohort been followed up, and have those lost to follow-up been described by their measurements at the start of the study?
2) How has the cohort been selected? Is the method of selection likely to influence the variables that are measured?
3) In a case–control study, are the cases likely to be typical of people with the disease? If the cases are not typical, how generalisable are the results likely to be?
4) In a matched case–control study, has allowance been made for matching in the analysis?
5) In any observational study, what are the possible biases? How have they been minimised and have the Bradford Hill criteria been considered?

14.12 Technical Details

Confidence Interval for a Relative Risk

Given the notation of Table 14.4 the standard error of the log relative risk for large samples is given by

$$\text{SE}(\log \text{RR}) = \sqrt{\left(\frac{1}{a} - \frac{1}{a+c} + \frac{1}{b} - \frac{1}{b+d}\right)}.$$

The reason for computing the standard error on the logarithmic scale is that this is more likely to be Normally distributed than the RR itself. It is important to note that when transformed back to the original scale, the confidence interval so obtained will be asymmetric about the RR. There will be a shorter distance from the lower confidence limit to the RR than from the RR to the upper confidence limit.

Worked Example

From the data of Table 14.5, RR = 1.20 and so log RR = 0.061, and

$$\text{SE(logRR)} = \sqrt{\left(\frac{1}{379} - \frac{1}{726} + \frac{1}{230} - \frac{1}{529}\right)} = 0.061.$$

Thus a 95% CI for log(RR) is 0.191−1.96 × 0.061 to 0.191 + 1.96 × 0.061 or 0.063 to 0.302. The corresponding 95% CI for the RR is exp(0.063) to exp(0.302) or 1.07 to 1.36

CI for an Odds Ratio

Using the notation of Table 14.6 the standard error of the log OR, in large samples, is given by

$$\text{SE(logOR)} = \sqrt{\left(\frac{1}{a} + \frac{1}{b} + \frac{1}{c} + \frac{1}{d}\right)}.$$

Worked Example

For the data of Table 14.7, OR = 1.01 and so log OR = 0.015, whilst

$$\text{SE(logOR)} = \sqrt{\left(\frac{1}{508} + \frac{1}{898} + \frac{1}{456} + \frac{1}{818}\right)} = 0.081.$$

This gives a 95% CI of −0.143 to 0.173.
The corresponding 95% CI for the OR is exp(−0.143) to exp(0.173) or 0.87 to 1.19.

CI for Matched Case Control Study

McNemar's test for matched pairs for testing independence between disease and exposure is:

$$\chi^2_{\text{McN}} = \frac{(f-g)^2}{f+g} \text{ or, for small studies,} \chi^2_{\text{McN-CC}} = \frac{[|f-g|-1]^2}{f+g}$$

which approximately follows a χ^2 distribution with one degree of freedom if the null hypothesis is true. A test-based 95% confidence interval (based on McNemar's test) for the odds ratio for the matched pairs is from $\text{OR}^{\left(1-1.96/\sqrt{\chi^2_{\text{McN}}}\right)}$ to $\text{OR}^{\left(1+1.96/\sqrt{\chi^2_{\text{McN}}}\right)}$. Note that this is an approximation and more accurate, but more complicated, formulas are given by Fagerland et al. (2017, Chapter 4).

Worked Example

For the data of Table 14.9 the odds ratio for an ACE as a risk for bilateral oophorectomy is given by

$$\text{OR} = f/g = 42/13 = 3.23 \text{ and } \chi^2_{\text{McN}} = \frac{(42-13)^2}{42+13} = 15.29.$$

The lower and upper 95% CI limits for the odds ratio are:

$$\text{OR}_{\text{Lower}} = 3.23^{\left(1-1.96/\sqrt{15.29}\right)} = 1.79 \text{ to } \text{OR}_{\text{Upper}} = 3.23^{\left(1+1.96/\sqrt{15.29}\right)} = 5.82.$$

14.13 Exercises

Table 14.11 shows the results of a prospective study of mortality in relation to smoking habits and 20 years' observations on a cohort of male British doctors. In 1951 the British Medical Association forwarded to all British doctors a questionnaire about their smoking habits, and 34 440 men replied. With few exceptions, all men who replied in 1951 were followed up for 20 years. The certified causes of all 10 072 deaths and subsequent changes in smoking habits were recorded (Doll and Peto 1976).

Table 14.11 Mortality in relation to smoking – 20 years' observations on male British doctors.

Died from any cause	Current or ex-smoker	Non-smoker	Totals
Yes	9132	940	10 072
No	19 495	4873	24 368
Total	28 627	5813	34 440

Source: data from Doll and Peto (1976).

14.1 From the data in Table 14.11 what proportion of subjects in the exposed (current or ex-smoker) group died from any cause in the 20-year follow-up?

A 0.162
B 0.292
C 0.319
D 0.681
E 0.838

14.2 From the data in Table 14.11 what is the risk of dying from any cause in the 20-year follow-up in the unexposed (non-smoker) group?

A 0.162
B 0.292
C 0.319
D 0.681
E 0.838

14.3 From the data in Table 14.11 what is the absolute risk difference (difference in proportions) for dying from any cause in the 20-year follow-up between current or ex-smokers and non-smokers?

A −0.162
B −0.139
C 0.019
D 0.157
E 0.319

14.4 From the data in Table 14.11 what is the relative risk for dying for current or ex-smokers compared to non-smokers?

    A 0.41

    B 0.51

    C 1.97

    D 2.03

    E 2.43

14.5 Using the data in Table 14.11 calculate the 95% confidence interval for the relative risk for dying for current or ex-smokers compared to non-smokers?

    A 0.61 to 0.74

    B 0.74 to 1.86

    C 1.17 to 2.10

    D 1.86 to 2.10

    E 5.97 to 26.55

Doll and Hill (1950) carried out a case–control study into the aetiology of lung cancer. Seven hundred and nine lung cancer patients and 709 controls drawn from the same hospitals were compared for their smoking history. The results are shown in Table 14.12.

Table 14.12 Results from a case–control study on lung cancer and smoking.

Smoking status	Cases	Controls
Smokers	688	650
Non-smokers	21	59
Total	709	709

Source: data from Doll and Hill (1950).

14.6 Using the data in Table 14.12 what is the odds ratio for lung cancer cases compared to controls for being a smoker?

    A 0.34

    B 1.05

    C 2.97

    D 11.02

    E 32.76

14.7 Using the data in Table 14.12 calculate the 95% confidence interval for the odds ratio for lung cancer cases compared to control for being a smoker?

    A 0.64 to 1.54

    B 0.68 to 1.66

    C 1.79 to 4.95

    D 2.86 to 4.10

    E 3.97 to 55

Table 14.13 shows the results of a matched case control study. Gazzuola Rocca et al. (2017) matched 128 women who underwent bilateral oophorectomy before age 46 years for a non-cancerous condition in 1988–2007 (cases) and 128 age-matched controls (±1 year). One variable of interest was whether or not women who suffered any abuse (verbal or emotional, physical, sexual) before age 19 are at increased risk of undergoing bilateral oophorectomy before menopause.

Table 14.13 Results of matched case control study to investigate the possible association between any abuse (verbal or emotional, physical, sexual) before age 19 and the occurrence of bilateral oophorectomy.

Cases (bilateral oophorectomy)	Controls (women without oophorectomy)		
Any abuse (verbal or emotional, physical, sexual) before age 19	Any abuse (verbal or emotional, physical, sexual) before age 19		
	Yes	No	Total
Yes	10	42	52
No	19	59	76
Total	29	99	128

14.8 From the data on Table 14.13; what is the odds ratio for cases compared to controls for any abuse (verbal or emotional, physical, sexual) before age 19?

A 0.18
B 0.45
C 2.21
D 3.23
E 5.70

14.9 Using the data in Table 14.13 calculate the value of McNemar's test statistic without continuity correction for investigating the association between an ACE and bilateral oophorectomy.

A 0.18
B 1.30
C 2.21
D 3.75
E 8.67

14.10 Using the data in Table 14.13 calculate the 95% confidence interval for the odds ratio for cases compared to controls for any abuse (verbal or emotional, physical, sexual) before age 19?

A 1.00 to 2.62
B 1.30 to 23.75
C 1.79 to 25.82
D 1.86 to 22.10
E 5.97 to 226.55

15 The Randomised Controlled Trial

Medical Statistics: A Textbook for the Health Sciences, Fifth Edition. Stephen J. Walters, Michael J. Campbell, and David Machin.
© 2021 John Wiley & Sons Ltd. Published 2021 by John Wiley & Sons Ltd.
Companion website: www.wiley.com/go/walters/medicalstatistics

Summary

This chapter emphasises the importance of randomised clinical trials in evaluating alternative treatments or interventions. The rationale for, and methods of, randomising patients are given. We delineate the 'ABC' of clinical trials: Allocation at random, Blindness, and Control. The value of a trial protocol is stressed. Different types of randomised trials, such as factorial, cluster, and cross-over trials are described. We distinguish between those trials conducted to establish superiority of one intervention over another from those that seek equivalence or non-inferiority. Checklists of points to consider when designing, analysing, and reading the reports describing a clinical trial are discussed.

15.1 Introduction

A clinical trial is defined as a prospective study to examine the relative efficacy of treatments or interventions in human subjects. In many applications, one of the treatments is a standard therapy (control) and the other a new therapy (test).

Even with well-established and effective treatments, it is well recognised that individual patients may react differently once these are administered. Thus, aspirin will cure some individuals of headache speedily whilst others will continue with their headache. The human body is a very complex organism, whose functioning is far from completely understood, and so it is not surprising that it is often difficult to predict the exact reaction that a diseased individual will have to a particular therapy. Even though medical science might suggest that a new treatment is efficacious, it is only when it is tried in practice that any realistic assessment of its efficacy can be made and the presence of any adverse side effects identified. Thus, it is necessary to do comparative trials to evaluate the new treatment against the current standard.

Although we are concerned with the use of statistics in all branches of medical activity, this chapter is focussed primarily on the randomised controlled clinical trial because it has a central role in the development of new therapies. It should be emphasised, however, that randomised controlled trials (RCT) are relevant to other medical problems and not just therapeutic interventions; for example, in the evaluation of screening procedures, alternative strategies for health education and contraceptive efficacy. For further details and examples, see Machin and Fayers (2010).

15.2 The Protocol

The protocol is a formal document specifying how the trial is to be conducted. It will usually be necessary to write a protocol if the investigator is going to submit the trial to a grant-giving body for support and/or to an ethical committee for approval. However, there are also good practical reasons why one should be prepared in any case. The protocol provides the reference document for clinicians entering patients into clinical trials. There are three fundamental aspects of study design that must be precisely defined at an early stage and included in the protocol. These are: (i) which patients are eligible; (ii) which treatments are to be evaluated; (iii) how each patient's response is to be assessed. Furthermore some medical journals insist that every trial they consider for publication should be pre-registered (and before patient entry) with an appropriate body such as the ISRCTN (International Standard Randomised Controlled Trial Number) registry http://www.isrctn.com. Further details of what should be included in a protocol are given by Machin and Fayers (2010) and, for cluster trials, by Campbell and Walters (2014). The SPIRIT (Standard Protocol Items: Recommendations for Interventional Trials) 2013 statement provides recommendations for a minimum set of scientific, ethical, and administrative elements that should be addressed in a clinical trial protocol http://www.spirit-statement.org. The recommendations are outlined in a 33-item checklist and figure.

15.3 Why Randomise?

Randomisation

Randomisation is a procedure in which the assignment of a subject to the alternatives under investigation is decided by chance, so that the assignment cannot be predicted in advance. It is probably the most important innovation that statisticians have given to medical science. It was introduced in agriculture by the founder of modern statistics, RA Fisher (1890–1962) and developed in medicine by Austin Bradford Hill (1897–1991). Chance could mean the toss of a coin, the draw of a card, or more currently a computer-generated random number. The main point is that the investigator does not influence who gets which of the alternatives. It may seem a perverse method of allocating treatment to a sick individual. In the early days of clinical trials, when treatment was expensive and restricted, it could be justified as being the only fair method of deciding who got treated and who did not. More recently it has been shown that it is the *only* method, both intellectually and practically, that can ensure there is no bias in the allocation process. In other methods an investigator has the potential, consciously or subconsciously, to bias the allocation of treatments. Bitter experience has shown that other methods are easily subverted, so that, for example, sicker patients get the new treatment. It is important to distinguish *random* from *haphazard* or *systematic* allocation. A typical systematic allocation method is where the patients are assigned to test or control treatment alternately as they enter the clinic. The investigator might argue that the factors that determine precisely which subject enters the clinic at a given time are random and hence treatment allocation is also random. The problem here is that it is possible to predict which treatment the patients will receive as soon as, or even before, they are screened for eligibility for the trial. This knowledge may then influence the investigator when determining which patients are admitted to the trial and which are not. Thus, including patients chosen in this way may lead to bias in the final treatment comparisons.

The main point of randomisation is that *in the long run* it will produce study groups comparable in *unknown* as well as *known* factors likely to influence outcome apart from the actual treatment being given itself. Sometimes one can balance treatment arms for known prognostic factors (see Section 15.4 on how to conduct randomisation). However, suppose after the trial, it was revealed that (say) red-headed people did better on treatment. Randomisation will ensure that in a large trial, red-headed people would be equally represented in each arm. Of course, any trial will only be of finite size, and one would always be able to find factors that don't balance, but at least randomisation enables the investigator to put 'hand-on-heart' and say that the design was as bias free as possible. Factors which are known to influence prognosis should, as far as possible, be balanced between treatment arms by design; randomisation controls the unknown but potentially biasing factors. Obvious variables to balance by design include: disease status; a baseline covariate that is also the main outcome variable; demographic factors known to influence prognosis such as age, gender, and address. All factors balanced by the design should be included in the analysis.

Randomisation also guarantees that the probabilities obtained from statistical tests will be valid, although this is a rather technical point.

Random Assignment and the Protocol

The trial protocol will clearly define the patient entry criteria for a particular trial. After the clinician has determined that the patient is indeed eligible for the study, there is one extra question to answer. This is: 'are each of the treatments under study appropriate for this particular patient?' If the answer is 'yes' the patient is then randomised. If 'no' the patient is not included in the trial and would receive treatment according to the discretion of the clinician. It is important that the clinician does not know, at this stage, which of the treatments the patient is going to receive if they are included in the trial. The randomisation list or random allocation sequence should therefore be prepared and held by separate members of the study team. The assignment of treatments to trial participants should be by a centralised or third-party telephone-based randomisation system or an online computer/internet-based randomisation system through a web browser. The decision to accept or reject a participant should be made, and informed consent should be obtained from the participant, in ignorance of the next assignment in the sequence.

The ethical justification for a clinician to randomise a patient in a clinical trial is his or her uncertainty as to the best treatment for the particular patient, so-called 'clinical equipoise'. There are situations where an individual clinician is convinced about the best method of treating a patient, whereas another clinician has a different conviction. Thus, one can justify randomisation when there is doubt within a community of clinicians. However, in such circumstances, getting individual clinicians to join the trial may be difficult.

Historical Controls

In certain circumstances, however, randomisation is not possible; one classical example was the first studies involving heart transplantation and the subsequent survival experience of the patients. At that time, it would have been difficult to imagine randomising between heart transplantation and some other alternative, and so the best one could do in such circumstances was to compare survival time following transplant with previous patients suffering from the same condition when transplants were not available. Such patients are termed historical controls. A second possibility is to make comparisons with those in which a donor did not become available before patient death. There are difficulties with either approach. One is that those with the most serious problems will die more quickly. The presence of any waiting time for a suitable donor implies only the less critical will survive this waiting time. This can clearly bias comparisons of survival experience in the transplanted and non-transplanted groups. For this reason, one should interpret studies that use historical controls with care.

15.4   Methods of Randomisation

Simple Randomisation

The simplest randomisation device is a coin which if tossed will land with a particular face upwards with probability one-half. Thus, one way to assign treatments of patients at random would be to assign treatment A whenever a particular side of the coin turned up, and B when the obverse arises. An alternative might be to roll a six-sided die; if an even number falls A is given, if an odd number, B. Such procedures are termed simple randomisation. It is usual to generate the randomisation list in advance of recruiting the first patient. This has several advantages: it removes the possibility of the clinician not randomising properly, it will usually be more efficient in that a list may be computer generated very quickly, and it also allows some difficulties with simple randomisation to be avoided.

To avoid the use of a coin or die for simple randomisation one can consult a table of random numbers such as Table T5 in the appendix. Although Table T5 is in fact computer generated, the table is similar to that which would result from throwing a 10-sided die, with faces marked 0–9, on successive occasions. The digits are grouped into blocks merely for ease of reading. The table is used by first choosing a point of entry, perhaps with a pin, and deciding the direction of movement, for example along the rows or down the columns. Suppose the pin chooses the entry in the 8th row and 13th column and it had been decided to move along the rows; the first 10 digits then give 534 55425 67; even numbers assigned to A and odd to B then generate BBA BBAAB AB. Thus of the first 10 patients recruited 4 will receive A and 6 B.

Although simple randomisation gives equal probability for each patient to receive A or B it does not ensure, as indeed was the case with our example, that at the end of patient recruitment to the trial equal numbers of patients received A and B. In fact, even in relatively large trials the discrepancy from the desired equal numbers of patients per treatment can be quite large. In small trials the discrepancy can be very serious perhaps, resulting in too few patients in one group to give acceptable statistical precision of the corresponding treatment effect.

Blocked Randomisation

To avoid such a problem, balanced or restricted randomisation techniques are used. In this case, the allocation procedure is organised in such a way that equal numbers are allocated to A and B for every block of a certain number of patients. One method of doing this, say for successive blocks of four patients, is to generate all possible combinations but ignoring those, such as AAAB, with unequal allocation. The valid combinations are:

1	AABB	4	BABA
2	ABAB	5	BAAB
3	ABBA	6	BBAA

These combinations are then allocated the numbers 1–6 and the randomisation table used to generate a sequence of digits. Suppose this sequence was 534 55425 67 as before, then reading from left to right we generate the allocation BAAB ABBA BABA BAAB for the first 16 patients. Such a device ensures that for every four successive patients recruited balance between A and B is maintained. Should a 0, 7, 8, or 9 occur in the random sequence then these are ignored as there is no associated treatment combination in these cases. It is important that the investigating clinician is not aware of the block size otherwise they will come to know, as each block of patients nears completion, the next treatment to be allocated. This foreknowledge can introduce bias into the allocation process since the clinician may then subconsciously avoid allocating certain treatments for particular patients. Such a difficulty can be avoided by changing the block size at random as recruitment continues.

Stratified Randomisation

In clinical trials that involve recruitment in several centres, it is usual to use a randomisation procedure for each centre to ensure balanced treatment allocation within centres. Another important use of this stratified randomisation in clinical trials is if it is known that a particular patient characteristic may be an important prognostic indicator, perhaps good or bad pathology, then equal allocation of treatments within each prognostic group or strata may be desirable. This ensures that treatment comparisons can be made efficiently, allowing for prognostic factors. Stratified randomisation can be extended to more than one stratum, for example, centre and pathology, but it is not usually desirable to go beyond two strata.

One method that can balance a large number of strata is known as minimisation. One difficulty with the method is that it requires details of all patients previously entered into the trial, before allocation can be made.

Carrying out Randomisation

Once the randomised list is made, and it is usually best done by an impartial statistical team and *not* by the investigator determining patient eligibility, how is randomisation carried out? One simple way is to have it kept out of the clinic but with someone who can give the randomisation over the telephone or electronically. The clinician rings the number, gives the necessary patient details, perhaps confirming the protocol entry criteria, and is told which treatment to give, or perhaps a code number of a drug package. Alternatively, if the investigators have access to the internet at the point of randomisation then online or internet-based randomisation can implemented. Investigators randomise patients by simply completing an on-screen form with patient details, inclusion and exclusion criteria. Investigators are immediately shown the treatment allocation. Once determined, treatment should commence as soon as is practicable.

The above discussion has used the example of a randomised control trial comparing two treatments as this is the simplest example. The method extends relatively easily to more complex designs, however. For example, in the case of a 2×2 factorial design involving four treatments, the treatments, labelled A, B, C and D, could be allocated the pair of digits 0-1, 2-3, 4-5 and 6-7 respectively. The random sequence 534 55425 67 would then generate CBC CCCBC DD; thus in the first 10 patients none would receive A, two B, six C and two D. Balanced arrangements to give equal numbers of patients per group can be produced by first generating the combinations for blocks of an appropriate size.

A series of short videos (at https://www.youtube.com/playlist?list=PL1mJ7IZ3qFxiYlJ-jGZ1cf__ZVC08mymM) introduces the main concepts (simple randomisation, blocked and stratified randomisation) and methodological approaches to randomised trials in health care.

15.5 Design Features

The Need for a Control Group

In Chapter 14 we discussed the hazards of conducting 'before-and-after' type studies, in which clinicians simply stop using the standard treatment and start using the new. In any situation in which a new therapy is under investigation, one important question is whether it is any better than the currently best available for the particular condition. If the new therapy is indeed better then, all other considerations being equal, it would seem reasonable to give all future patients with the condition the new therapy. But how well are the patients doing with the current therapy? Once a therapy is in routine use it is not generally monitored to the same rigorous standards as it was during its development. So although the current best therapy may have been carefully tested many years prior to the proposed new study, changes in medical practice may have ensued in the interim. There may also be changes in patient characterisation or doctors' attitudes to treatment. It could well be that some of these changes have influenced patient outcomes. The possibility of such changes makes it imperative that the new therapy be tested alongside the old. In addition, although there may be a presumption of improved efficacy, the new therapy may turn out to be not as good as the old. It therefore becomes very important to re-determine the performance of the standard treatment under current conditions.

Treatment Choice and Follow-up

When designing a clinical trial, it is important to have firm objectives in view and be sure that the therapeutic question concerned is of sufficient importance to merit the undertaking. Thus, clearly different and well-defined alternative treatment regimens are required. The criteria for patient entry should be clear and measures of efficacy should be pre-specified and unambiguously determined for each patient. All patients entered into a trial and randomised to treatment should be followed up in the same manner, irrespective of whether or not the treatment is continuing for that individual patient. Thus, a patient who refuses a second injection in a drug study should be monitored as closely as one who agreed to the injection. From considerations of sample size (see Chapter 16) it is often preferable to compare at most two treatments, although, clearly, there are situations in which more than two can be evaluated efficiently.

Blind Assessment

Just as the clinician who determines eligibility to the study should be blind to the actual treatment that the patient would receive, any assessment of the patient should preferably be 'blind'. Thus, one should separate the assessment process from the treatment process if this is at all possible. To obtain an even more objective view of efficacy it is desirable to have the patient 'blind' to which of the treatments they are receiving. It should be noted that if a placebo or standard drug is to be used in a double-blind trial, it should be packaged in exactly the same way as the test treatment. Clinical trials are concerned with real and not abstract situations so it is recognised that the ideal 'blind' situation may not be possible or even desirable in all circumstances. If there is a choice, however, the maximum degree of 'blindness' should be adhered to. In a 'double-blind' trial, in which neither the patient nor the clinician know the treatment, careful monitoring is required since treatment-related adverse side-effects are a possibility in any trial and the attendant clinician may need to be able to have immediate access to the actual treatment given should an emergency arise.

Pilot Trials and Feasibility Studies

Clinical trials can cost huge amounts of money, and it is sensible to try to design them is such a way that they produce a result that can answer a useful clinical question. It is common to carry out feasibility studies prior to the main trial to decide questions such as the number of patients eligible for the trial, the willingness of clinicians to randomise patients and the likely length of the trial (Whitehead et al. 2014). An important decision is which outcome variable is to be the primary one. Once these questions have been answered, it may be sensible to conduct a *pilot trial*. This to some extent will mimic the intended main trial, but is much smaller, and can be used, for example, to check whether patients are willing, in actuality rather than hypothetically, to enter the trial, and to estimate the variability of the main outcome variable, which may be used in sample size calculations for the main trial. Pilot trials may be *external* or *internal*. External pilot trials are carried out when the investigators expect the design features to alter in the main trial, and so the results from the pilot cannot be used in the main trial. Internal pilot trials occur when the design features are fixed, but there may be uncertainty about how many centres will contribute patients, or the variability of the outcome variable. Usually, internal pilots have a point at which decisions about whether to continue the trial, or extend it, have to be made. This is commonly after about a year, when realistic estimates of recruitment rates and outcome variability can be ascertained.

The main point about external pilots is that they are *not* designed to test treatment efficacy, since they are too small to have reasonable power for a sensible effect size. Thus testing of the statistical significance of treatment effects is discouraged, (Eldridge et al. 2016). The size of a pilot trial can vary from 24 (12 per arm (Julious 2005)) to 75 (Whitehead et al. 2016) to 120 (for binary outcomes, Teare et al. 2014).

Design Features of Feasibility Studies and Pilot Trials

- The endpoint for feasibility studies and pilot trials is a decision about a forthcoming main trial, not whether a treatment works or not.
- Tests of significance have limited value in pilot and feasibility studies.

*Example – External Pilot Trial – Physiotherapy Management of Lumbar Radicular Syndrome (LRS)
– The POLAR Trial*

Reddington et al. (2018) undertook an external pilot RCT, in patients with lumbar radicular syndrome (LRS), to investigate the feasibility of undertaking a definitive RCT. Participants were randomised into early intervention physiotherapy or usual care (UC) with the former receiving their treatment within two weeks after randomisation and the latter at six week post-randomisation. Outcomes included process measures to determine the feasibility of the study and an exploratory analysis of patient self-reported outcomes, including disability, pain, and general health, these were collected at baseline, 6, 12 and 26 weeks post-randomisation. Eighty participants were recruited in 10 GP practices over 34 weeks, a recruitment rate of 2.4 participants per week, and randomised to UC ($n = 38$) or early intervention physiotherapy ($n = 42$). Follow-up rates at 26 weeks were 84% (32/38) in the UC and 86% (36/42) in the early intervention physiotherapy group. The authors concluded that the results of the external pilot study suggested that a full RCT is feasible and will provide evidence as to the optimal timing of physiotherapy for patients with LRS.

*Example – External Pilot Trial – Early Pulmonary Rehabilitation (EPR) in Patients with Chronic
Obstructive Pulmonary Disease (COPD)*

Cox et al. (2018) undertook an external pilot RCT, in patients with chronic obstructive pulmonary disease (COPD), to assess the feasibility of recruiting patients, collecting data and delivering early pulmonary rehabilitation (EPR) to patients with acute exacerbations of COPD compared with UC. Participants were randomised to EPR or UC. Main outcomes included: the feasibility of recruiting 76 participants in seven months at two centres; intervention delivery; views on intervention/research acceptability; clinical outcomes including the six-minute walk distance (6MWD).

Over seven months 449 patients were screened, of whom most were not eligible for the trial or felt too ill and declined entry. In total, 58 participants (76%) of the target 76 participants were recruited. The primary clinical outcome (6MWD) was difficult to collect with only 21 participants providing data. Hospital EPR was difficult to deliver over five days because of patient discharge or staff availability, with only 34% of the scheduled sessions delivered. The authors concluded that a full-scale RCT using the protocol would not be feasible.

*Example – Internal Pilot Trial – Endometrial Trauma in Women Undergoing
in vitro Fertilisation (IVF)*

Pye et al. (2018) undertook a multicentre, parallel group, RCT with a nine-month internal pilot phase to investigate the effect of performing an endometrial scratch (ES) in the mid-luteal phase prior to a first-time in vitro fertilisation (IVF) in women with a history of infertility problems wanting to have a baby. Participants were randomised to receive the ES procedure in the mid-luteal phase of the preceding cycle prior to first-time IVF treatment or usual IVF treatment (control). The primary outcome was live-birth rate after completing 24 weeks gestation. The trial intended to recruit 1044 women from 16 fertility units.

The trial consisted of two phases – an internal pilot to assess feasibility of recruitment and delivery of the intervention, and a two-year main recruitment phase. The trial commenced, using the same trial procedures as for the planned main RCT, with a nine-month internal pilot recruitment phase across eight fertility units to justify whether or not the recruitment strategy and the scheduling of the ES procedure were feasible. The trial would be considered to be infeasible, and so would be stopped, if either of the following applied:

1) Lack of feasibility to recruit to the main trial: defined as recruitment of fewer than 108 participants (75% of the 144 target) during the internal pilot phase.
2) Unsatisfactory scheduling of the ES procedure: defined as fewer than 75% of women scheduled to receive ES have received their ES at the correct time point.

The internal pilot demonstrated feasibility in that by nine-months 231 were recruited and 85% (99/116) received their ES procedure at the correct time-point. The RCT then continued recruitment to its target sample size of 1044 women.

Protocol Violations

In many trials some participants will not have followed the protocol, either on purpose or by mistake. Included here are patients who actually receive the wrong treatment (that is, not the one allocated) and patients who do not take their treatment, known as non-compliers. In addition, it is sometimes discovered after the trial has begun that a patient was not after all eligible. The only safe way to deal with all of these circumstances is to keep all randomised patients in the trial and to *analyse as you randomise*. The analysis is thus based on the groups as randomised, and is known as an *intention-to-treat* (ITT) analysis. Any other approach towards protocol violations will involve subjective decisions and will thus create an opportunity for bias (Machin and Fayers 2010, pp. 35–36). It is sometimes useful to perform an additional analysis of only those patients adhering to the protocol, a *per-protocol* analysis. However, the analysis of the groups as randomised must be considered the main analysis for the trial (Altman 1991).

'Pragmatic' and 'Explanatory' Trials

One can draw a useful distinction between trials that aim to determine the exact pharmacological action of a drug ('explanatory' trials) and trials that aim to determine the efficacy of a drug as used in day-to-day clinical practice ('pragmatic' trials). There are many factors besides lack of efficacy that can interfere with the action of a drug; for example, if a drug is unpalatable, patients may not like its taste and therefore not take it.

Explanatory trials often require some measure of patient compliance, perhaps by means of blood samples, to determine whether the drug was actually taken by the patient. Such trials need to be conducted in tightly controlled situations. Patients found not to have complied with the prescribed dose schedule may be excluded from analysis.

On the other hand, pragmatic trials lead to analysis by ITT. Thus once patients are randomised to receive a particular treatment they are analysed as if they have received it, whether or not they did so in practice. This will reflect the likely action of the drug in clinical practice, where even when a drug is prescribed there is no guarantee that the patient will take it. In general, we would recommend that trials be analysed on an ITT basis although there are situations where a so-called 'per protocol' analysis is best. For example, a trial in which blood levels of the drugs were also to be monitored where it is important that only those actually taking the drugs (rather than allocated to the drug and possibly not taking it) are used to summarise the profiles.

Superiority and Equivalence Trials

Implicit in a comparison between two treatments is the presumption that if the null hypothesis is rejected then there is a difference between the treatments being compared. Thus, one concludes that one treatment is 'superior' to the other irrespective of the magnitude of the difference observed. However, in certain situations, a new therapy may bring certain advantages over the current standard, possibly in a reduced side-effects profile, easier administration or cost but it may not be anticipated to be better with respect to the primary efficacy variable. For example, if the treatments are for an acute (but not serious) condition then perhaps a cheaper but not so efficacious (within quite wide limits) alternative to the standard treatment may be acceptable. However, if the condition was life threatening then the limits of 'equivalence' would be narrow as any advantages of the new approach must not be offset by an unacceptable increase in (say) death rate. Under such conditions, the new approach may be required to be at least 'equivalent' to the standard in relation to efficacy if it is to replace it in future clinical use. This implies that 'equivalence' is a pre-specified maximum difference between treatments that, if observed to be less after the clinical trial is conducted, would render the two treatments equivalent.

One special form of equivalence trial is termed a 'non-inferiority' trial. Here we only wish to be sure that one treatment is 'not worse than' or is 'at least as good as' another treatment: if it is better, that is fine (even though superiority would not be required to bring it into common use). All we need is to get convincing evidence that the new treatment is not worse than the standard.

Design Features of Equivalence Trials

Decide on whether equivalence or non-inferiority is required.
Decide the limits for equivalence or non-inferiority.
Ensure very careful attention to detail in trial conduct especially patient compliance.
Plan for a per protocol analysis.

Although analysis and interpretation can be quite straightforward, the design and management of equivalence trials is often much more complex. In general, careless or inaccurate measurement, poor follow-up of patients, poor compliance with study procedures and medication all tend to bias results towards no difference between treatment groups. This implies that an ITT analysis is not likely to be appropriate since we are trying to offer evidence of equivalence, poor study design and logistical procedures may therefore actually help to hide treatment differences. In general, therefore, the quality of equivalence trials needs especially high compliance of the patients with respect to the treatment protocol. Reporting guidelines for non-inferiority and equivalence RCTs recommend that it should be clearly indicated whether the conclusion relating to non-inferiority or equivalence is based on ITT or per-protocol analysis or both and whether those conclusions are stable with respect to the different types of analyses (Piaggo et al. 2012); ideally both approaches should support non-inferiority/equivalence.

Example – Non-inferiority – Adjuvant Treatment of Postmenopausal Women with Early Breast Cancer
The ATAC Trialists' Group (2002) conducted a three-group randomised trial of anastrozole, *A*, tamoxifen, *T*, and the combination, *AT*, in postmenopausal women with early breast cancer. The trial was designed to test two hypotheses. One was that that the combination *AT* was superior

to T alone. The second A was either non-inferior or superior to T. This latter comparison comprises the 'equivalence' component to the trial.

The trial report quotes: 'Disease-free survival at 3 years was 89.4% on anastrozole and 87.4% on tamoxifen (hazard ratio 0.83 [95% CI 0.71–0.96] $p = 0.8$)'. Thus, with a better disease-free survival (DFS) at three-years, there was no evidence of inferiority with A as compared to T. One can be confident of non-inferiority but this does not imply a conclusion of superiority even though the three-year DFS rate is higher by 2.0%.

Early and Late Phase Trials

Clinical trials testing new treatments, particularly pharmaceutical treatments such as a new drug, are sometimes divided into different stages, called phases. The phases of clinical research are the steps in which scientists conduct experiments with a health intervention in an attempt to find enough evidence for the intervention which would be useful as a medical treatment. In the case of a pharmaceutical study, the phases start with drug design and drug discovery then proceed on to animal testing. If this is successful, the clinical phase of development begins by testing for safety in a few human subjects and expands to test in many study participants if the treatment is safe. Clinical trials involving new drugs are commonly classified into five main phases, although some individual trials may cover more than one phase. The earliest phase trials look at whether a drug is safe or the side effects it causes. Later phase trials aim to test whether a new treatment is better than existing treatments. Therefore, it may be easier to think of early phase trials and later phase trials. Thus, Phase I trials are the earlier trials and Phase III the later phase trials. Some trials even have an earlier stage called Phase 0, and there are some Phase IV trials done after a drug has been licenced. Some trials are randomised. Table 15.1 shows the main trial phases. Note that researchers distinguish between *efficacy*, which means: does the drug work on patients in ideal circumstances, who have confirmed disease, confirmed drug consumption and short term (often surrogate) outcomes; and *effectiveness*, which means: does the drug work in the real world, where patients might not take the treatment, and where the outcome is one that matters to the patient. Efficacy is measured with an explanatory trial and effectiveness in a pragmatic trial. Often efficacy refers to a drug working better than placebo, whereas effectiveness means working better than the best alternative or usual care.

15.6 Design Options

Parallel Designs

In a parallel design, one group receives the test treatment, and one group the control as represented in Figure 15.1.

Example from the Literature – Parallel Group Trial – Reduced Nicotine Cigarettes
Allen et al. (2017) plan to randomly allocate 200 adult smokers with a current or lifetime unipolar mood and/or anxiety disorder to receive either usual nicotine (UN) cigarettes or reduced nicotine (RN) cigarettes with the nicotine reduced in five steps over 18 weeks. The subjects will smoke regular nicotine cigarettes for two weeks prior to randomisation. The primary outcome will be blood cotinine, and secondary outcomes include anxiety and depression measures. Participants and study staff will be blind to the experimental cigarette allocation from the randomisation visit to the last

Table 15.1 Phases of pharmaceutical clinical trials.

Phase	Main aims of trial	Dose	Is it randomised?	Typical number of people taking part
Preclinical	Testing of the drug in non-human subjects (animals), to gather efficacy, toxicity, and pharmacokinetic information (what the drug does to the animal).	Unrestricted	Sometimes	Not applicable (in vitro and in vivo only).
Phase 0	Testing a low (sub-therapeutic) dose of the drug/treatment in humans to check it is not harmful.	Very low, sub-therapeutic	Sometimes	Small – often about 10–20 people.
Phase I	Testing the drug in healthy volunteers for safety and finding out about side effects, and what happens to the treatment in the body such as the time for the drug to be excreted (pharmacokinetics) and what the drug does to the body (pharmacodynamics). May involve testing multiple doses (dose-ranging).	Often sub-therapeutic, but with ascending doses	Sometimes	6–100 normal healthy volunteers (or for cancer drugs, cancer patients).
Phase II	Testing the drug on patients to assess efficacy and finding out more about side effects, and what happens to the treatment in the body. Determines whether drug can have any efficacy; at this point, the drug is not presumed to have any therapeutic effect whatsoever.	Therapeutic dose	Sometimes	100–300 patients with specific diseases.
Phase III	Testing the drug on patients to assess efficacy, effectiveness and safety by comparing the new drug treatment to the standard treatment. Determines a drug's therapeutic effect; at this point, the drug is presumed to have some effect.	Therapeutic dose	Usually	Large – hundreds or thousands of people with specific diseases.
Phase IV	Post marketing surveillance – watching drug use in public and finding out more about long-term benefits and side effects.	Therapeutic dose	No	Anyone seeking treatment and prescribed the drug. Large – hundreds or thousands of people.

Source: adapted from Cancer Research UK (2019).

visit. The RN cigarettes will be identical in appearance to the UN cigarettes. A previous paper found a difference of 127 ng mL^{-1} of cotinine for an experimental group with an average SD of 118 ng mL^{-1}. With a sample size of 70 participants per group, they are able to detect the difference in plasma cotinine concentration level between the two groups as small as 58 ng mL^{-1} (SD 118) with a 5% significance level and at least 80% power (and 68 ng mL^{-1} with at least 90% power). Allowing

Figure 15.1 Stages of a parallel two group randomised controlled trial.

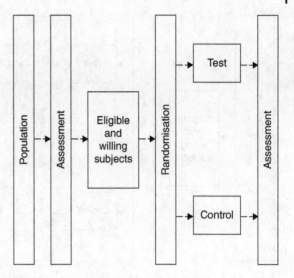

for a 30% participant withdrawal rate, they planned to recruit 100 participants for each group (200 in total).

The trial report of Allen et al. (2017) displays the usual good and poor practices of reporting parallel group trials. The method of randomisation is not described but the sample size is reproducible and shows the usual 'half a standard deviation' effect size (see Chapter 16). To their credit, the authors do attempt to blind the study. The usual problem with blinding is that one might expect the participants on the intervention arm to notice the effects of the intervention (in this case withdrawal symptoms from tobacco). There is no way to combat this, but the reader should look for effects of unblinding, such as being more likely to drop out of the study with RN, and the reporting of smoking of cigarettes purchased outside of the study. A pragmatic approach would be to measure cotinine at 18 weeks, even in those who dropped out or bought their own cigarettes, and analyse the data by the group the participants were randomised to.

Cross-over Designs

In a cross-over design the subjects receive both the test and the control treatments in a randomised order over two periods as in Figure 15.2. This contrasts with the parallel group design in that *each* subject now provides an estimate of the difference between test and control. Situations where crossover trials may be useful are in chronic diseases that remain stable over long periods of time, such as diabetes or arthritis, where the purpose of the treatment is palliation and not cure.

Example from the Literature – Cross-over Trial – Nutrition in Diabetes
Berkowitz et al. (2019) conducted a crossover trial of a home delivery of 10 meals per week for 12 weeks (M) against usual diet and a healthy eating brochure (U). The primary outcome was the Healthy Eating Index 2010 score (HEI) (range 1–100). This was measured three times during each period and the score averaged in each of the two periods of the design. With at least 40 participants, they claimed that the study had greater than 80% power to detect a difference of five points or more in the total HEI score, but did not provide enough information to verify this.

They recruited 42 subjects of whom 20 were randomised to M followed by U, and 22 were randomised to the opposite order of U followed by M. They found the HEI score for M was 71.3,

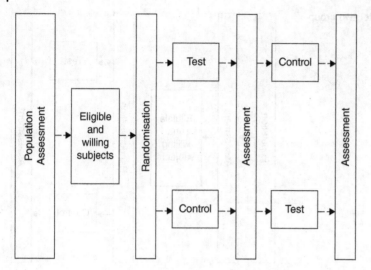

Figure 15.2 Stages of a two group two period cross-over randomised controlled trial.

whereas for U it was 39.9. This is a difference of 31.4 points ($p < 0.0001$), but no confidence interval (CI) for this effect was quoted.

The two-period, two-treatment (2×2) cross-over trial has the advantage over a parallel group design testing the same hypothesis in that, because subjects act as their own controls, the number of subjects required is considerably less.

There are, however, a number of problems. One difficulty with cross-over designs is the possibility that the effect of the particular treatment used in the first period will carry over to the second period. This may then interfere with how the treatment scheduled for the second period will act, and thus affect the final comparison between the two treatments (the carry-over effect). To allow for this possibility, a washout period, in which no treatment is given, should be included between the successive treatment periods. Other difficulties are that the disease may not remain stable over the trial period, and that because of the extended treatment period, more subject drop-outs will occur than in a parallel group design.

A cross-over study results is a paired (or matched) analysis. It is incorrect to analyse the trial ignoring this pairing, as that analysis fails to use all the information in the study design.

Cluster Randomised Controlled Trials

In some cases, because of the nature of the intervention planned, it may not be possible to randomise on an individual subject basis. In these situations, random assignment to groups of people (such as communities, families, or medical practices) may be possible. Reasons for group assignment include the possibility of 'contamination' (the unintentional spill-over of intervention effects from one treatment group to another) of the interventions if individual randomisation is used. Trials with this design are variously known as field, community based, group randomised, place based or, more generally, cluster randomised trials.

Cluster trials, randomise interventions to groups of patients, for example, families or medical practices. Thus, an investigator may have to randomise communities to evaluate different types of health promotion or different types of vaccine, when problems of contamination or logistics, respectively, mean that it is better to randomise a group. Alternatively, one may wish to compare different ways of counselling patients, and it would be impossible for a health professional once trained to a new approach to switch between counselling methods for different patients following randomisation. For example, 10 health professionals may be involved and these are then randomised, five to each group, to be trained or not in new counselling techniques. The professionals each then recruit a number of patients who form the corresponding cluster all receiving counselling according to the training (or not) of their health professional. The simplest way to analyse these studies is by group, rather than on an individual subject basis. Further details are given in Campbell and Walters (2014).

Example from the Literature – Cluster Design – Diabetes
REPOSE (2017) is a cluster randomised trial of training courses designed to teach adults with type 1 diabetes different methods of administering insulin. Forty-six training courses were randomised: 23 where subjects were trained in using multiple dose injectors (MDI; and 23 where they were trained to use an insulin pump (IP). Their HbA1c was measured at baseline and at 24 months. The sample size was based on a difference in HbA1c between groups of 0.5% which is believed to be clinically important. A total of 248 participants (128 IP, 120 MDI) made up the analysis set. Both groups reduced their HbA1c and the difference in groups was found to be −0.24% (95% CI −0.53 to 0.05) in favour of pumps.

The REPOSE (2017) study was by necessity clustered since the subjects are taught to use MDIs or IP in groups. It should be noted the CI for the difference between arms of the trial includes the value for a clinically important difference. Thus, this trial does not provide enough evidence to say the interventions are different, but neither can we conclude that they are equivalent.

Stepped Wedge Cluster Randomised Trials

Another grouped randomised design is known as a Stepped Wedge Design cluster randomised design (SW-CRT), in which subjects all start on the control (time zero) and are gradually randomised to the test intervention under study. Time is usually divided into a number of periods and each cluster is randomised to a *sequence* which defines in which period the intervention starts for that cluster. This design can be more powerful than a parallel group cluster trial, since it contains a within-subject element that can increase power. Unlike a cross-over design, clusters cannot revert to the control after having had the intervention. Cohort SW-CRTs follow individuals from clusters over time starting at time zero. In cross-sectional designs, the individuals in one cluster in one time period differ from those in the same cluster but a different time period. Open designs are a mixture of the previous two, whereby individuals may appear in more than one period and may join the trial after time zero. They are beyond the scope of this book but for further details see Hemming et al. (2018) and Campbell et al. (2019).

Example for the Literature – Stepped Wedge Cluster Randomised Trial – SHAREHD
The SHAREHD study of Fotheringham et al. (2017) aimed to assess the effectiveness of a structured programme to support patient involvement in centre-based haemodialysis. It implemented a programme of Shared Haemodialysis Care (SHC) that aimed to improve experience and outcomes for those who are treated with centre-based haemodialysis, and give more patients the confidence to dialyse independently both at centres and at home. Following a six-month set up or baseline period, a phased implementation programme was initiated across 12 dialysis centres (the clusters) using a

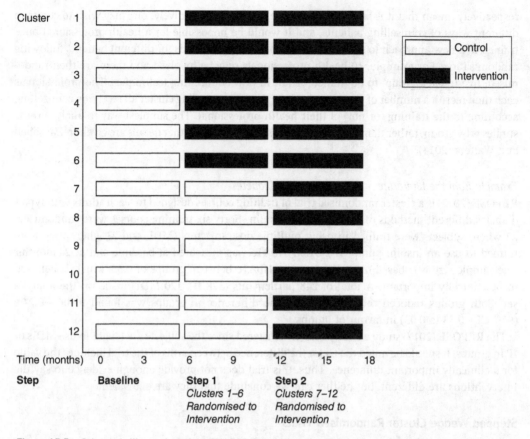

Figure 15.3 Schematic illustration of the SHARED Stepped Wedge Cluster Randomised Trial (with 12 clusters, 3 periods, and 2 steps).

SW-CRT with 6 dialysis centres participating in each of two steps, each lasting six months as illustrated in Figure 15.3. The 12 centres were randomised to receive the SHAREHD intervention in step 1 or step 2. The primary outcome measure was the number of patients performing at least five dialysis-related tasks collected using three-monthly questionnaires at 0, 3, 6, 9, 12 and 15 months.

Factorial Trials

A factorial trial is used to evaluate two or more interventions simultaneously. In general, the treatments in a factorial design are known as factors and usually they are applied at only one level, that is, a particular factor is either present or absent. For example, one factor may be radiotherapy for patients with a certain cancer and the options are to give or not give. Factorial designs are useful in two situations: first the clinician may believe that the two treatments together will produce an effect that is over and above that anticipated by adding the effects of the two treatments separately (synergy), and is often expressed statistically as an interaction. Alternatively, the clinician may believe that an interaction is very unlikely. In this case, one requires fewer patients to examine the effects of the two treatments, than the combined number of patients from two separate parallel group trials, each one examining the effect of one of the treatments.

Example from the Literature – 2 × 2 Factorial Design – AspECT Trial

Jankowski et al. (2018) describe The Aspirin and Esomeprazole Chemoprevention in Barrett's metaplasia Trial (AspECT). A total of 2557 patients with Barrett's oesophagus of 1 cm or more were randomised 1 : 1 : 1 : 1 to receive (first factor) high-dose (40 mg twice daily) or low-dose (20 mg once daily) proton pump inhibitor (PPI), (second factor) with or without aspirin (300 mg per day) for at least eight years, in an unblinded manner. The investigators did not expect the treatments to interact. They found that high-dose PPI and aspirin chemoprevention therapy, especially in combination, significantly, and safely improved outcomes. Thus, the investigators were able to answer two different questions within a single trial and show that effects of the two factors was additive. The use of this 2 × 2 factorial design enabled two questions to be asked simultaneously.

15.7 Meta-analysis

In many circumstances RCTs have been conducted that are unrealistically small, some unnecessarily replicated whilst others have not been published as their results have not been considered of interest. It has now been recognised that, to obtain the best current evidence with respect to a particular therapy, all pertinent clinical trial information needs to be obtained, and if circumstances permit, the overview is completed by a formal combination of all the trials by means of a (statistical) meta-analysis of all the trial data (see Chapter 18). This recognition has led to the Cochrane Collaboration, and a worldwide network of overview groups, to address numerous therapeutic questions https://www.cochrane.org/about-us. In certain situations this has brought definitive statements with respect to a particular therapy. For others it has led to the launch of a large-scale confirmatory trial.

Although it is not appropriate to review the methodology here, it is clear that the 'overview' process has led to many changes to the way in which clinical trial programmes have developed. They have provided the basic information required in planning new trials, impacted on an appropriate trial size (see Chapter 16), publication policy and very importantly raised reporting standards. They are an integral part evidence based medicine and are impacting directly on decisions that affect patient care and questioning conventional wisdom in many areas. Reviewers have long been aware that not all trials are published. There may be many reasons for this, but cynics might claim that drug companies may not publish trials that do not show their product in a favourable light and academics and journals may lack the incentive to publish negative trials. This has led to the 'all trials' movement, which is trying to ensure all trials are published (http://www.alltrials.net).

15.8 Checklists for Design, Analysis and Reporting

A whole variety of checklists to aid critical reading of trials and other studies is given by the EQUATOR network (http://www.equator-network.org) and the Critical Appraisal Skills Programme (CASP) Checklists (https://casp-uk.net/casp-tools-checklists).

Design

The main consideration here is that should the design not be suitable to answer the trial question(s) posed, no amount of 'statistical juggling' at the analysis stage can correct any basic faults. For example, if a cross-over trial design is used without an adequate washout period then this cannot be rectified by the analysis. A major consideration at the planning stage is whether there is a reasonable expectation that sufficient patients can be recruited to the proposed trial. Most of the points covered here should be clearly answered in the protocol and should also be made very explicit in any subsequent publication.

Checklist of Design Features

1) Are the trial objectives clearly formulated?
2) Are the diagnostic criteria for entry to the trial clear?
3) Is there a reliable supply of patients?
4) Are the treatments (or interventions) well defined?
5) Is the method and reason for randomisation well understood?
6) Is the treatment planned to commence immediately following randomisation?
7) Is the maximum degree of blindness being used?
8) Are the outcome measures appropriate and clearly defined?
9) How has the study size been justified?
10) What arrangements have been made for collecting, recording, and analysis of the data?
11) Has appropriate follow-up of the patients been organised?
12) Are important prognostic variables recorded?
13) Are side-effects of treatment anticipated?
14) Are many patient drop-outs anticipated?

Analysis and Presentation

Provided a good design is chosen, then once completed the statistical analysis may be relatively straightforward and will have been anticipated at the planning stage. However, there are always nuances and unexpected features associated with data generated from every clinical trial that will demand careful detail at the analysis stage. Perhaps there are more missing values than anticipated, or many more censored survival observations through patient loss in one group than the other, or many of the assumptions made at the design stage have not been realised. In contrast to the choice of a poor design, a poor analysis can be rescued by a second look at the same data, although this necessity will be wasteful of time and resource and delay dissemination of the 'true' trial results.

In many situations, the final trial report published in the medical literature can only concentrate on the main features and there may be a limit on the detail that can be presented. This may lead to difficult choices of exactly what to present. However, guidance for the 'key' features should be in the trial protocol itself.

Checklist for Analysis and Presentation

1) Are the statistical procedures used adequately described or referenced?
2) Are the statistical procedures appropriate?
3) Have the potential prognostic variables been adequately considered?
4) Is the statistical presentation satisfactory?
5) Are any graphs clear and the axes appropriately labelled?
6) Are CIs given for the main results?
7) Are the conclusions drawn from the statistical analysis justified?

15.9 CONSORT

It is widely recognised that RCTs are the only reliable way to compare the effectiveness of different therapies. It is thus essential that RCTs be well designed and conducted, and it is important that they be reported adequately. In particular, readers of trial reports should not have to infer what was probably done – they should be told explicitly. To facilitate this, the modified CONSORT Statement of Schultz et al. (2010) has been published and includes a list of 25 items that should be covered in any trial report and a suggested flow chart to describe the patient progress through the trial (http://www.consort-statement.org). The checklist applies principally to trials with two parallel groups. Some modification is needed for other situations, such as cross-over trials and those with more than two treatment groups. A number of extensions of the CONSORT Statement have been developed to give additional guidance for RCTs with specific designs (such as non-inferiority and equivalence trials, cluster trials, pragmatic trials, pilot and feasibility trials), data and interventions (herbal medicine, acupuncture and non-pharmacologic treatments).

In essence, the requirement is that authors should provide enough information for readers to know how the trial was performed so that they can judge whether the findings are likely to be reliable.

The CONSORT recommendations have been endorsed by many of the major clinical journals, and together with the use of checklists similar to those above, these will influence the design and conduct of future trials by increasing awareness of the requirements for a good trial.

15.10 Points When Reading the Literature About a Trial

1) Go through the checklists described in Section 15.7.
2) Check whether the trial is indeed truly randomised. Alternate patient allocation to treatments is not randomised allocation.
3) Check the diagnostic criteria for patient entry. Many treatments are tested in a restricted group of patients even though they could then be prescribed for other groups. For example, one exclusion criterion for trials of non-steroidal anti-inflammatory drugs (NSAIDs) is often extreme age, yet the drugs once evaluated are often prescribed for elderly patients.
4) Was the analysis conducted by 'intention to treat' or 'per protocol'?
5) Is the actual size of the treatment effect reported, and the associated CI reported?
6) Does the abstract correctly report what was found in the paper?
7) Have the CONSORT suggestions been followed?

15.11 Exercises

15.1 The Allen et al. (2017) trial planned to randomly allocate 200 adult smokers with a current or lifetime unipolar mood and/or anxiety disorder to receive either UN cigarettes or RN cigarettes with the nicotine reduced in five steps over 18 weeks. With reference to this trial which of the following statements, if any, are true?
   A The trial is a 'within-subjects' trial because it measures a baseline and an outcome.
   B The trial is double-blind.

C   The trial is overpowered to detect the effect size given by previous literature.
D   The trial is a superiority trial.
E   One can say the trial is properly randomised.

15.2   Berkowitz et al. (2018) conducted a trial of a home delivery of 10 meals per week for 12 weeks against usual diet and a healthy eating brochure. With reference to this cross-over trial which of the following statements, if any, are true?
A   The cross-over design is a 'within subjects' study design.
B   The sample is not prone to selection bias since subjects are compared to themselves.
C   The cross-over trial is prone to a carry-over effect.
D   The cross-over trial would be expected to take longer than the equivalent parallel groups design.
E   The cross-over trial design is more efficient than a comparable parallel groups design.

15.3   With reference to the REPOSE trial (2017) of Section 15.6 which of the following statements, if any, are true
A   The subjects were blind to treatment.
B   The subjects were randomised individually to MDIs or pumps.
C   All subjects got pumps in the end.
D   The trial showed a clear benefit of pumps compared with MDIs.
E   The cluster size was about five.

16   Sample Size Issues

Medical Statistics: A Textbook for the Health Sciences, Fifth Edition. Stephen J. Walters, Michael J. Campbell, and David Machin.
© 2021 John Wiley & Sons Ltd. Published 2021 by John Wiley & Sons Ltd.
Companion website: www.wiley.com/go/walters/medicalstatistics

Summary

We cover the rationale for sample size calculations. Calculations when the objective is to estimate a prevalence, or to compare two groups with binary or continuous outcomes are described.

16.1   Introduction

Why Sample Size Calculations?

There are a number of reasons for requiring investigators to perform a (so-called) power-based sample size calculation before the start of a study. A study that is too small may be unethical, since it exposes participants to procedures that may turn out to be of no value, if the study is not powerful enough to demonstrate a worthwhile difference. Similarly, a study that is too large may also be unethical since one may be giving patients a treatment that could already have been proven to be inferior. On more pragmatic grounds, funding agencies will require a sample size estimate since the cost of a study is usually directly proportional to the size, and the agency will want to know that its money is well spent. Many journals now have checklists that include a question on whether a sample size calculation is included (and to be reassured that is was carried out *before* the study and not in retrospect!). For example, the *Delta²* project of Cook et al. (2018) states: '*Central to the design of an RCT is an a-priori sample size calculation, which ensures the study has a high probability of achieving its pre-specified objectives*'. Such a question often forms part of measures which assess the quality of study outcome reports.

Why Not Sample Size Calculations?

A cynic once said that sample size calculations are a guess masquerading as mathematics. To perform such a calculation we often need information on factors such as the standard deviation of the outcome which may not be available. Moreover, the calculations are quite sensitive to some of the assumptions made.

One could argue that any study, whatever the size, contributes information, and therefore could be worthwhile as several small studies, pooled together in a meta-analysis (see Chapter 18), are more generalisable than one big study. Rarely is a single study alone going to answer a clinically important question. Often the size of studies is determined by practicalities, such as the number of available patients, resources, time, and the level of finance available. Finally, studies, including randomised controlled trials (RCTs), often have several outcomes, such as benefit and adverse event measures, each of which will require a different sample size and yet sample size calculations are often focussed on a single outcome.

Summing Up

Our experience is that sample size calculations are invaluable in forcing the investigator to think about a number of issues before the study commences. The mere fact that a calculation has been made suggests that a number of fundamental issues have been thought about: (i) What is the main outcome variable and when it is to be measured? (ii) What is the size of effect judged clinically or practically important? (iii) What is the method and frequency of data analysis? Some medical journals now require protocols to be lodged in advance of the study being conducted, and it can be instructive to see whether the outcomes eventually reported coincide with those highlighted in the protocol. A trial may declare two treatments equivalent, but a glance at the protocol may show that the confidence interval for the difference between them actually includes values that were deemed clinically important prior to the study commencing.

An investigator should not expect a single number carved in stone as 'the sample size' from a medical statistician, rather the statistician would supply two answers. One, whether the study is worth attempting, given the time and resources available. Secondly, a range of numbers that would indicate what size sample would be required under different scenarios.

It is important to know that the number of patients required depends on the type of summary statistic being utilised. In general, studies in which the outcome data are continuous, and can be summarised by a mean, require fewer patients than those in which the response can be assessed only as either a success or failure. Survival time studies (see Chapter 11) often require fewer events to be observed than those in which the endpoint is 'alive' or 'dead' at some fixed time after allocation to treatment.

16.2 Study Size

In statistical terms the objective of any medical study is to estimate from a sample the corresponding population parameter or parameters. Thus if we were concerned with blood pressure measurements, the corresponding population mean is μ, which is estimated by $\bar{x}$, whereas if we were concerned with the response rate to a drug the population parameter is π, which we estimate by p. When planning a study, we clearly do not know the population values and neither do we have the corresponding estimates. However, what we do need is some idea of the *anticipated* values that the population parameters may take. We denote these with the subscript 'Plan' in what follows. These anticipated values need to be derived from detailed discussions within the design team by extracting relevant information from the medical literature and their own experience. In some cases, the team may be reasonably confident in their knowledge whilst in other circumstances the 'Plan' values may be very tentative.

For illustrative purposes, we will assume we are planning a two-group randomised trial of test (T) versus control (C) treatments and we consider the situations of continuous (say blood pressure) and binary (response rate) outcomes. In either case the main parameter of interest is the true difference in efficacy of the treatments, δ, which we anticipate to be δ_{Plan}.

The appropriate number of patients to be recruited to a comparative study is dependent on four components, each of which requires careful consideration by the investigating team.

Fundamental Ingredients for a Sample Size Calculation

1) Type I error rate α.
2) Type II error rate β.
3) i) For continuous outcomes – the anticipated standard deviation of the outcome measure, σ_{Plan}, usually assumed the same in the test and control groups.
   ii) For binary outcomes – the proportion of events anticipated in the control group $\pi_{Plan,C}$.
4) i) For continuous outcomes, the target or anticipated effect size $\delta_{Plan} = \mu_{Plan,T} - \mu_{Plan,C}$.
   ii) For binary outcomes, the target or anticipated effect size $\delta_{Plan} = \pi_{Plan,T} - \pi_{Plan,C}$.

Type I and Type II Error Rates

In Chapter 6 we discussed the definition of Type I and Type II errors. The error rates are usually denoted by α and β and are the false positive and false negative error rates respectively. We argued earlier, and it is worth repeating, against the rigid use of statistical significance tests. Thus, we have discouraged the use of statements such as: 'the null hypothesis is rejected P-value < 0.05', or worse, 'we accept the null hypothesis P-value > 0.05'. However, in calculating sample size it is convenient to think in terms of a significance test and to specify the test size (and Type I error rate) α in advance. It is conventional to set $\alpha = 0.05$. We also require the acceptable false negative rate, β, that is judged to be reasonable. This is the probability of not rejecting the null hypothesis of no difference between treatments, when the anticipated benefit in fact exists. The *power* of the study is defined by $1 - \beta$, which is the probability of rejecting the null hypothesis when it is indeed false. Experience of others suggests that in practice the Type II error rate is often set at a maximum value of $\beta = 0.2$ (20%). More usually this is alternatively expressed as setting the *minimum* power of the test as $1 - \beta = 0.8$ (80%). One may ask: why is the allowable Type I error (0.05) less than the Type II error (0.20) error? Investigators are innately conservative so, in general, they would prefer to accept an established treatment against the evidence that a new treatment is better, rather than risk going over to a new treatment, with all its possible attendant problems such as long-term side effects, and different procedures.

Standard Deviation of the Outcome Measure

For continuous data it is necessary to specify the standard deviation of the outcome measure, σ_{Plan}. This may be obtained from previous studies that used this measure. Note that we need the standard deviation, not the standard error, and that it is the standard deviation of the outcome measure. When comparing two treatments, as here, it is commonly assumed that the standard deviation is the same in the two groups.

Tips on Finding the Anticipated Standard Deviation of an Estimate

- Often papers only give estimate of an effect with a 95% CI.
- We need the standard deviation, s.
- Let U be upper limit of the CI and L the lower limit.
- Use fact that $U - L$ is about four times the standard error, SE.
- Use fact that SE = $s/\sqrt{n}$ to obtain s = SE $\times \sqrt{n}$.
- Some papers give an estimate of the treatment difference, d, plus its associated 95% CI. Assuming equal numbers of subjects, n per group, and the same standard deviation in both groups then the SE(d) = $\sqrt{\dfrac{s^2}{n} + \dfrac{s^2}{n}} = \sqrt{\dfrac{2s^2}{n}} = \dfrac{\sqrt{2}s}{\sqrt{n}}$, from which s = $\dfrac{SE(d) \times \sqrt{n}}{\sqrt{2}}$.

Control Group Response

For binary data it is necessary to postulate the response of patients to the control or standard therapy. As already indicated, we denote this by $\pi_{Plan,C}$ to distinguish it from the value that will be obtained from the trial, denoted p_C. Experience of other patients with the particular disease or the medical literature may provide a reasonably precise value for $\pi_{Plan,C}$ in many circumstances.

The (Anticipated) Effect Size

The effect size is the most important variable in sample size calculations. Broadly speaking, two different approaches can be taken to specify the target difference for a trial. Either a difference that is considered to be important to one or more stakeholder groups or a realistic (plausible) difference, based on either existing evidence, or expert opinion.

The *Delta*^{2} project of Cook et al. (2018) outlines a very large literature which exists on defining and justifying a (clinically) important difference. In a similar manner, discussions of the relevance of estimates from existing studies are also common. However, there are a number of potential pitfalls to their use, which require careful consideration of how they should inform the choice of the target difference (Cook et al. 2014). In a sample size calculation for an RCT, the target difference between the treatment groups, strictly relates to a group level difference for the *anticipated* study population. Nevertheless, the difference in an outcome that is important to an individual might differ from the corresponding value at the population level. More extensive consideration of the variations in approach is provided elsewhere by Hislop et al. (2014).

For a binary outcome we must postulate the size of the anticipated response or event rate in patients receiving the new treatment, which we denote by $\pi_{\text{Plan,T}}$. Thus, one might know that approximately 40% of patients are likely to respond to the control therapy, and if this could be improved to 50% by the new therapy then a clinically worthwhile benefit would have been demonstrated. Thus, the anticipated benefit or effect size $\delta_{\text{Plan}} = \pi_{\text{Plan,T}} - \pi_{\text{Plan,C}} = 0.50 - 0.40 = 0.10\ (10\%)$. Of course, it is not yet known if the new therapy will have such benefit, but the study should be planned so that if such an advantage does exist there will be a good chance of detecting it.

Relationship Between Type I Error, Type II Error and Effect Size

In a trial, with a continuous and Normally distributed outcome, to compare two treatments with n patients in each group, the true difference in means is $\delta = \mu_T - \mu_C$, and this is estimated by the difference in sample means, $d = \bar{x}_T - \bar{x}_C$, with standard error $\text{SE}(d) = \sqrt{\dfrac{s^2}{n} + \dfrac{s^2}{n}} = \sqrt{\dfrac{2s^2}{n}} = s\sqrt{\dfrac{2}{n}}$, assuming the standard deviations, s, are the same in both groups.

Figure 16.1 shows the distribution of the difference in means, d, under the null (H_0: $\delta = 0$) and alternative hypothesis (H_A: $\delta \neq 0$). If the difference in means exceeds a certain value determined

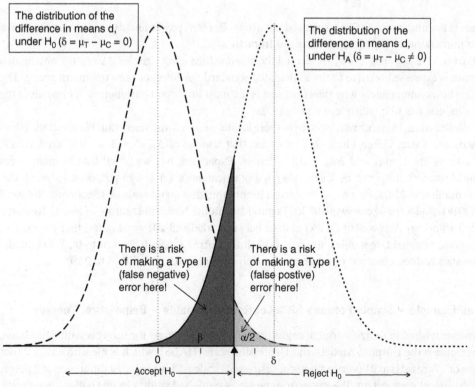

Figure 16.1 Distribution of the difference in means, d, under the null ($\delta = 0$) and alternative hypothesis ($\delta \neq 0$).

by the test statistic then we reject the null hypothesis, and accept the alternative. Where does the sample size come in? The width of the curves is determined by the standard error of the estimate, SE(d), which is proportional to the inverse of the square root of the sample size. Thus, as the sample size gets bigger the curves become narrower and therefore more peaked. In which case, if α and δ remain the same, the value of β will diminish and so the power will increase. If we keep the sample size fixed, but increase δ then again β will diminish and the power increase.

Directions of Sample Size Estimates

- Goes up for smaller α.
- Goes up for smaller β (that is, larger power).
- Goes up for smaller δ_{Plan}.
- Goes *down* for smaller σ_{Plan}.

16.3   Continuous Data

A simple formula, for comparing the mean difference in outcomes between two groups, for two-sided significance of 5% and power of 80% is given by

$$n = 16\left(\frac{\sigma_{\mathrm{Plan}}}{\delta_{\mathrm{Plan}}}\right)^2 = \frac{16}{\Delta_{\mathrm{Plan}}^2}, \tag{16.1}$$

where n is the number of patients required per group. For 90% power and two-sided significance of 5% the numerator, in Eq. (16.1), is changed from 16 to 21.

In Eq. (16.1), $\Delta_{\mathrm{Plan}} = \delta_{\mathrm{Plan}}/\sigma_{\mathrm{Plan}}$ is termed the *standardised effect size* (*SES*) since the anticipated difference is expressed relative to the anticipated standard deviation of each treatment group. The formula shows immediately why the effect size is the most important parameter – if one halves the effect size, one has to quadruple the sample size.

For clinical trials, in circumstances where there is little prior information available about the (standardised) effect size, Cohen (1988) has proposed that a value of $\Delta_{\mathrm{Plan}} \leq 0.2$ is considered 'small', $\Delta_{\mathrm{Plan}} \approx 0.5$ as 'moderate', and $\Delta_{\mathrm{Plan}} \geq 0.8$ as 'large'. Experience has suggested that in many areas of clinical research these can be taken as a good practical guide for design purposes, although this rule of thumb should not be used as an excuse for not thinking about realistic effect sizes. Rothwell et al. (2018) conducted a review of 107 RCTs published in the National Institute of Health Research Health Technology Assessment (HTA) journal between 2006 and 2016 and found that the median standardised planned target effect size was 0.30 (interquartile range, IQR: 0.20 to 0.38), whilst the median standardised observed effect size was much smaller at 0.11 (IQR 0.05 to 0.29).

Worked Example – Simple Formula for a Continuous Variable – Behavioural Therapy

Suppose we wished to design a trial of cognitive behavioural therapy for subjects with depression. The outcome is the Hospital Anxiety and Depression scale (HADS), which is measured on a 0 (not anxious or distressed) to 21 (very anxious or distressed) scale and we regard a difference of 2 points as being clinically important. We know from previous published studies in this patient population that the standard deviation of HADS score is 4 points.

Thus, the anticipated SES is, $\Delta_{Plan} = \delta_{Plan}/\sigma_{Plan} = 2/4 = 0.5$ which Cohen would suggest is a 'moderate' effect. Using Eq. 16.1, for 80% power and two-sided 5% significance, we would require $n = 64$ patients per group or 128 patients in all.

As this calculation is based on 'anticipated' values the calculated sample size should be rounded upwards sensibly – in this case certainly to 130 patients or possibly even 150 depending on circumstances.

Example from the Literature of a Sample Size for a Continuous Outcome – The IPSU Trial

The IPSU trial of Jha et al. (2018) was designed to compare the effectiveness of electric stimulation plus standard pelvic floor muscle training (intervention) compared to standard pelvic floor muscle training alone (control) in women with urinary incontinence and sexual dysfunction. The primary outcome for the trial was the mean Prolapse and Incontinence Sexual function Questionnaire (PISQ-31) physical dimension score at six-months post randomisation. The 10-item physical dimension of the PISQ-31 is scored on a 0–40 scale with higher scores indicating better sexual functioning.

From a previous study of sexual function, in 54 women, following surgery for urodynamic stress incontinence the mean PISQ-31 Physical score pre-operation was 31.0 (SD 6.2) and 35.2 (SD 4.8) post-surgery a mean improvement in sexual functioning of 4.2 points following surgery (Jha et al. 2007). The investigators assumed a three-point difference (δ_{Plan}) was of clinical and practical importance and a standard deviation of five-points ($\sigma_{Plan} = 5$) giving a SES of $\Delta_{Plan} = \delta_{Plan}/\sigma_{Plan} = 3/5 = 0.6$. Then, to have an 80% power of detecting a three-point difference in mean PISQ-31 physical dimension scores at six months between the intervention and control groups as statistically significant at the 5% (two-sided) level, using Eq. 16.1, would require 45 patients per group (90 in total).

16.4 Binary Data

For binary data, Table 16.1 shows how the number of patients required per treatment group changes as $\pi_{Plan,C}$ (denoted π_{Plan1}) changes for fixed $\alpha = 0.05$ and $1 - \beta = 0.8$.

Thus, for $\pi_{Plan1} = 0.5$ (50%), the number of patients to be recruited to each treatment decreases from approximately 400, 100, 40, and 20 as δ_{Plan} (denoted $\delta_{Plan} = \pi_{Plan2} - \pi_{Plan1}$) increases from 10, 20, 30 to 40%. If α or β are decreased then the necessary number of subjects increases. The eventual study size depends on these arbitrarily chosen values in a critical way.

Example from the Literature of Sample Size Calculation for Binary Outcomes – Corn Plaster Trial

The corn plaster trial of Farndon et al. (2013) was designed to investigate the effectiveness of salicylic acid plasters (P) compared with usual scalpel (S) debridement for treatment of foot corns. The primary outcome was the presence, at three month post randomisation, of an unhealed or recurrent corn that required further or on-going treatment. The investigators at the design or planning stage assumed that there could be a three-month recurrence rate of up to 40% with P and 60% with S and that a 20% difference in corn recurrence rates between the groups was of clinical and practical importance. These provide the anticipated response rate for the control treatment as $\pi_{Plan,C} = 0.40$ and an expected benefit, $\delta_{Plan} = \pi_{Plan,T} - \pi_{Plan,C} = 0.60 - 0.40 = 0.20$.

Setting $\alpha = 0.05$ and $1-\beta = 0.8$, then Table 16.1 suggests approximately $n = 97$ patients per group. Thus, a total of 194 (2×97) patients would be required for the trial study. For the protocol the investigators rounded the target sample size up to 100 participants in each treatment arm.

Table 16.1 Sample size n per group for the comparison of two anticipated or planned proportions π_{Plan1} and π_{Plan2} with 80% power $(1 - \beta = 0.80)$ and 5% $(\alpha = 0.05)$ two-sided significance.

π_{Plan2}	π_{Plan1}																	
	0.05	0.10	0.15	0.20	0.25	0.30	0.35	0.40	0.45	0.50	0.55	0.60	0.65	0.70	0.75	0.80	0.85	0.90
0.10	432																	
0.15	138	683																
0.20	73	197	903															
0.25	47	97	248	1092														
0.30	33	59	118	291	1248													
0.35	24	40	70	136	326	1374												
0.40	19	29	47	79	150	354	1468											
0.45	15	22	33	52	86	160	373	1531										
0.50	12	17	25	36	55	91	167	385	1562									
0.55	10	14	19	27	38	58	94	171	389	1562								
0.60	8	11	15	20	28	40	59	95	171	385	1531							
0.65	6	9	12	16	21	29	40	59	94	167	373	1468						
0.70	5	7	9	12	16	21	29	40	58	91	160	354	1374					
0.75	4	6	7	10	12	16	21	28	38	55	86	150	326	1248				
0.80	3	5	6	7	10	12	16	20	27	36	52	79	136	291	1092			
0.85	3	4	5	6	7	9	12	15	19	25	33	47	70	118	248	903		
0.90	2	3	4	5	6	7	9	11	14	17	22	29	40	59	97	197	683	
0.95	1	2	3	3	4	5	6	8	10	12	15	19	24	33	47	73	138	432
1.00	1	1	2	2	3	4	5	6	7	8	10	12	15	19	24	32	45	71

The cells in the table give the number of patients required in each group.

Formulae for more precise calculations for the number of patients required to make comparisons of two proportions and for the comparison of two means are given in Section 16.8. The book by Machin et al. (2018) gives extensive examples, tables and computer software for this and other situations.

It is usual at the planning stage of a study to investigate differences that would arise if the assumptions used in the calculations are altered. In particular we may have over-estimated the response rate of the controls. If $\pi_{\text{Plan,C}}$ is set to 0.45 rather than 0.40, but keeping $\pi_{\text{Plan,T}} = 0.60$ then $\delta_{\text{Plan}} = 0.15$. As a result, there is now a major change in our estimate of the required number of patients from $n = 97$ to approximately 173 per group. As a consequence, we may have to be concerned about the reliability of the planning value utilised.

In certain situations, an investigator may have access only to a restricted number of patients for a particular trial. In this case the investigator reasonably asks: 'with an anticipated response rate $\pi_{\text{Plan,C}}$ in the controls, a difference in efficacy postulated to be δ_{Plan}, and assuming $\alpha = 0.05$, what is the power $1-\beta$ of my proposed study?' If the power is low, say 50%, the investigator should decide not to proceed further with the trial, or seek the help of other colleagues, perhaps in other centres, to recruit more patients to the trial and thereby increase the power to an acceptable value. This device of encouraging others to contribute to the collective attack on a clinically important question is used by, for example, the British Medical Research Council, the US National Institutes of Health, and the World Health Organization.

16.5 Prevalence

We described surveys in Chapter 14 and one might be designed to find out, for example, how many people wear dentures. Such a study is non-comparative and therefore does not involve hypothesis testing, but does require a sample size calculation. Here, what we need to know is how accurately should we estimate the prevalence of people wearing dentures in the population. Recall from Chapter 5 that, if N (rather than n) is the sample size, then the estimated standard error of the proportion p estimated from a study is $\text{SE}(p) = \sqrt{\dfrac{p(1-p)}{N}}$. This expression can be inverted to give

$$N = \frac{p(1-p)}{\text{SE}(p)^2}.$$

Thus, if we state that we would like to estimate a prevalence, which is anticipated to have a particular value π_{Plan}, and we would like to have a 95% confidence interval of $\pi_{\text{Plan}} \pm 1.96\text{SE}_{\text{Plan}}$. Now we have the ingredients for a sample size calculation if we specify a required magnitude for the SE in advance. Specifically

$$N = \frac{\pi_{\text{Plan}}(1 - \pi_{\text{Plan}})}{\text{SE}_{\text{Plan}}^2}.$$

Here, there is no explicit power value. The Type I error is reflected in the width of the confidence interval. If we do carry out a survey of the prescribed size, N, *and* the prevalence is about the size of π_{Plan} we specified, then we would expect our calculated confidence interval to be wider than specified 50% of the time, and narrower than specified 50% of the time.

Worked Example – Sample Size – Prevalence

Suppose we wished to estimate the prevalence of left-handed people in a population, using a postal questionnaire survey. We believe that it should be about 10% and we would like to have a final 95% confidence interval of 4 to 16%.

Here $\pi_{\text{Plan}} = 0.1$ and the anticipated width of the confidence interval is 0.16 to 0.04 = 0.12, suggesting $\text{SE}_{\text{Plan}} = 0.12/(2 \times 1.96) \approx 0.03$. Thus $N = [0.1(1 - 0.1)]/(0.03^2) = 100$. This implies the upper

Table 16.2 Sample size N required to estimate the anticipated prevalence (π_{Plan}) with upper and lower confidence limits of ±0.01, ±0.02, ±0.05, ±0.06, or ±0.10 away from the anticipated value.

π_{Plan}	Required precision for the upper and lower confidence limits for the anticipated prevalence π_{Plan}				
	±0.01	±0.02	±0.05	±0.06	±0.10
0.05	1825	457	73		
0.10	3458	865	139	97	35
0.15	4899	1225	196	137	49
0.20	6147	1537	246	171	62
0.25	7203	1801	289	201	73
0.30	8068	2017	323	225	81
0.35	8740	2185	350	243	88
0.40	9220	2305	369	257	93
0.45	9508	2377	381	265	96
0.50	9604	2401	385	267	97
0.55	9508	2377	381	265	96
0.60	9220	2305	369	257	93
0.65	8740	2185	350	243	88
0.70	8068	2017	323	225	81
0.75	7203	1801	289	201	73
0.80	6147	1537	246	171	62
0.85	4899	1225	196	137	49
0.90	3458	865	139	97	35
0.95	1825	457	73	–	–

and lower limits of the confidence interval are ±0.06 away from the estimated prevalence, π_{Plan}. Using Table 16.2, this leads to a more accurately estimated sample size of $N = 97$.

Note N is the number of responders to the survey. We may have to survey more patients to allow for non-response. If we assume a 50% response rate to the postal survey then we actually need to mail out $2 \times 100 = 200$ questionnaires in order to get the required number of responders.

16.6 Subject Withdrawals

One aspect of a clinical trial, which can affect the number of patients recruited, is the proportion of patients who are lost to follow-up during the course of the trial. These withdrawals are a particular problem for trials in which patients are monitored over a long period of follow-up time.

In these circumstances, as a precaution against such withdrawals, the planned number of patients is adjustment upwards to $N_W = N/(1-W)$ where W is the anticipated withdrawal proportion. The estimated size of W can often be obtained from reports of studies conducted by others. Walters et al. (2017) following a review of 151 RCTs published by the UK's National Institute for Health Research (NIHR) HTA Programme found that the median retention rate (proportion of participants with valid primary outcome data at follow-up) was estimated at 89% (IQR 79 to 97%), that is, an attrition or withdrawal rate of 11%. If there is no such experience to hand, then a pragmatic value may be to take $W = 0.1$.

Example from the Literature – Withdrawals – The IPSU Trial

For the IPSU trial of Jha et al. (2018) the sample size calculations from Eq. 16.1 suggested approximately $n = 45$ patients per group (90 in total). The investigators assumed an anticipated a $W = 0.2$ (20%) withdrawal rate so the trial needed to recruit and randomise in total $N_W = 90/(1 - 0.8) = 112.5$ or 114 patients.

16.7 Other Aspects of Sample Size Calculations

Pilot Studies

A RCT is a major and expensive undertaking and one should not embark on one lightly. One sensible step is to start with feasibility and pilot studies. These are conducted to inform a later definitive study. Their aim is to fill gaps in knowledge that need to be clarified before progressing to a full trial. The intention is that by resolving points of uncertainty at an early stage the ultimate study is more likely to succeed. A developed framework suggests the following definitions: a feasibility study asks whether something can be done, should we proceed with it, and if so, how. A pilot study asks the same question but has a specific design feature in mind: in a pilot study a future trial, or a component of an intended future trial, is conducted but on a smaller scale (Eldridge et al. 2016).

The corollary of these definitions is that all pilot studies are feasibility studies but not all feasibility studies are pilot studies. Avery et al. (2017) define internal and external pilot studies as follows: an external pilot is a rehearsal of the main study where the outcome data are not included as part of the main trial outcome data set whereas in an internal pilot, the pilot phase forms the first part of the trial and the outcome data generated may contribute to the final analysis.

The choice of design (internal or external) should be pre-specified to avoid bias. External pilot studies allow for greater flexibility to change the trial design for the main study once the pilot is complete, whereas internal pilot studies may be seen as more efficient. The CONSORT extension for pilot trials can be used for designing and planning a pilot trial, not just when reporting (Eldridge et al. 2016).

The sample size for an external pilot or feasibility study should be adequate to estimate the uncertain critical parameters (SD for continuous outcomes; consent/recruitment rates, event rates, attrition rates for binary outcomes) needed to inform the design of the full RCT with sufficient precision. The usually relatively small sample size of the external pilot study will affect the accuracy of the resulting SD, s_{Pilot}. The small sample size introduces some imprecision that should be allowed for when deciding the corresponding planning value, σ_{Plan}, which is then to be used as a key element when estimating the sample size for the main trial. Two different methods, the upper confidence limit (UCL) and the non-central t (NCT) approach, have been developed to deal with the issue of imprecise SD estimates. Both methods allow for the imprecision of s_{Pilot} by automatically inflating its observed value. It is this inflated estimate σ_{Main} that is then used for the main trial sample size calculation (Machin et al. 2018). There are several flat rules of thumb (see Table 16.3) for sample sizes for two-armed external pilot trials ranging from 24 in total to as many as 150 depending on the inflation method characteristics chosen.

Example from Literature of Sample Size for a Pilot or Feasibility Study – The POLAR Trial
The POLAR trial of Reddington et al. (2017, 2018) was an external pilot RCT, in patients with lumbar radicular syndrome (LRS), designed to investigate the feasibility of undertaking a definitive trial to compare the effectiveness of early intervention physiotherapy or usual care. They used the Teare

Table 16.3 Flat rules of thumb for external pilot trial sample sizes (for a two-armed trial) with a continuous Normally distributed outcome.

Author	Type of calculation	Inflation method	Recommended total sample size
Browne (1995)	Precision based		30
Julious (2005)	Precision based		24
Sim and Lewis (2012)	Drop in main trial power	90% UCL	60
	Drop in main trial power	95% UCL	50
Teare et al. (2014)	Precision based		70
Whitehead et al. (2016)	NCT, SES $\Delta = 0.1$		150
	NCT, SES $\Delta = 0.2$		50
	NCT, SES $\Delta = 0.5$		30
	NCT, SES $\Delta = 0.8$		20

NCT – non-central t, UCL – upper confidence limit, SES – standardised effect size.

et al. (2014) rule of thumb that recommend that an external pilot study has at least 70 measured subjects (35 per group) when estimating the SD for a continuous outcome.

Post-hoc Sample Size Calculations

Sample size estimation and power calculation are essentially a priori, that is, before the data is collected. After a trial has been carried out, it is the *observed* data that will determine the size and direction of the treatment effect and the corresponding width of any confidence interval. Thus, it is the size (with the width of the associated confidence interval) of the treatment effect and its interpretation that are important. The value set by the a priori power at the design stage is immaterial to this. The width of the confidence interval depends on the precision or standard error of the estimated treatment effect, which is itself dependent on the variability of the outcome and the study sample size. The only parameter we need to consider from the initial power calculation is the size of the effect we considered to be clinically/practically meaningful, δ_{Plan}, and how our observed treatment effect and associated confidence intervals appear in relation to this Walters (2008).

Other Designs

This chapter is only intended to cover the basics of sample size calculations. Further examples of sample size calculations for a wide variety of other designs and outcomes are covered by Machin et al. (2018).

Summary

A sample size calculation and any such estimate (with all its attendant assumptions) is better than no sample size calculation at all. The mere fact of a sample size calculation means that the investigators have thought about a number of fundamental issues. In particular: what is the main outcome variable? What is a clinically/practically important effect? How is it measured? What methods (and with what frequency) are to be used for data analysis? Thus, protocols that are explicit about sample size are easier to evaluate in terms of their scientific quality and the likelihood of achieving their objectives.

16.8   Points When Reading the Literature

1) Check if there is a power-based assessment of the sample size, which was done before the study was conducted, or if the sample size was based on availability of subjects. If neither then consider the report to be of lower quality.
2) Check if the variable used in the sample size calculation is the main outcome in the analysis.
3) If a study is not statistically significant, and the authors are claiming equivalence, look at the size of the effect considered clinically important in the sample size calculation and see if the confidence intervals reported in the analysis contain this effect. If so, the equivalence claim is not proven.
4) Check that the key items in the sample size calculation are given, namely: Type I and Type II error rates, the effect size and the variability of the outcome if the outcome is continuous, or the control arm prevalence if the outcome is binary.

16.9   Technical Details

As described earlier, to compute sample sizes we need to specify a two-sided significance level α and a power $1 - \beta$. The calculations depend on a function $(z_{1-\alpha/2} + z_{1-\beta})^2$, where $z_{1-\alpha/2}$ and $z_{1-\beta}$ are the values from the standard Normal distribution (corresponding to areas or probabilities under the Normal distribution curve of $1 - \alpha/2$ and $1 - \beta$ respectively). Some convenient values of $z_{1-\alpha/2}$ and $z_{1-\beta}$ are given in Table 16.4.

Continuous Outcomes – Comparison of Two Means

Suppose in the control treatment group we expect the mean outcome to be $\mu_{\text{Plan,C}}$ and in the test treatment group we expect the mean outcome to be $\mu_{\text{Plan,T}}$, a planned or target difference of $\mu_{\text{Plan,T}} - \mu_{\text{Plan,C}} = \delta_{\text{Plan}}$. If the standard deviation, σ_{Plan}, of the outcome is assumed to be the same in both groups, then for a two-sided significance level α and power $1 - \beta$ the approximate number of patients per group, is:

$$n_{\text{Cont}} \text{ per group} = \frac{2\sigma_{\text{Plan}}^2 (z_{1-\alpha/2} + z_{1-\beta})^2}{\delta_{\text{Plan}}^2} \text{ or } \frac{2(z_{1-\alpha/2} + z_{1-\beta})^2}{\Delta_{\text{Plan}}^2}. \tag{16.4}$$

Worked Example – Comparison of Two Means

Suppose we are planning a two-group RCT of new type of cognitive behavioural therapy for treating depression in stroke patients compared to usual stroke care (USC). The primary outcome measure will be the Patient Health Questionnaire-9 (PHQ-9) six-months post-randomisation. The PHQ-9 is a nine-item self-completed questionnaire used as a screening and diagnostic tool for mental health disorders, scored on a 0–27 scale with higher scores indicating more depressive symptoms. Suppose we regard a difference of three points as being clinically or practically important.

Table 16.4 Table of Z values from the Normal distribution for various α and $1 - \beta$.

α		$1 - \beta$	Z
Two sided	One sided		
0.001	0.0005	0.9995	3.2905
0.005	0.0025	0.9975	2.8070
0.010	0.0050	0.9950	2.5758
0.020	0.0100	0.9900	2.3263
0.025	0.0125	0.9875	2.2414
0.050	0.0250	0.9750	1.9600
0.100	0.0500	0.9500	1.6449
0.200	0.1000	0.9000	1.2816
0.300	0.1500	0.8500	1.0364
0.400	0.2000	0.8000	0.8416
0.500	0.2500	0.7500	0.6745
0.600	0.3000	0.7000	0.5244
0.700	0.3500	0.6500	0.3853
0.800	0.4000	0.6000	0.2533

Thomas et al. (2019) describe the results of a RCT to comparing behavioural activation (BA) to USC for four months for patients with post-stroke depression. They report the mean difference in PHQ-9 scores at six-month post-randomisation between the BA and USC as 4.3 points (95% CI: 0.4 to 8.2) for 39 stroke patients. The width of the CI is 8.2 to 0.4 = 7.8, which is four standard errors. So, one SE = 7.8/4 = 1.95. If we assume an equal sample size of 39/2 = 19.5 or 20 per group then the estimated SD of the PHQ-9 outcome in this sample is $(SE \times \sqrt{n})/\sqrt{2} = (1.95 \times \sqrt{20})/\sqrt{2} = 6.2$. Given this is an estimate from a relatively small trial then to be conservative this is rounded to the nearest larger whole number to give an SD of seven points for the PHQ-9 outcome.

Suppose one planned a trial to detect a difference of three-points, with SD = 7, power 90% and 5% two-significance level. Here $\delta_{Plan} = 3$, $\sigma_{Plan} = 7$ giving $\Delta_{Plan} = 3/7 = 0.43$. Use of Table 16.4 with $\alpha = 0.05$ and $\beta = 0.1$ gives $z_{1 - \alpha/2} = 1.96$ and $z_{1 - \beta} = 1.2816$, hence

$$n = \frac{2 \times 7^2 \times (1.96 + 1.2816)^2}{3^2} = 114.4 \text{ or (rounding up to the nearest whole number) 115 per}$$

group or $N = 230$ patients in total.

Binary Outcomes – Comparison of Two Proportions

Suppose we wished to detect a planned difference in proportions $\delta_{Plan} = \pi_{Plan,T} - \pi_{Plan,C}$ with two-sided significance level α and power $1 - \beta$. For a χ^2 test, the number in each group should be at least

$$n_{Binary} \text{ per group} = \frac{(z_{1-\alpha/2} + z_{1-\beta})^2 [\pi_{T,Plan}(1 - \pi_{T,Plan}) + \pi_{C,Plan}(1 - \pi_{C,Plan})]}{\delta_{Plan}^2}. \tag{16.5}$$

We can also use Table 16.1, if we only require a significance level of 5% and a power of 80%.

Worked Example – Comparison of Two Proportions

In a clinical trial suppose the anticipated placebo response is 0.25, and a worthwhile response to the drug is 0.50. How many subjects are required in each group so that we have an 80% power at 5% significance level?

With $\alpha = 0.05$ and $\beta = 0.2$, then from Table 16.4, gives $z_{1 - \alpha/2} = 1.96$ and $z_{1 - \beta} = 0.8416$. The investigators suggest $\delta_{Plan} = \pi_{Plan,T} - \pi_{Plan,C} = 0.25$, $n = \frac{(1.96 + 0.8416)^2 [0.5(1 - 0.5) + 0.25(1 - 0.25)]}{(0.25)^2} = 54.9$ or 55 per group after rounding to the nearest whole number. Thus, we need at least $N = 2n = 2 \times 55 = 110$ patients in all. From Table 16.1, we would be able to say that the required number of patients is 55 per group.

16.10 Exercises

16.1 When calculating the required sample size for a two-group superiority RCT with a continuous outcome which of ONE of the following pieces of information is NOT required?

    A The probability of a Type I error.
    B The probability of a Type II error.
    C The variability or standard deviation of the outcome.
    D The proportion in the control group with a positive outcome.
    E The anticipated or target effect size.

16.2 Which ONE of the following statements about how the required sample size for a study changes is INCORRECT?

    A Goes up with a smaller Type I error.
    B Goes up with smaller Type II error.
    C Goes up with a larger power.
    D Goes down with a larger power.
    E Goes down with a larger effect size.

16.3 Which ONE of the following statements about the Type I error is INCORRECT?

    A The Type I error is the probability of rejecting the null hypothesis when it is true.
    B The Type I error is the probability of a false positive result.
    C The usual level for Type I error rate in sample size calculations is 0.05.
    D The Type I error is the probability of rejecting the null hypothesis when it is false.
    E We can reduce the risk of a Type I error by increasing the level of statistical significance we demand.

16.4 Which ONE of the following statements about the Type II error is INCORRECT?

    A The Type II error is the probability of rejecting the null hypothesis when it is true.
    B The Type II error is the probability of a false negative result.
    C The usual level for Type II error rate in sample size calculations is 0.10 or 0.20.
    D To make a Type II error is to reject the alternative hypothesis when it is true.
    E We can reduce the risk of a Type II error by increasing the power of the study.

16.5 When calculating the required sample size for a two-group superiority RCT with a binary outcome which of ONE of the following pieces of information is NOT required?

A   The probability of a Type I error.

B   The probability of a Type II error.

C   The variability or standard deviation of the outcome.

D   The proportion in the control group with a positive outcome.

E   The anticipated or target effect size.

16.6 Which ONE of the following statements about the SES Δ_{Plan} used in the sample size formula for continuous data is INCORRECT?

A Δ_{Plan} is calculated as the difference in means divided by the standard deviation of the outcome.

B   Goes down with a larger standard deviation

C   Goes up with a larger standard deviation.

D   Goes up with a larger mean difference.

E   A Δ_{Plan} of 0.5 is equivalent to a difference of half a standard deviation between the group means.

Suppose we are planning a new RCT in patients with venous leg ulcers to see if a new treatment with a special chemically impregnated dressing called 'Quickheal' will lead to improved outcomes compared to a standard dressing (control). The primary outcome for the trial will be the number of weeks the patients are ulcer free over the 12-month post-randomisation follow-up period. We know from published data that the mean number of ulcer-free weeks is 20 (with a standard deviation of 20 weeks). Suppose the effect of the new dressing on ulcer healing will be considered important if it increases the number of ulcer-free weeks, at one-year post-randomisation, by at least eight weeks.

16.7 The SES for the sample size calculation is:

A   0.20

B   0.30

C   0.33

D   0.35

E   0.40

16.8 Work out how many patients (in total in both groups combined) need to be recruited to the 'Quickheal' trial with a 5% (two-sided) significance level and a power of 80%?

A   100

B   193

C   132

D   200

E   264

16.9 How many patients in each group would need to be recruited to the 'Quickheal' trial with a 5% (two-sided) significance level and a power of 90%?

A   100

B   193

C   132

D   200

E   264

16.10 Suppose the effect of the new dressing on ulcer healing will be considered important if it increases the number of ulcer-free weeks, at one-year post-randomisation, by at least 10 weeks. The SES for the sample size calculation is:

A   0.20
B   0.30
C   0.30
D   0.40
E   0.50

16.11 Suppose the primary outcome for the study is changed to a binary outcome of whether or not the ulcer had healed at three month post-randomisation. Published data on ulcer healing rates in this population suggest an ulcer healing rate of 20%. Suppose the effect of the new dressing will be considered important if it increases the ulcer healing rate from 20% to 30%, at three month post-randomisation.

Use the appropriate sample size formula to work out how many patients in each group need to be recruited to such a trial with a 5% (two-sided) significance level and a power of 80%?

A   291
B   389
C   582
D   778
E   1251

16.12 Use the appropriate sample size formula to work out how many patients in each group need to be recruited to such a trial with a 5% (two-sided) significance level and a power of 90%?

A   291
B   389
C   582
D   778
E   1251

17   Other Statistical Methods

Medical Statistics: A Textbook for the Health Sciences, Fifth Edition. Stephen J. Walters, Michael J. Campbell, and David Machin.
© 2021 John Wiley & Sons Ltd. Published 2021 by John Wiley & Sons Ltd.
Companion website: www.wiley.com/go/walters/medicalstatistics

Summary

This chapter will describe some methods not covered elsewhere in this book. These include: analysis of longitudinal data (particularly summary measures such as the area under the curve [AUC]); imputation of missing data; bootstrap methods; and Poisson regression.

   This chapter will describe how outcome data from longitudinal studies can be summarised, tabulated, and graphically displayed. It will also show how repeated measures for each subject can be reduced to a single summary measure for statistical analysis and how standard statistical methods of analysis can then be used. Finally, it will describe two extensions of the linear regression model, marginal and random effects models, which allow for the fact that successive measurements assessments by a particular patient are likely to be correlated.

17.1   Analysing Serial or Longitudinal Data

Recall that one of the main purposes of a statistical analysis is to generalise from the sample to the population. Measuring one individual repeatedly does not tell us what measurements on other individuals are likely to be. One needs some measure of the variation between individuals to be able to generalise. Thus it is important to distinguish between different sorts of variation. Imagine measuring blood pressure. The purpose may be to decide on a person's true blood pressure, or it may be to see the effects of treatment on blood pressure. There is variation due to measurement error, there is variation of the measurement over time on the same person and variation between people. Often a study will measure individuals repeatedly and there are sound reasons for doing this. If the measurement error is thought to be high, then measures made close in time can be averaged to give a better estimate of the true value for an individual. Thus GPs recommend measuring blood pressure in the morning and evening for seven days to determine an individual's true blood pressure. If the measures are thought to vary over time; for example if the patient is improving in health, then measures spaced in time can estimate the rate of progress. Finally, to generalise to the population, we need to take measurements on a number of individuals. These repeated measurements, on the same individual subject, are likely to be related or correlated. This means that the usual statistical methods for analysing such data (such as the two independent samples *t*-test and multiple linear regression described in Chapters 7 and 9 respectively) which assume independent outcomes may not be appropriate. In particular, if different numbers of measurements are made for different individuals, these need to be accounted for. One cannot treat one individual measured 100 times the same as 100 individuals measured once. This section will show how repeated measures for each subject can be reduced to a single summary measure for statistical analysis and how standard statistical methods of analysis can then be used. Finally, the section will describe a more complex modelling approach, based on an extension of the linear regression model that allows for the fact that successive outcomes assessments by a particular patient are likely to be correlated.

Three Broad Approaches to Analysing Repeated Measurements

For data that comprise repeated measurements, there are several different approaches to analysis that can be adopted. Three broad approaches described by Everitt (2002) are:

1) Time by time analysis

2) Response feature analysis – the use of summary measures
3) Modelling of longitudinal data.

To illustrate some of the methods we will use data from the low back pain trial (Thomas et al. 2006). The primary objective of the trial was to determine the effect of a short course of acupuncture compared with usual care (usual) for the treatment of persistent non-specific low back pain. The trial design was a pragmatic unblinded individually randomised controlled trial with 24 month follow-up. The primary outcome was self-reported pain as measured by the SF-36 bodily pain outcome measured at baseline, 3, 12 and 24 months post-randomisation. Figure 17.1 shows that 241 patients were randomised but by 24 months follow-up there were only 76% (182/241) with outcome data for analysis.

Summarising Repeated Measurements

An important initial step, prior to analysing the repeated measurements, is to tabulate the data and/or graphically display it (Walters 2009a), as this will give an idea of how the outcomes change over time. In the low back pain trial, the patients' pain was assessed four times; at baseline (0), and 3, 12 and 24 months after randomisation using part of the quality of life (QoL) measure, the SF-36. The SF-36 pain dimension is scored on a 0 (poor) to 100 (good health) scale. Table 17.1 shows one way of presenting such data. Note that differences between the acupuncture and usual care groups in the mean SF-36 pain scores are not tested at each time point. The results of the hypothesis test and confidence intervals are only presented for two summary measures, in the last two rows of the table, the mean follow-up and the AUC. These summary measures are described later. The sample size at each of the follow-up time points varies and therefore it is important to report the sample size for each row of the data.

Table 17.2 is in the same format as Table 17.1 but this time gives the results for only those patients who completed all four QoL assessments. This makes it easier to see how the mean pain scores vary over time. We can plot such data as a line graph of Figure 17.2a, with a separate line for each group. This clearly shows how the pain outcome varies over the two-year period. The acupuncture group appears to have slightly better pain scores at all three follow-up time points compared to the usual care group. Because the same numbers of subjects are included at each time point, it is legitimate to join the mean pain scores together with a solid line. However, if the data in Table 17.1 were presented in a similar figure it would be misleading to join the observed means at each time point by solid lines, since we are not measuring the same people at each time point. Figure 17.2b shows how the mean SF-36 pain scores varies over time using all available QoL data. The number of valid QoL observations per group at each assessment time point are included just below the horizontal axis. This makes clear how the number of valid QoL observations at the various follow-up assessment points declines over time and on how many subjects the calculation of each mean summary measure is based. Again, the mean profiles and pattern are similar to the complete case analysis with the acupuncture group having slightly better pain scores at all three follow-up time points compared to the usual care group.

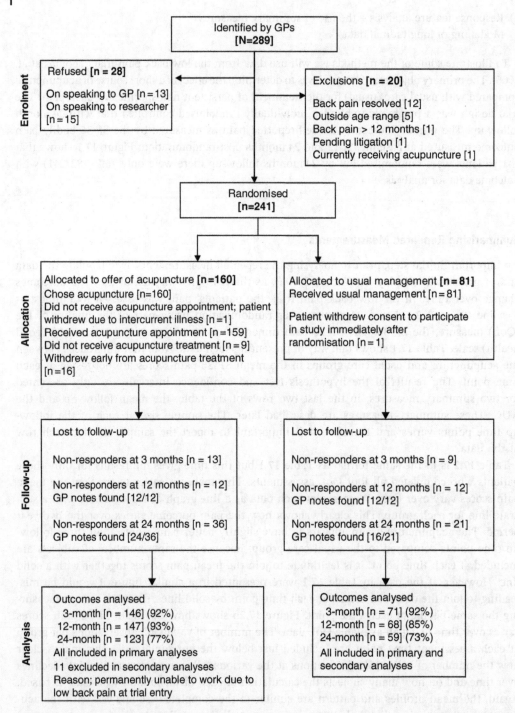

Figure 17.1 Patient progress through the trial – CONSORT flow chart for low back pain study. (*Source:* data from Thomas et al. 2006).

Table 17.1 Mean SF-36 pain scores over time by treatment group with all valid patients at each time point.

SF-36 pain outcome[a]	Treatment group						Difference in means[b]	95% CI		P-value[c]
	Usual care			Acupuncture				Lower	Upper	
Time (months)	n	Mean	SD	n	Mean	SD				
0	80	30.4	(18.0)	159	30.8	(16.2)				
3	71	55.4	(25.4)	146	60.9	(23.0)				
12	68	58.3	(22.2)	147	64.0	(25.6)				
24	59	59.5	(23.4)	123	67.8	(24.1)				
Mean of 3, 12 and 24 month follow-ups	76	57.2	(19.8)	153	63.4	(20.9)	6.3	0.6	12.0	0.030
AUC	59	113.2	(36.7)	123	124.8	(38.9)	11.5	−0.4	23.5	0.058

CI: confidence interval; AUC: area under the curve.
[a] The SF-36 pain dimension is scored on a 0 (poor) to 100 (good health) scale.
[b] A positive mean difference indicates the acupuncture group has the better QoL.
[c] P-value from two independent samples *t*-test.
Source: data from the low back pain trial (Thomas et al. 2006).

Table 17.2 Mean SF-36 pain scores over time by treatment group with patients who completed all four QoL assessments.

SF-36 pain outcome[a]	Treatment group						Difference in means[b]	95% CI		P-value[c]
	Usual care			Acupuncture				Lower	Upper	
Time (months)	n	Mean	SD	n	Mean	SD				
0	55	29.9	(18.5)	118	31.5	(16.6)				
3	55	57.4	(26.9)	118	62.3	(22.4)				
12	55	57.8	(21.8)	118	64.1	(25.4)				
24	55	59.4	(23.7)	118	68.1	(23.8)				
Mean of 3, 12 and 24 month follow-ups	55	58.2	(19.5)	118	64.8	(20.1)	6.7	0.3	13.1	0.042
AUC	55	112.7	(36.7)	118	125.2	(39.4)	12.6	0.1	25.0	0.048

CI: confidence interval; AUC: area under the curve.
[a] The SF-36 pain dimension is scored on a 0 (poor) to 100 (good health) scale.
[b] A positive mean difference indicates the acupuncture group has the better QoL.
[c] P-value from two independent samples *t*-test.
Source: data from Thomas et al. (2006).

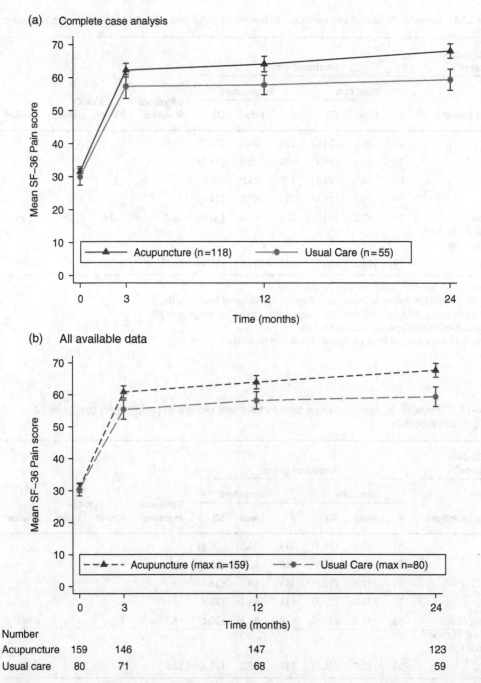

(a)   Complete case analysis

(b)   All available data

Number
Acupuncture   159   146   147   123
Usual care   80   71   68   59

Figure 17.2 Profile of mean SF-36 pain scores over time by treatment group (*Source:* data from Thomas et al. 2006). The points on the graph are means, the bars are ±1 SEM (standard error of mean). (a) Complete case analysis. (b) All available data.

Time by Time Analysis

A series of two independent samples t-tests (or the non-parametric equivalent), could be used to test for differences in outcomes, between the two groups at each time point. For example, in the low back pain trial we could compare mean SF-36 pain scores between the acupuncture and usual care groups at 3, 12 and 24 month post-randomisation using a series of three independent sample t-tests. The procedure is straightforward but has a number of serious flaws and weaknesses as pointed out by Everitt (2001). In particular, the measurements in a subject from one time point to the next are not independent, so interpretation of the results is difficult. The large number of hypothesis tests carried out implies that we are likely to obtain significant results purely by chance. We lose information about the within-subject changes in the measurement over time. Consequently, we will not describe this method any further here.

Response Feature Analysis – The Use of Summary Measures

Here the repeated measures for each participant are summarised into a single number considered to capture some important aspect of the participant's response (Matthews et al. 1990).

A simple and often effective strategy is to:

1) Reduce the repeated measurements into one or two summaries;
2) Analyse each summary as the main outcome measure.

Examples of summary measures include the AUC or the overall mean of the post-randomisation measures. Other possible summary measures are listed in Matthews et al. (1990) and are shown in Table 17.3. Having identified a suitable summary measure, a simple t-test (or ANOVA) can be applied to assess between group differences. If the data for each patient can effectively be summarised by a pre-treatment mean and a post-treatment mean, then the analysis of covariance (ANCOVA) is the preferred method of choice (Frison and Pocock 1992). It is superior to both the analysis of post-treatment means or analysis of mean changes. Diggle et al. (2002) suggested that provided the data are complete, then the method of derived variables or summary measures can give a simple and easily interpretable analysis with a strong focus on particular aspects of the mean response.

The Area Under the Curve (AUC)

The AUC is a useful way of summarising the information from a series of measurements on one individual (Matthews et al. 1990). The AUC can also be used to *summarise* repeated observations over time into a single measure for each patient.

Table 17.3 Response features suggested in Matthews et al. (1990).

Type of data	Property to be compared between groups	Summary measure
Peaked	Overall value of response	Mean or area under the curve (AUC)
Peaked	Value of most extreme response	Maximum (minimum)
Peaked	Delay in response	Time to maximum or minimum
Growth	Rate of change of response	Linear regression coefficient
Growth	Final level of response	Final value or (relative) difference between first and last observation
Growth	Delay in response	Time to reach a particular value

Calculating the AUC

The area (see Figure 17.3) can be split into a series of trapeziums. The areas of the separate individual trapeziums are calculated as the sum of their two parallel sides multiplied by the time interval between them. These are then summed for each patient to obtain the AUC for that patient.

Thus if Q_j represent the response variable observed at times $t_1 = 0$, t_2, t_3, ..., t_{T-1}, $t_T = T$ on a particular subject, then the set of repeated outcomes for that subject can be collected into a single row of length $T + 1$, that is, $\boldsymbol{Q} = (Q_0, Q_1, Q_2, ...,Q_T)$. The AUC for that subject is calculated by

$$AUC = \frac{1}{2} \sum_{j=0}^{T-1} (t_{j+1} - t_j)(Q_{j+1} + Q_j) \qquad (17.1)$$

When the time points are equally spaced, the intervals concerned, $\delta_t = (t_{j+1} - t_j)$, are constant of width (say) Δ. Eq. (17.1) then reduces to $AUC = \Delta \left(\frac{Q_0 + Q_T}{2} + \sum_{j=1}^{T-1} Q_j \right)$.

The AUC can be calculated for an individual even when there are some missing data, except when the first and final observations are missing. The units of AUC are the product of the units used for Q and t, and may not be easy to understand. Also, it may be useful to divide the AUC by the total time, T, to obtain a weighted average level of the response over the time period. If there are N patients to consider, then the overall AUC is the mean of the AUCs obtained from each individual.

In the low back pain trial, the patients' pain was assessed four times. If the time for each QoL assessment is represented in years then the AUCs represent the weighted average level of QoL over the two-year period. An AUC of 200 would correspond to no pain or 'good health' over the period, conversely an AUC of 0, corresponds to 'poor health' or high levels of pain over the period. If we divide by the total time (of two years) then we get back to the 0 to 100 scale of the original SF-36 pain scale measurement which makes interpretation of the results somewhat easier.

Consider a patient in the low back pain trial, with SF-36 pain scale scores of 33.3, 44.4, 55.6 and 77.8 at 0, 0.25, 1 and 2 years, then the AUC for this patient is:

$$AUC = 0.5 \times \{[(0.25 - 0) \times (33.3 + 44.4)] + [(1 - 0.25) \times (44.4 + 55.6)]$$
$$+ [(2 - 1) \times (55.6 + 77.7)]\} = 113.9.$$

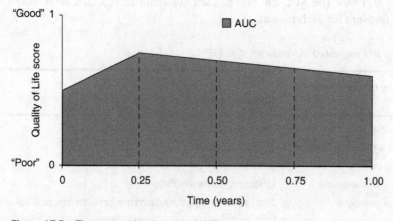

Figure 17.3 The area under the curve (AUC).

Confidence intervals for the difference in mean AUC between groups can be readily calculated as the AUCs are more likely than the original observations to be plausibly Normally distributed. Multiple linear regression methods can be used to adjust AUCs for other covariates such as age and gender.

Table 17.1 shows that the mean AUC was 124.8 (standard deviation [SD] 38.9) and 113.2 (SD 36.7) in the acupuncture and usual care groups respectively, a difference in means of 11.5 (95% CI: −0.4 to 23.5; $P = 0.058$); with a positive difference in means indicating the acupuncture group has the better QoL on average.

Example from the Literature – AUC and the POLAR Trial

Reddington et al. (2018) undertook an external pilot RCT, in 80 patients with lumbar radicular syndrome (LRS), to investigate the feasibility of undertaking a definitive RCT. Participants were randomised into early intervention physiotherapy (early) or usual care (usual) with the former receiving their treatment within two weeks and the latter at six week post-randomisation. Patients were asked to complete self-report outcome measures at four-time points: first, at the time of consent and then at 6, 12 and 26 weeks post-randomisation. The main outcome was the Oswestry Disability Index (ODI) which is scored 0 to 100, where a higher score indicates higher level of self-rated disability. For the ODI the results showed a mean AUC (SD) for usual care of 16.6 (11.4) and for early intervention 16.0 (14.0), difference −0.6 (95% CI −6.8 to 5.6). Such a small difference suggests that the investigators should re-examine the details of their proposed intervention before initiating a main trial.

Other Summary Measures

Figures 17.2a and b and 17.3 and Tables 17.1 and 17.2 from the low back pain trial suggest that the mean SF-36 pain scale scores at 3, 12 and 24 month follow-up are fairly similar (the lines in the graph appear to be almost horizontal at these time points). Therefore, another sensible summary measure would be the mean post-randomisation follow-up SF-36 pain scale score. For this summary measure, patients need only to have one valid follow-up SF-36 pain scale score.

A simple analysis would be to use the two-independent sample *t*-test to compare mean follow-up SF-36 pain scale score scores between the acupuncture and usual care groups. The correlation between baseline and mean follow-up pain scores is 0.30 so a more powerful statistical analysis, is an ANCOVA or multiple regression (Frison and Pocock 1992). This involves a multiple regression analysis with the average follow-up pain score (the mean of the 3-, 12- and 24-month assessments) as the dependent variable, $\overline{Y}_i$, and the baseline pain (x_{Base_i}) and treatment group, x_{Group_i}, (coded usual care = 0, acupuncture = 1) as covariates.

The linear regression model for the *i*th subject is:

$$\overline{Y}_i = \beta_0 + \beta_{\text{Group}}x_{\text{Group}_i} + \beta_{\text{Base}}x_{\text{Base}_i} + \varepsilon_i \tag{17.2}$$

where β_0 is a constant and ε_i is a random error term that is assumed Normally distributed with expected value of zero and a variance σ^2.

Table 17.4 shows the results on the fitting the ANCOVA model to the data. The adjusted difference is smaller than the unadjusted difference and the confidence intervals for the adjusted analysis are narrower; but both the simple and adjusted analysis suggest that the acupuncture group has the better average QoL over the follow-up period.

Table 17.4 Unadjusted and adjusted differences in mean follow-up SF-36 pain outcome scores between acupuncture and usual care groups.

SF-36 dimension[b]	Usual			Acupuncture			Unadjusted difference[c] 95% CI	P-value	Adjusted[a] difference[c] (95% CI)	P-value
	n	Mean	SD	n	Mean	SD				
Mean follow-up pain score	76	57.2	(19.8)	153	63.4	(20.9)	6.3 (0.6to 12.0)	0.030	6.1 (0.7 to 11.6)	0.027

[a] N = 229 difference adjusted for baseline pain score.
[b] The SF-36 pain dimension is scored on a 0–100 (no pain) scale.
[c] Improvement is indicated by a positive difference on the SF-36 pain dimension.
Source: data from Thomas et al. (2006).

Longitudinal Models

In longitudinal studies, multiple assessments on the same subject at different time points are taken and these within subject responses are therefore correlated. This correlation must be accounted for by analysis methods appropriate to the data. A random effects model for longitudinal data with a continuous outcome y_{it} for the *ith* subject measured at time t is

$$y_{it} = \beta_0 + \alpha_i + \beta_1 x_{1_{it}} + \beta_2 x_{2_{it}} + \ldots + \beta_p x_{p_{it}} + \varepsilon_{it}. \tag{17.3}$$

In this model, each subject i is assumed to have an additive effect α_i on the outcome, which is assumed to have a Normal distribution with mean zero and variance σ^2_α. The random error term ε_{it} is also assumed to have a Normal distribution with mean zero and variance σ^2.

This model makes a number of assumptions which should be checked.

1) The variance σ^2 is independent of subject, i.e. once we allow for subject effects the variability within subjects is expected to be the same for each subject.
2) The correlation is only introduced by the term α_i. Observations on different subjects are correlated by $\sigma^2_\alpha / (\sigma^2 + \sigma^2_\alpha)$, the intra-class correlation coefficient (ICC).
3) The ICC is positive or zero. Thus. if there are differences between subjects, the variability can only increase. This means that there cannot be negative correlation within subjects.
4) Conditional on subject i the errors terms ε_{it} are independent and uncorrelated, i.e. the correlation (corr) between the error terms for subject i at times s and t is $\mathrm{corr}(\varepsilon_{is}, \varepsilon_{it}) = 0$ if $s \neq t$.

The last assumption is called the exchangeable correlation model, that is the order of the times within a subject does not matter. An alternative model is the first order autocorrelation model in which $\mathrm{correlation}(\varepsilon_{is}, \varepsilon_{it}) = r^{|t-s|}$.

Random-effects models are also called generalized linear mixed models, multilevel models or conditional models. These are analysed using maximum likelihood, where the random effects are integrated over the probability distribution. An alternative method of analysing the data is a so-called marginal model, which uses an iterative technique called generalized estimated equations (GEEs). This latter method does not model the correlation structure explicitly, but rather uses the data structure to estimate and allow for it in the model estimates. The choice of one or the other depends on the objectives of the study. Note that model (17.3) is also used in cluster randomised trials (Campbell and Walters 2014).

17.2   Poisson Regression

In any longitudinal study which investigates the occurrence of an event (such as death or disease or admission to hospital), we should take into account the fact that subjects are usually followed for different lengths of time. This may be because some subjects drop out of the study or because subjects are entered into the study at different times, and therefore at the close of the study the follow-up times from different subjects will vary. As subjects with longer follow up times are more likely to experience the event than those with shorter follow-up, we consider the rate at which the event occurs per person per period of time. Often the unit which represents a convenient period of time is a year (but it could be a minute or a day). *Poisson regression* is used to analyse the rate of some event when individuals have different follow-up. In Poisson regression we assume that the rate of the event amongst individuals with the same explanatory variables is constant over the whole study period.

This contrasts with logistic regression (Chapter 10), which is concerned only with whether or not the event occurs and is used to estimate odd ratios. The Poisson regression model takes a similar form to the logistic regression model but here we use the natural logarithm transformation ($\log_e$) of the expected rate, λ, to produce an estimated regression Eq. (17.4):

$$\log_e(\lambda) = \beta_0 + \beta_1 x_1 + \beta_2 x_2 + \ldots + \beta_p x_p. \tag{17.4}$$

Thus the observed count is assumed to have a Poisson distribution with parameter λ, which is the expected rate, β_0 is the constant term providing the log rate when all x_is in the equation have the value of zero (the log of the baseline rate); β_1, β_2,...,β_p are the Poisson regression coefficients to be estimated (which when back-transformed are rate ratios) for an individual with a particular set of values of x_1, x_2, ... ,x_p.

The exponential of a particular coefficient, for example, $\exp(\beta_1)$, is the estimated relative rate or rate ratio associated with the relevant variable. For a particular binary predictor (1 – exposed, 0 – not exposed) it is the ratio of the rates for exposed versus unexposed individuals whilst adjusting for all the other x_is in the model. For a continuous predictor x_1, it is the estimate rate of disease for a value ($x_1 + 1$) relative to the estimate rate of disease for value x_1, and assumes this ratio remains the same for all values of x_i (the linearity assumption). If the rate ratio (RR) is equal to one (unity) then the event rates do not change when x_1 changes and indicates no relationship between the outcome and the predictor. A value of the RR > 1 indicates an increased event rate; and a value of RR < 1 indicates a decreased event rate, with increasing x_1. Further details are given by Campbell (2006).

Use of an Offset

The dependent variable is the observed count, for an individual O_i with parameter λ_i. The parameter λ_i comprises an expected count E_i divided by the follow-up or exposure time T_i. Thus the model becomes

$$\log_e(E_i) = \log_e(T_i) + \beta_1 x_{1i} + \beta_2 x_{2i} + \ldots + \beta_b x_{bi}. \tag{17.5}$$

Note that the coefficient associated with $\log_e(T_i)$ is not estimated, but fixed at unity. This is based on the linear assumption that the risk is directly proportional to the time exposed. Because this coefficient is not estimated, it is known as an *offset* and must be coded separately from the other covariates.

Calculating the Probability of an Event

We can rearrange the Poisson regression equation, with estimated coefficients $b_0, b_1, b_2, \ldots, b_p$, to calculate the event rate for an individual with a particular combination of values of $x_1, x_2, \ldots, x_p$. For each set of covariate values $x_1, x_2, \ldots, x_p$ we calculate

$$z = b_0 + b_1x_1 + b_2x_2 + \ldots + b_px_p.$$

Then, the event rate for that individual is estimated as $\exp(z)$.

Example from the Literature – Cystic Fibrosis the ACTif Trial

Hind et al. (2019) looked at the incidence of intravenous (IV) treated exacerbations in patients with cystic fibrosis as part of an external pilot RCT to assess the feasibility and acceptability of a new complex intervention, linking a nebuliser with data recording and transfer capability to a software platform, and strategies to support self-management with trained interventionists (intervention) or usual (usual) care. The pilot trial randomised 33 to Intervention and 31 to usual care. They observed 86 exacerbations in the 64 patients (24 patients had no exacerbations; 14 had one; 13 two, 9 three and 2 four, 1 five and 1 six) who were followed up for between 13 and 314 days post-randomisation. The mean exacerbation rates per month were 0.17 (SD 0.16) and 0.20 (SD 0.28) for patients in the usual care and intervention groups respectively. They compared the exacerbation rates between the two groups using Poisson regression with the number of days of follow-up included as offset in the model and also adjusted for the site and number of IV days in the previous year. The results are shown in Table 17.5 and suggest no overall effect of the intervention with an incidence rate ratio of 0.95 (95% CI: 0.62 to 1.46) after adjustment for covariates.

Extra-Poisson Variation

Poisson regression assumes the number of events follows a Poisson distribution. A quick check for this is that the mean and variance are similar as would be expected from a Poisson distribution (see Chapter 4). If the variance is much larger than the mean, there is said to be 'over-dispersion'. This can often be caused by the omission of an important predictor variable, or perhaps because an outlier is present or the data are clustered. Under a Poisson assumption, the estimated standard errors

Table 17.5 Poisson regression of the number of exacerbations treated with IV antibiotic that occurred with the number of days of data collection included as an offset in the model. Adjusted for site and number of IV days in the previous year ($N = 64$).

Number of exacerbations	b	SE(b)	Z	P-value	IRR (exp b)	95% CI Lower	95% CI Upper
Group (usual =0, intervention =1)	−0.05	0.22	−0.24	0.809	0.95	0.62	1.46
Site	0.23	0.22	1.02	0.309	1.25	0.81	1.94
IV days	0.02	0.004	5.7	<0.001	1.02	1.01	1.03
Constant	−0.35	0.39	−0.91	0.365			
log(time)	1	(exposure)					

IRR: incidence rate ratio.

(SEs) are usually underestimated in this case and consequently, the confidence intervals for the parameters are too narrow and the P-values are too small. In these circumstances it may be best to fit a regression model based on the negative Binomial distribution (another type of probability distribution that can use for counts) instead of the Poisson distribution.

When a sample of individuals is followed up from a natural starting point, such as the date of randomisation, until that person develops an endpoint of interest, we could use survival analysis (Chapter 11); which in contrast to Poisson regression does not assume that the rate of the events in a small interval (termed the 'hazard') is constant over time.

17.3 Missing Data

Missing data are common, particularly in longitudinal data. For example, for QoL measures this can be individual questions, termed missing items, or missing questionnaires, as might occur if a patient did not attend an assessment. *Item non-response* arises when there are single missing item(s) from an otherwise complete questionnaire. *Unit non-response* is when the whole QoL questionnaire is missing when one was anticipated from the patient. There are two important potential consequences of missing data (Bell and Fairclough 2014). The first is the decrease in precision (wider confidence intervals) and power caused by the reduction in data for analysis. The second, and more serious, is the potential for bias in the estimation of both between group (for example, the effect of treatment) and within group effects (such as changes over time). However, if the proportion of missing data is small then little bias will result. If it not small then a crucial question is: are the characteristics of patients with missing data different from those for whom complete data are available? If the answer is yes, then the study results will be biased and may not reflect the truth (Walters 2009a). Table 17.1 shows that of the 239 patients with valid baseline SF-36 pain data only 76% (182/239) had valid SF-36 pain outcome data at 24 month follow-up. That is 24% of the possible outcome data is potentially missing.

Types and Patterns of Missing Data

There are essentially three types of missing data.

1) Missing completely at random (MCAR). When the probability of a specific response at time t is independent of both the previously observed values and the potential (but unobserved) value at time t. For example, in the low back pain trial this would mean that missing values at say three month post-randomisation follow-up are not associated with say the baseline value of quality life and other factors such as age and gender as well as the patient's current unobserved SF36 pain score.

2) Missing at random (MAR). When the probability of response at time t depends on the previously observed values but not the unobserved values at time t. For example, in the low back pain trial this would mean that missing values at say three month post-randomisation follow-up would depend on the baseline value of quality life and other factors such as age and gender but not the current unobserved SF36 pain score.

3) Not missing at random (NMAR). When the probability of response at time t depends on the actual (but unobserved) values at time t. For example, low back pain trial this would mean that missing values at say three month post-randomisation follow-up would depend on the current unobserved SF36 pain score, perhaps because the patient's back pain had worsened and their (unreported) current level of pain was considerably worse than their baseline value.

Table 17.6 Missing data pattern from the low back pain trial.

	Time (month)				Number of participants		
	0	3	12	24	Total	Acupuncture	Usual care
Baseline only	X				10	6	4
Complete data to 3 months	X	X			14	6	8
Intermittent data up to 12 months	X		X		3	2	1
Complete data to 12 months	X	X	X		30	22	8
Intermittent data up to 24 months	X		X	X	9	5	4
Complete data to 24 months	X	X	X	X	173	118	55
					239	159	80

X = valid outcome data.

If a patient drops out of the study or dies, their data from a certain point onwards will be unobserved. This pattern of missingness is termed *monotone*. *Intermittent missingness* is defined to be when an outcome is unobserved at one assessment but is observed at a following assessment. Intermittent missing data are more typical in studies of individuals with chronic conditions. In contrast, monotone missing data occur in studies of populations with significant morbidity or mortality, and in trials where monotonicity occurs as the result of the design. Table 17.6 shows the patterns of missing data in the low back pain trial. The data appears to show an intermittent missing data pattern.

Describing the Extent and Patterns of Missing Data

After the study has been conducted and it is time to report results, the first step is to describe how many participants were in the study at each time-point. A table, such as Table 17.1, or a CONSORT flow diagram of Figure 17.1 are a good way to achieve this.

To explore mechanisms of missingness, a good place to start is a graph of the QoL outcome versus time, stratified by dropout time, as shown in Figure 17.4 for the low back pain trial. If the trajectories over time are substantially different, the data are not MCAR. For example, are patients who have lower baseline values more likely to drop out, or are steeper rates of increase or decrease over time associated with dropout? In Figure 17.4 there is little separation between the missingness patterns providing some evidence that the data are likely to be MCAR.

We can explore missing data mechanisms by comparing those who dropout versus those who do not via: *t*-tests to compare means (for example by comparing the mean age of those drop out versus those who do not); cross-tabulations; logistic regression (to look at multiple predictors of those who drop out). Survival analysis can be used to look at predictors of time to dropout.

Incomplete Data

From the CONSORT flow diagram in Figure 17.1, 241 patients were randomised in the low back pain trial but only 182 (75% of the original cohort) provided outcomes at 24 months that could be

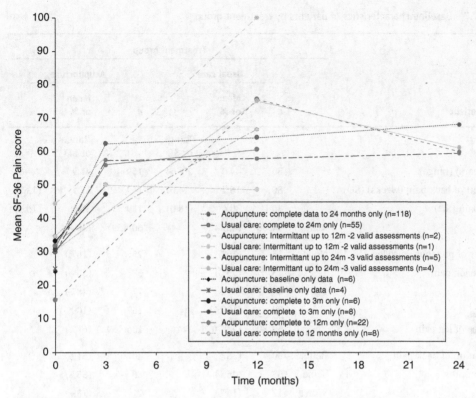

Figure 17.4 Profile of mean SF-36 pain scores over time stratified by drop out time from the low back pain trial (*Source:* data from Thomas et al. 2006).

analysed. Two patients dropped out immediately after randomisation and provided no data. Ideally the reasons for patients dropping out should be recorded. In the original 239 patients, Table 17.7 clearly shows that the two groups were well matched at baseline in terms of their characteristics. However, withdrawal may be caused by treatment related side effects. Whatever the reason, the incomplete data, may compromise the initial baseline balance between the two treatment groups (as seen in Table 17.7).

Table 17.8 compares the baseline characteristics of those patients who dropped out (non-responders) with those who were actually analysed (responders). It is a useful table, but one rarely reported in RCTs. The table helps us see if the baseline characteristics of the patients who are the basis for the analysis are similar to those patients who dropped out. It shows that in fact those subjects actually analysed were similar between the acupuncture and usual care groups at baseline, and the subjects analysed were similar to those who dropped out. For example, of subjects who responded at baseline 10/59 (17%) subjects in the usual care arm had no previous episodes of back pain compared with 20/123 (16%) in the acupuncture arm. This suggests that the drop-out for this variable is independent of randomisation.

In the low back pain trial none of the participants died within the two-year post-randomisation follow-up. However, the question of how to deal with patients who die is a 'vexing issue' that has not been resolved (Bell and Fairclough 2014). Some researchers impute a score of 0 (or whatever is the minimum possible score on the scale). Whilst this is reasonable for some scales where 0 is explicitly anchored to death (e.g. utility scales such as the EQ-5D and SF-6D), it does not make sense for

Table 17.7 Baseline characteristics of patients by treatment group.

Characteristic		Usual care n	Usual care Mean or %	Usual care Range or SD	Acupuncture n	Acupuncture Mean or %	Acupuncture Range or SD
Age (years) (range)		80	44.0	20–64	159	41.9	26–64
Duration of back pain (weeks) (SD)		80	16.7	(14.6)	159	17.1	(13.5)
SF-36 pain (SD)		80	30.4	(18.0)	159	30.8	(16.2)
Gender	Male	34/80	(43%)		60/159	(38%)	
Number of previous episodes	None	13	(16%)		25	(16%)	
of low back pain	1–5	23	(29%)		57	(36%)	
	>5	44	(55%)		77	(48%)	
		80	(100%)		159	(100%)	
Presence of leg pain	Yes	59/80	(74%)		106/159	(67%)	
Expectation of back pain	Better	30	(38%)		80	(51%)	
in six months	Same	37	(46%)		56	(35%)	
	Worse	12	(16%)		21	(13%)	
		79	(100%)		157	(100%)	

Source: data from Thomas et al. (2006).

others such as symptom and physical scales, where a 0 could mean that the deceased patient is experiencing severe nausea, vomiting, and pain.

Analyses which assume the outcome data are MCAR are: complete case analysis; repeated univariate (time-by-time) analysis; marginal models with coefficients estimated by GEE; and summary measures, such as AUC. On the other hand, analyses that assume the outcome data are MAR are: random effects models (maximum likelihood methods); multiple imputation (MI); and marginal models with coefficients estimated by extensions to GEE with inverse probability weights (IPW), MI or both (doubly robust estimation – DR-GEE). Different assumptions are required for the two models regarding missing data. The marginal model using the GEE requires a missing data process completely at random (MCAR). Under this assumption, missingness does not depend on individual characteristics (observed or not). In contrast, random effects models only need the less stringent assumption of MAR. In this process, the probability of missingness depends only on observed variables (previous covariates or outcomes).

What if we Think the Data Is MNAR?

Unfortunately, we cannot test whether or not the data are missing not at random (MNAR). We have not observed the missing outcome, so it is not possible to formally test the hypothesis that the 'missingness' does not depend on the value of the outcome at the time the assessment is missing. The data we need to test the hypothesis are missing! More complex models are required.

In trials of cancer patients at the end of life or being treated with palliative care the statistical analysis can be problematic due to high levels of missing data, attrition, and response shift

Table 17.8 Baseline characteristics of all randomised patients (N = 239) by treatment group and response status at 24 months with outcomes for analysis (N = 182).

	Treatment group						Acupuncture					
	Usual care											
	Response at 24 months											
	No (n = 21)			Yes (n = 59)			No (n = 36)			Yes (n = 123)		
Characteristic	n	Mean	SD	n	Mean	SD	n	Mean	SD	n	Mean	SD
Age (years)	21	40.0	(8.9)	59	45.5	(10.6)	36	39.9	(11.2)	123	42.5	(10.7)
Duration of back pain (weeks)	21	18.7	(15.9)	59	16.0	(14.1)	36	17.3	(14.1)	123	17	(13.3)
Baseline SF-36 pain	21	31.7	(16.2)	59	29.9	(18.7)	36	30.9	(14.6)	123	30.8	(16.6)
	n	%		n	%		n	%		n	%	
Gender												
Male	11	52%		23	39%		16	44%		44	36%	
Female	10	48%		36	61%		20	56%		79	64%	
Total	21	100%		59	100%		36	100%		123	100%	
Number of previous episodes of low back pain												
None previously	3	14%		10	17%		5	14%		20	16%	
1–5 episodes	7	33%		16	27%		15	42%		42	34%	
More than 5 episodes	11	52%		33	56%		16	44%		61	50%	
Total	21	100%		59	100%		36	100%		123	100%	
Presence of leg pain												
No back only	8	38%		13	22%		12	33%		41	33%	
Yes	13	62%		46	78%		24	67%		82	67%	
Total	21	100%		59	100%		36	100%		123	100%	
Expectation of back pain in six months												
Better	5	24%		25	43%		23	64%		57	47%	
Same /worse	16	76%		33	57%		13	36%		64	53%	
Total	21	100%		58	100%		36	100%		121	100%	

Source: data from Thomas et al. (2006).

(a change over time in an individual's basis on which they perceive, judge, and value their own QoL) as disease progresses. For palliative care and end-of-life care studies, it is likely that data are MNAR since the likelihood of a patient of not responding to a QoL questionnaire at a particular time point is likely to depend on the unobserved values for their QoL at that time point (Preston et al. 2013). Analyses that assume the outcome data are MNAR are: mixture models (MM) and pattern mixture models (which are a special case of MM); shared random effects parameter models; joint multivariate models; and selection models. These complex models are beyond the scope of this book, but the interested reader is referred to the article by Bell and Fairclough (2014) or the text books by Fairclough (2010) and Diggle et al. (2002) for more details.

Imputation of Missing Data

In statistics, imputation is the technique of replacing missing data with substituted or imputed values. Imputation is seen as a way to overcome the problems involved with listwise deletion of cases that have missing values. That is to say, when one or more values are missing for a case, most statistical packages default to discarding any case that has a missing value, which may introduce bias or affect the representativeness of the results. Imputation retains all cases, in the analysis, by replacing missing data with an estimated value based on other available information. Once all missing values have been imputed, the data set can then be analysed using standard techniques for complete data. New methods of imputation are regularly being developed and requires consistent attention to new information regarding the subject. Commonly used techniques for imputing missing data include: mean imputation; regression imputation; last observation carried forward (LOCF); hot deck imputation; stochastic imputation; and multiple imputation (Fayers and Machin 2016; Walters 2009a).

Example – Imputation of Missing Data – IPSU Trial

Jha et al. (2018) undertook a single centre two arm parallel group RCT, to evaluate the clinical effectiveness of electric stimulation plus standard pelvic floor muscle training compared to standard pelvic floor muscle training alone in women with urinary incontinence and sexual dysfunction. Participants were randomised to electric stimulation (intervention) or standard pelvic floor muscle training (usual care control). The primary outcome was the self-reported Prolapse and Incontinence Sexual function Questionnaire (PISQ) physical function dimension at post-treatment. One-hundred and fourteen women were randomised (intervention $n = 57$; control group $n = 57$) and 64/114 (56%) participants had valid primary outcome data at follow-up (intervention 30; control 34). Table 17.9 shows the mean PISQ-PF dimension scores at follow-up were 33.1 (SD 5.5) and 32.3 (SD 5.2) for the intervention and control groups respectively; with the control group having a higher (better) score. After adjusting for baseline score, BMI, menopausal status, time from randomisation and baseline Oxford scale score the mean difference was −1.0 (95% CI: −4.0 to 1.9; $P = 0.474$).

A variety of imputation methods were used to make up or 'impute' the missing primary outcome data in the IPSU trial. These imputed results are reported alongside the observed trial results in Table 17.9 as part of a sensitivity analysis to check the robustness of the observed results to missing data. The authors used a variety of imputation methods including:

1) LOCF where the baseline score was carried forward.
2) Assuming a one-point decrease from baseline in subjects with missing follow up data.

Table 17.9 Observed and imputed Prolapse and Incontinence Sexual function Questionnaire (PISQ) physical function dimensions scores post-treatment in the IPSU trial.

| Outcome | Treatment group | | | | N analysis | Unadjusted Difference in means | 95% CI | P-value | N analysis | Adjusted Difference in means[a] | 95% CI | P-value |
| | Control | | Intervention | | | | | | | | | |
	n	Mean (SD)	n	Mean (SD)								
Observed data	34	33.1 (5.5)	30	32.3 (5.2)	64	−0.8	−3.5 to 1.9	0.572	60	−1	−4.0 to 1.9	0.474
LOCF imputed data	55	31.3 (6.1)	52	30.0 (6.0)	107	−1.3	−3.6 to 1.0	0.28	76	−0.8	−3.1 to 1.5	0.494
Assuming −1 point decrease	55	30.9 (6.3)	52	29.6 (6.3)	107	−1.3	−3.7 to 1.1	0.29	76	−0.9	−3.3 to 1.5	0.443
Regression imputed data	41	33.0 (5.1)	40	32.1 (4.6)	81	−0.9	−3.0 to 1.2	0.407	76	−0.7	−2.9 to 1.4	0.494
Multiple imputation[b]	57	32.7 (6.1)	57	31.7 (6.0)	114	−1	−3.6 to 1.6	0.453	114	−0.6	−3.1 to 1.9	0.64

A positive mean difference implies the Intervention group had the better outcome; whereas a negative mean difference the converse that the control group had the better outcome.

[a] Adjusted for baseline score, BMI, menopausal status, time from randomisation and Oxford scale score.

[b] 20 imputations using baseline score, follow-up, menopausal status, time from randomisation, body mass index, diastolic blood pressure, SF36 physical score, SF36 mental score and Oxford scale score.

3) Regression imputation in subjects with missing follow up data.
4) Multiple imputation.

Multiple imputation was used to impute missing data on the primary outcome. Data were imputed using chained equations (regression) with 20 imputations using baseline, follow-up, menopausal status, time from randomisation, body mass index, diastolic blood pressure, SF36 physical score, SF-36 mental score, and baseline Oxford scale. This shows similar results to the primary analysis suggesting the observed results are consistent and fairly robust to the missing outcome data and loss to follow-up.

17.4   Bootstrap Methods

The *bootstrap* is a computer-intensive simulation method for statistical analysis (Efron and Tibshirani 1993). It involves repeatedly drawing random samples from the original data, with replacement. It seeks to mimic in an appropriate manner the way the sample is collected from the population in the bootstrap samples from the observed data. The *with replacement* means that any observation can be sampled more than once. Bootstrap methods can be used for hypothesis tests and regression analyses, but are usually used for calculating non-parametric confidence intervals when we do not want to make assumptions about the sampling distribution of the estimate (e.g. Normal distribution for sample mean). Efron and Tibshirani (1993) suggest that 1000 or more bootstrap resamples are needed for estimating bootstrap confidence intervals.

Jackknifing is a similar technique to bootstrapping. However, rather than creating random samples of the original sample, we remove one observation from the original sample of size n and then compute the estimated parameter (e.g. mean) of the remaining $(n-1)$ observations. This process is repeated, removing each observation in turn, giving rise to n estimates of the parameter.

A Simple Example of the Bootstrap

The difference in the distance walked, in metres, on a six-minute walking test (6MWT) in 13 patients with multiple myeloma awaiting stem cell transplantation before and after a six-week duration pre-transplant exercise programme (prehabilitation) is shown in Table 17.10 (data from Keen et al. 2018). The research question here was: does a pre-transplant exercise programme (prehabilitation) change the distance walked of patients with multiple myeloma awaiting autologous haematopoietic stem cell transplantation? Suppose we wish to estimate a confidence interval for the difference in distance walked and are concerned that the difference is not Normally distributed and does not satisfy the assumptions for estimating a confidence interval using the t-distribution described in Chapter 7.

The first bootstrap random sample (of size 13) has a mean of 143.9 m and subject L for example (with a value of 195 m) is selected or resampled three times in this bootstrap sample. The second bootstrap sample has a different mean of 137.5 m; the 1000th bootstrap sample has a mean of 87.7 m. The distribution of the 1000 bootstrap means is shown in Figure 17.5. The mean of the 1000 bootstrap means is 104.46 m. This compares to the observed mean of 104.92 m.

Bootstrap Methods for Confidence Interval Estimation

The best estimate of the statistic is the observed mean from the original data, not the mean of the bootstrap means, which is biased. The difference between the observed mean in the

Table 17.10 Distance walked, in metres, on a six-minute walking test (6MWT) in 13 patients with multiple myeloma awaiting stem cell transplantation before and after a six-week duration pre-transplant exercise programme.

Subject	Observed data	Bootstrap		
		Sample$_1$	Sample$_2$	Sample$_{1000}$
A	15	15	25	15
B	15	25	25	15
C	25	98	53	25
D	53	98	83	25
E	60	135	98	53
F	83	135	98	83
G	98	135	135	98
H	135	165	145	98
I	135	195	165	98
J	145	195	240	135
K	165	195	240	135
L	195	240	240	165
M	240	240	240	195
Mean	104.92	143.92	137.46	87.69
SD	71.41	71.85	82.35	59.12

Source: data from Keen et al. (2018).

original data and the mean of the bootstrap means is the *bias* (i.e. 104.92 – 104.46 = 0.46). The SD of the 1000 or so bootstrap means is the bootstrap SE. In Figure 17.5 the standard deviation of the means or SE is 19.01. This SE can be used to calculate CIs using standard methods, i.e. *estimate ± 1.96 SE(estimate)*. These bootstrap CIs are called 'Normal'. Alternatively, non-parametric bootstrap CIs based on the percentiles of the cumulative distribution of the 1000 bootstrap means can be calculated. That is, a percentile based 95% CI is given by the 2.5 and 97.5% percentiles of the distribution of the bootstrap means. This is known as the *percentile method*, and although it is an obvious choice, it is not the best method for bootstrapping confidence intervals, because it can have a bias, which one can estimate and correct for. This leads to methods such as the *bias corrected method* and the *bias corrected and accelerated* (BC$_a$) method, the latter being the preferred option (Davison and Hinckley 1997; Efron and Tibshirani 1993). Carpenter and Bithell (2000) provide a useful practical guide on bootstrap confidence intervals.

Table 17.11 shows various bootstrap confidence intervals, for the mean difference in distance walked, in metres, on a six-minute walking test (6MWT) in 13 patients with multiple myeloma awaiting autologous haematopoietic stem cell transplantation before and after a six-week duration pre-transplant exercise programme, based on 1000 bootstrap samples. Table 17.11 shows that the estimates and lengths of the CIs are similar with the normal bootstrap confidence interval producing the narrowest interval and the BC$_a$ method producing the widest interval. Table 17.11 also shows that the percentile, BC and BC$_a$ are non-symmetric about the point estimate of the mean difference.

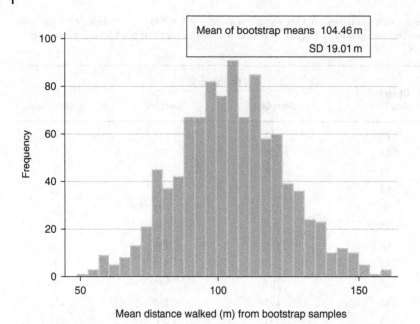

Figure 17.5 Histogram of mean distance walked (in metres) from 1000 bootstrap samples of size 13.

Table 17.11 Bootstrap 95% confidence intervals for the mean difference in distance walked, in metres, on a six-minute walking test (6MWT) in 13 patients with multiple myeloma awaiting autologous haematopoietic stem cell transplantation before and after a six-week duration pre-transplant exercise programme.

Number of bootstrap resamples	Observed mean	Bias	Standard error	95% CI Lower	Upper	Method
1000	104.9	−0.5	19.0	67.7	142.2	(N)
				67.9	143.9	(P)
				69.2	145.5	(BC)
				69.8	146.8	(BC$_a$)

(N) Normal, (P) percentile, (BC) bias-corrected, (BC$_a$) bias-corrected and accelerated.
Source: data from Keen et al. (2018).

Using the bootstrap method, valid bootstrap confidence intervals can be constructed for all common estimators such as the sample mean, median, proportion, difference in means, and difference in proportions. The bootstrap can be applied to data with a more complex structure than the simple single sample example considered above. The bootstrap can also be used for other statistics (such as ratios) and more complex datasets. With a two group RCT, we should randomly sample with replacement separately for each group. In economic evaluations alongside clinical trials both cost and effect data is measured for each individual patient. Therefore, we randomly sample with replacement each patient and their paired cost and effect data. This takes into account the correlations between cost and effect outcomes.

Example from the Literature

Morrell et al. (2000) calculated bootstrap percentile based confidence intervals for the mean difference in SF-36, Edinburgh Postnatal Depression Scale and Duke scores at six weeks postnatally between a group of new mothers randomly allocated to receive extra postnatal support or usual care (control) in a RCT to establish the effectiveness of community postnatal support workers. They quoted the bootstrap CI rather than the parametric CI because of concerns with the distribution of the data. For the primary outcome, the SF-36 general health dimension, the difference between intervention and control was found to be −1.6 with bootstrap percentile 95% CI of (−4.7 to 1.4), whereas the parametric estimate was −1.6 (95% CI −4.8 to 1.5) which is very similar.

17.5   Points When Reading the Literature

For longitudinal data, do any tables and figures clearly state the sample size at each time point and whether this is an available data or listwise deletion of cases?

For a randomised controlled trial is the number of participants with valid primary outcome data reported? How does this compare with the number randomised?

Is a complete case analysis likely to lead to biases, i.e. is there evidence that the missing data are not MAR.

In a Poisson regression, is there evidence of over dispersion? Has this been accounted for?

If bootstrap methods are used, are the number of bootstrap resamples reported and the method of calculating the confidence interval described (e.g.: normal, percentile, bias corrected or BC_a)?

17.6   Exercises

17.1 Which if any of the following statements about types and patterns of missing data IS CORRECT?

   A Data is MCAR when the probability of a response at time t is independent of both the previously observed values and the unobserved values at time t.

   B Data is MAR when the probability of response at time t depends on the previously observed values but not the unobserved values at time t.

   C Data is NMAR when the probability of response at time t depends on the unobserved values at time t.

   D Intermittent missingness is when a patient drops out of the study or dies, their data from a certain point onwards will be unobserved.

   E Monotone missingness is defined to be when an outcome is unobserved at one assessment but is observed at a following assessment.

17.2 Which if any of the following statements about the analysis of missing data IS CORRECT?

   A We cannot test whether or not the data are MNAR

   B Complete case analyses assumes the missing outcome data are MNAR.

   C Multiple imputation assumes the missing outcome data are MNAR.

D Pattern mixture models can be used to analyse data that are MNAR

E Imputation is the technique of replacing missing data with substituted or imputed values.

17.3 Which if any of the following is not a method of imputing missing data?

A Multiple imputation

B One at a time imputation

C Hot deck imputation

D Mean imputation

E Last observation carried forward imputation

17.4 Which if any of the following statements about the bootstrap method is INCORRECT?

A The bootstrap method involves repeatedly drawing random samples from the original data

B The bootstrap method involves repeatedly drawing random samples from the original data, with replacement

C Bootstrap methods can be used for hypothesis tests and regression analyses and for calculating non-parametric confidence intervals

D 1000 or more bootstrap samples are typically needed for estimating bootstrap confidence intervals.

E The best estimate of the statistic (e.g. sample mean) is the observed mean from the original data.

17.5 Which if any of the following IS NOT a recognised method of estimating bootstrap confidence intervals?

A Percentile

B Bias corrected and accelerated

C Bias corrected

D Normal

E Jackknife

18   Meta-analysis

Medical Statistics: A Textbook for the Health Sciences, Fifth Edition. Stephen J. Walters, Michael J. Campbell, and David Machin.
© 2021 John Wiley & Sons Ltd. Published 2021 by John Wiley & Sons Ltd.
Companion website: www.wiley.com/go/walters/medicalstatistics

Summary

A systematic review attempts to collate all relevant evidence that fits pre-specified eligibility criteria to answer a specific research question. It uses explicit, systematic methods to minimise bias in the identification, selection, synthesis, and summary of studies. Meta-analysis is the statistical analysis of the data from a collection of studies in order to synthesise the results. The rationale for meta-analysis is to increase the precision of estimates of treatment effects or exposure risks and to examine whether the estimates are heterogeneous and if so, to examine reasons why this may be so. The PICOTS (Populations, Interventions, Comparators, Outcomes, Time frame, and Setting/Study design) framework is used for conducting systematic reviews and looking for clinical heterogeneity in the studies. This chapter describes how outcomes from different studies can be summarised and combined using a fixed or random effects statistical model to produce an overall summary measure of the treatment effect, pooled across all the studies. The chapter also shows how these effect sizes can be graphically displayed as forest plots to display the results of each of the studies and the combined result and funnel plots to investigate heterogeneity.

18.1 Introduction

A systematic review is a formalised and stringent process of combining the information from all relevant studies (both published and unpublished) of the same health condition. These studies are usually RCTs of the same or similar treatments but may be observational studies. Often single clinical trials and observational studies have a number of limitations: they may be restricted in size; they may be restricted to a single population and to a particular place and time. The hallmark of good science is that it is replicable, and so when studies are repeated a meta-analysis will examine whether the outcomes are consistent and, if so, combine them. A meta-analysis is a series of statistical techniques to examine the heterogeneity of outcomes and combine results from different studies. The reason for adding a meta-analysis to a systematic review is to obtain the best overall estimate of the effect of an intervention or treatment and by combining the results of all the studies available we increase the power to detect important treatment effects.

A systematic review is an integral part of evidence-based medicine (EBM) which applies the results of the best available evidence, together with clinical expertise, to the care of patients. So important is the role of systematic reviews in EBM that it has become the focus of an international network of clinicians, methodologists, and consumers who have formed the Cochrane Collaboration. http://www.cochrane.org. This has produced the Cochrane Library which comprises regularly updated evidence-based healthcare databases that contain different types of high-quality, independent evidence to inform healthcare decision-making http://www.cochranelibrary.com. The Cochrane Handbook for Systematic Reviews of Interventions (http://handbook.cochrane.org) is the official guide that describes in detail the process of preparing and maintaining Cochrane systematic reviews on the effects of healthcare interventions.

18.2 What is a Meta-analysis?

A meta-analysis is a particular type of systematic review that focusses on the numerical results. The main aim of a meta-analysis is to combine the results from several independent studies to produce,

---

Box 18.1   Meta-analysis: What Does it Achieve?

- Large numbers of studies are reduced to a simple summary.
- A systematic review is generally cheaper and faster to carry out than a new study. It may prevent others embarking on unnecessary studies, and can shorten the time lag between medical developments and their implementation.
- Results can often be generalised to a broader patient population in a wider setting than would be possible from a single study. Consistencies in the results from different studies can be assessed, and any inconsistencies determined.
- The systematic review aims to reduce errors, and so tends to improve the reliability and accuracy of recommendations when compared with haphazard reviews or single studies.
- The quantitative systematic review has greater power to detect effects of interest and provides more precise estimates than a single study.

---

if appropriate, an estimate of the overall or average effect of interest. The direction and size of this average effect, together with its associated confidence interval (CI) and hypothesis test result, may be used to make decisions about the therapy or intervention under investigation. The purposes of meta-analysis are described in Box 18.1.

Traditionally, when seeking advice in controversial or novel areas, clinicians and scientists have relied heavily on 'informed' editorials or narrative reviews. There is now good evidence to suggest that these methods are subject to bias and inaccuracy (Begley and Ioannidis 2015). Reviewers using traditional methods are less likely to detect a small but significant effect or difference compared with reviewers using formal statistical techniques. As most current medical reviews do not use scientific methods to assess and present data, different reviewers often reach different conclusions based on the same data. For these reasons some formal statistical process of review should replace the informal approach. Meta-analysis can be used to resolve uncertainty when reports, editorials or reviews disagree.

The major limitation of meta-analysis is that it can only work with what is available. Thus, a meta-analysis can only include studies that are published or in some other way retrievable. The available studies may be non-comparable or give inadequate data. They may vary in design, quality, outcome measure or population studied. Publication bias is the main concern regarding the availability of studies. Authors are more likely to submit, and editors more likely to publish, studies with significant results. This is also called the 'file drawer problem'; those doing a meta-analysis wonder about the influence the studies tucked away in file drawers might have on their results. In particular, pharmaceutical companies may simply not bother to publish trials that do not reflect favourably on their product. This problem of non-publication is not only a commercial one, many academic trials which fail to show an effect are also not published either because the authors could not be bothered to write them up, or the publisher deemed the results not to be of interest. A campaign Alltrials (www.alltrials.net) has been launched to try and ensure all trials are published and is having some success. In particular, it is now required that all trials should be registered with their protocol before they start, so they can be identified, and a check made on whether they were subsequently published. All meta-analyses summarise information up to the date they are conducted and they should be updated as more studies become available, in order to maintain their usefulness.

18.3   Meta-analysis Methods

Is a Meta-analysis Appropriate? The PICOTS Approach

We need to ask two questions:

1) Can the results of each of the studies be expressed as an 'effect measure', (such as an odds ratio, risk ratio, rate difference or difference in means) which has a numerical value and can then be combined into a single estimate?
2) More importantly, does it make sense to combine the results of the different studies into a single estimate?

The answer to the latter question should only be 'yes' if the following are sufficiently similar across all studies:

The populations receiving the interventions (P)
The intervention (I)
The comparison intervention (C)
The outcomes being measured (O)
The timing or duration of follow-up or data collection (T)
The setting or the study design (S)

These are known as the elements of the PICOTS model to formulate a search question for a systematic review. A meta-analysis can be justified only if both questions are answered in the affirmative.

Fixed Effects and Random Effects Meta-analysis

A fixed effects meta-analysis assumes that the true effect is the same for all studies, whereas a random effects meta-analysis assumes that the individual studies have different effect sizes that vary randomly around the overall mean effect. Thus, the random effects meta-analysis specifically allows for between study heterogeneity and within study variability. When the research question is specifically about the studies in question, then a fixed effects analysis is appropriate. However, between study variation is an important source of variation that cannot be ignored and so should be incorporated if it is unlikely to be simply due to random variation between studies. In contrast to a fixed effect model, the result from a random effects model is taken to be an estimate of the average of the effect from all possible studies, i.e. ones not observed as well as those observed. The estimate will naturally be of lower precision. However, although a random effects model incorporates studies heterogeneity in its estimates, it does not 'control for' or 'adjust for' heterogeneity, i.e. an investigator cannot just fit a random effects model as a safety precaution, and then proceed to ignore the heterogeneity of results. It is incumbent on the investigator to examine the sources of heterogeneity. It is possible the treatment effect varies in different populations, with different applications of treatments, or different stages of disease. These should be investigated before producing a single summary measure.

Combining the Results of Different Studies

A systematic review of the literature is conducted to identify relevant studies, the quality of the studies assessed and, where possible, ranked or graded. These quality assessments are usually used in a qualitative way to assess whether the study should be included. Then the investigators choose a suitable outcome measure and a standardised measure (an effect size) to summarise the outcome of each trial. This may be an odds ratio or risk ratio in the case of binary outcomes, or a difference in means divided by the pooled standard deviation for continuous measures. The results of the individual studies are then represented on a graph known as a *forest plot* which shows a point estimate of each study's effect size, with its CI indicated by a horizontal line on either side of the point. Much of the benefit from the review can be obtained simply from examining the forest plot. One can see if the results are consistent and if there are any obvious outliers. The plot usually includes an estimate of the weight that each study contributes to the overall estimate, so one can see which studies are influential in the final estimate.

The results are then combined using methods described in the technical appendix. The output is a combined weighted effect size or standardised mean difference (SMD) with a CI. The output also typically produces a test for heterogeneity and a test for an overall effect.

Finally, one can use a *funnel plot* to look for publication bias. This is a plot of some measure of the size of the study such as the standard error of the estimate against the estimate. If all studies are supposedly a random sample from all possible trials then one would expect a unimodal distribution, centred around the true effect. Large studies will be expected to be closer to the true effect and to have a small standard error. Smaller studies will have more variability and so be expected to vary more widely around the true effect. If, for example, small studies that fail to show an effect in the expected direction are not published, then one would anticipate a plot with one side truncated. Included in the plot is usually some error region as described in the technical appendix. One would expect most study estimates to be within this region, so any outside it deserves special scrutiny.

Heterogeneity

Most programs will also provide statistics to describe the heterogeneity. The two most common are the Q statistic and the I^2 statistic which are described in the technical details (Section 18.6). Under the null hypothesis that there are no differences in the intervention effect amongst the studies then the Q statistic follows a chi-squared distribution with $k - 1$ degrees of freedom, where k is the number of studies in the meta-analysis. The I^2 statistic measures the extent of the inconsistency amongst the studies results and is derived from the Q statistic. It is interpreted as approximately the proportion of the total variation in the study estimates that is due to heterogeneity rather than sampling error. Rules of thumb for the I^2 statistic are: <50%: low heterogeneity; 50–75%: moderate heterogeneity; and $\geq$ 75%: high heterogeneity. One can also plot an area on the funnel plot so that one would expect 95% of all studies to be within the area, and this is simplest using the standard error, where the area is constrained by straight lines and is recommended (see Sterne and Egger 2001).

18.4   Example: Mobile Phone Based Intervention for Smoking Cessation

Whittaker et al. (2016) described a meta-analysis of trials of mobile phone based interventions to encourage smokers to give up smoking. They found 12 trials that fitted the PICOTS criteria.

(P) Populations receiving the interventions – any smokers who want to quit smoking.
(I) Intervention – any type of mobile phone based intervention for smoking cessation.

(C) Comparison intervention – control programmes varied widely from: nothing to fortnightly or daily text messages; written/internet untailored materials; and untailored messages to standard cessation advice and treatment.

(O) Outcomes – smoking abstinence at six months or longer from the start of the intervention.

(T) Timing or duration of follow-up or data collection – smoking abstinence up to six months or longer from the start of the intervention.

(S) Setting or the study design-randomised or quasi-randomised trials. (A quasi-randomised trial is one where the allocation of treatments to subjects is not random, but is one that is plausibly free from allocation bias. For example, one heath authority adopts a screening procedure and another does not, perhaps because of different priorities. Then the subjects living in one authority get different treatment to those living in another, but not because of any inherent differences in the subjects except for geography.) In the Whittaker et al. (2016) meta-analysis the settings and recruitment methods, and therefore the participants, varied considerably across studies. The 12 trials in this meta-analysis were performed between 2005 and 2015.

The data are shown in Table 18.1. Since the data are counts of events, numbers of subjects abstinent from smoking for six months, with total number of smokers, in each arm, the best summary measure is the risk and the standardised effect size is the risk ratio. The data were analysed using the R programme METAFOR (Viechtbauer 2010). The funnel plot is given in Figure 18.1. The left-hand plot uses the risk ratio and it can be seen that it is dominated by study 1 which has wide CIs and so it is difficult to see the details of the other studies. It is better to use the log risk ratio (RR) given in the right-hand side of the figure. One can see that study 12 gives the greatest weight to the overall estimate, 46%, and that only 4 studies have CIs that exclude the null or no effect value. The FE term in the graph means that model was a fixed effect model and the best estimate using a fixed effects model is a RR of 1.63 (95% CI 1.42 to 1.86). Table 18.2 shows the output from the

Table 18.1 Mobile phone based interventions for smoking cessation.

Study	Intervention		Control	
	Events	Total	Events	Total
1	6	30	1	30
2	2	54	2	53
3	3	236	5	238
4	29	262	12	241
5	13	142	15	142
6	34	299	19	303
7	15	102	19	98
8	36	372	26	383
9	29	110	32	116
10	68	755	26	422
11	64	852	39	853
12	268	2991	124	38.1

Source: from Whittaker et al. (2016).

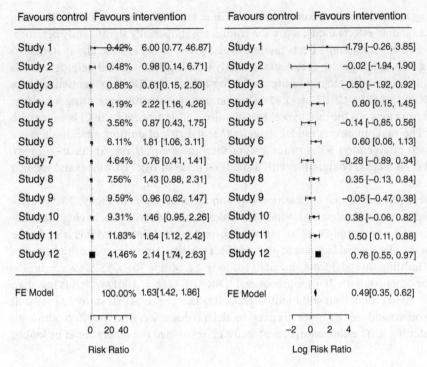

Figure 18.1 Forest plot of data from Table 18.1 with weights, point estimates and 95% confidence intervals for the Risk Ratio and Log Risk Ratio.

Table 18.2 Output from meta-analysis programme.

Fixed effects
Test for heterogeneity:
Q (df = 11) = 26.8059, p-value = 0.0049

Model results:

Estimate	SE	Z-value	P-value	95% CI lower	95% CI upper
0.4867	0.0679	7.1723	< 0.0001	0.3537	0.6197

Random effects
tau^2 (estimated amount of total heterogeneity): 0.0804 (SE = 0.0687)
tau (square root of estimated tau^2 value): 0.2836
I^2 (total heterogeneity / total variability): 55.37%

Test for heterogeneity:
Q (df = 11) = 26.8059, P-value = 0.0049

Model results:

Estimate	SE	Z-value	P-value	95% CI lower	95% CI upper
0.3567	0.1219	2.9270	0.0034	0.1179	0.5956

meta-analysis program. The test for heterogeneity is $Q(\text{df} = 11) = 26.8059$, $p = 0.0049$. This suggests we may try a random effects model since the studies are statistically significantly heterogeneous. The analysis using a random effects method is also given in Table 18.2. The I^2 statistic is 55.37% suggesting that although the Q statistic is highly significant the actual heterogeneity is moderate to low. However, the program outputs the log RR not the RR. Exponentiating these results gives a RR of 1.43 (95% CI 1.13 to 1.81). One can see that the estimate using a random effects model is shrunk towards the null hypothesis of unity, and as expected, the CI is wider with a random effect. The random effects model suggests that the risk of quitting smoking using a mobile phone-based intervention is 1.4 times greater than the control/comparator treatments. The 95% CI for the estimate is compatible with a small increase in risk (1.1 times) and a larger increase (1.8 times).

We need to investigate the source of heterogeneity and the funnel plot of Figure 18.2 is quite symmetric suggesting no publication bias. Study 12, which can be identified as having the smallest standard error, is the only study with an estimate beyond normal limits and this is by far the largest trial. From the plot it would appear to give an effect which is larger than one might expect from the others. Omitting this trial from the analysis, we get a $Q(\text{df} = 10) = 15.2845$, $p = 0.1220$ suggesting that the other trials are homogeneous and a RR of 1.34 ($p = 0.001$) which is less than that of the random effects model but still highly significant. This suggests that study 12 may well be different to the others and using a random effects model has down-weighted its effect, although not as much as omitting it. The characteristics of study 12, relative to the others could be looked into in more detail.

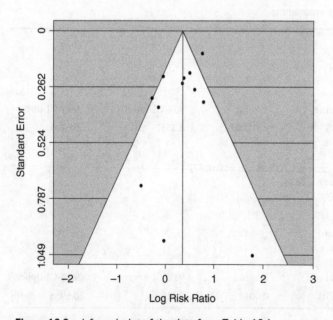

Figure 18.2 A funnel plot of the data from Table 18.1.

18.5 Discussion

The Main Problems with Meta-analysis

The following main problems should be investigated before a meta-analysis is performed and reported.

1) *Publication bias*. The tendency to include in the analysis only the results from published papers; these favour statistically significant findings.
2) *Clinical heterogeneity*. Differences in the PICOTS of the studies included in the analysis create problems of non-compatibility.
3) *Quality differences*. The design and conduct of the studies may vary in their quality.
4) *Dependence*. The results from studies included in the meta-analysis may not be independent, for example, when results from a study are published on more than one occasion.

Presentation of Results

Moher et al. (2009) describe the Preferred Reporting Items for Systematic Reviews and Meta-Analyse (PRISMA) Statement (http://www.prisma-statement.org). PRISMA is an evidence-based minimum set of 27 items for reporting in systematic reviews and meta-analyses. It focuses on the reporting of reviews evaluating randomised trials, but can also be used as a basis for reporting systematic reviews of other types of research.

Further Reading

For up-to-date information about systematic reviews and meta-analysis the interested reader is referred to the Cochrane Collaboration website http://www.cochrane.org. The Cochrane Collaboration website includes the Cochrane Library which contains high-quality, independent evidence to inform healthcare decision-making. It includes reliable evidence from Cochrane and other systematic reviews, clinical trials and more. The Cochrane Handbook for Systematic Reviews of Interventions is the official document that describes in detail the process of preparing and maintaining Cochrane systematic reviews on the effects of healthcare interventions. The handbook is available for browsing online (or downloading) at http://training.cochrane.org/handbook. The browsable handbook is also available from the help menu in Review Manager 5 (software for composing Cochrane Reviews) which is available to download at http://tech.cochrane.org/revman. There are also a number of useful books that cover meta-analysis, for example Sutton et al. (2000), Egger et al. (2001), Whitehead (2002), and Cleophas and Zwinderman (2017).

18.6 Technical Details

Fixed Effects

Meta-analysis is readily carried out using freely available software such as Revman (https://community.cochrane.org/help/tools-and-software/revman-5). For each trial one has to input the basic summary measures for each treatment arm: for continuous outcomes the mean, standard deviation and sample size; for binary data using an odds ratio the number of events and non-events and, for binary data using a risk ratio, the number of events and the total sample size. More complicated summary measures such as hazard ratios require an estimate and its standard error. From these the summary measure or effect size, termed the SMD, is calculated. This is the estimate of the treatment effect over the control, divided by the standard error of this estimate.

Suppose we have outcomes in k studies which are to be combined. We denote the SMD estimate for the ith study by $\hat{\theta}_i$ and its standard error by $SE\{\hat{\theta}_i\}$. The individual study effect sizes are weighted according to the reciprocal of their variances

$$w_i = \frac{1}{(SE\{\hat{\theta}_i\})^2}.$$

The pooled Inverse Variance (IV) estimate of the effect size is given by

$$\hat{\theta}_{IV} = \frac{\sum_{i=1}^{k} w_i \hat{\theta}_i}{\sum_{i=1}^{k} w_i}.$$

The standard error of the pooled estimate of the effect size is given by

$$SE\{\hat{\theta}_{IV}\} = \frac{1}{\sqrt{\sum_{i=1}^{k} w_i}}.$$

The $100(1 - \alpha)\%$ CI for $\hat{\theta}_{IV}$ is given by $\hat{\theta}_{IV} - z_{1-\alpha/2}SE\{\hat{\theta}_{IV}\}$ to $\hat{\theta}_{IV} + z_{1-\alpha/2}SE\{\hat{\theta}_{IV}\}$, where $z_{1-\alpha/2}$ are the appropriate values from the standard Normal distribution for the $100(1 - \alpha/2)$ percentiles (see Table T1 in the appendix).

One can test whether the SMDs plausibly come from the same population using the heterogeneity statistic

$$Q = \sum_{i=1}^{k} w_i (\hat{\theta}_i - \hat{\theta}_{IV})^2.$$

Under the null hypothesis that there are no differences in intervention effect amongst studies this follows a chi-squared distribution with $k - 1$ degrees of freedom.

The I^2 statistic measures the extent of the inconsistency amongst the studies' results and is calculated as

$$I^2 = \max\left\{100\% \times \frac{Q - (k - 1)}{Q}, 0\right\}.$$

As stated in the main text, this is interpreted as approximately the proportion of the total variation in the study estimates that is due to heterogeneity rather than sampling error. Rules of thumb for the I^2 statistic are: $<50\%$: low heterogeneity; $50–75\%$: moderate heterogeneity; and $\geq75\%$: high heterogeneity.

The test for the presence of an overall intervention effect is given by

$$Z = \frac{\hat{\theta}_{IV}}{SE\{\hat{\theta}_{IV}\}}.$$

Under the null hypothesis that there is no overall effect of the intervention, Z, follows a standard Normal distribution.

Random Effects

The expected value of Q under the assumption that the true treatment effect does not vary from trial to trial is $k - 1$. DerSimonian and Laird (1986) described a method of using this to estimate the overall treatment effect and additional variance of this effect if in fact the treatment effect varied from trial to trial.

The additional variance of the treatment effect is given by

$$\hat{\tau}^2 = \max\left\{\frac{Q - (k-1)}{\sum w_i - (\sum w_i^2)/\sum w_i}, 0\right\}.$$

The study effect size weight is modified to

$$w_i^{RE} = \frac{1}{w_i^2 + \hat{\tau}^2}.$$

The random effect (RE) pooled effect size is given by

$$\hat{\theta}_{RE} = \frac{\sum w_i^{RE}\hat{\theta}_i}{\sum w_i^{RE}}.$$

The standard error of the pooled estimate of the effect size is

$$SE\{\hat{\theta}_{RE}\} = \frac{1}{\sqrt{\sum_{i=1}^{k} w_i}}.$$

The $100(1 - \alpha)\%$ CI for $\hat{\theta}_{RE}$ is given by

$$\hat{\theta}_{RE} - z_{1-\alpha/2}SE\{\hat{\theta}_{RE}\} \text{ to } \hat{\theta}_{RE} + z_{1-\alpha/2}SE\{\hat{\theta}_{RE}\}.$$

A funnel plot graphs $\frac{1}{w_i^2 + \hat{\tau}^2}$ versus $\hat{\theta}_i$ for each study i. The control limits are calculated so that one might expect 95% of trial SMDs to lie within them if there were no heterogeneity. Trials with SMDs outside of the control limits are viewed as possible outliers where the treatment effect is different, and these trials should be scrutinised carefully.

18.7 Exercises

The results of a meta-analysis of four randomised trials to evaluate the efficacy of motivation interviewing (MI) for smoking cessation are shown in Table 18.3 (Lindson et al. 2019). The meta-analysis included randomised controlled trials in which MI or its variants were offered to smokers to assist smoking cessation. The outcome was smoking cessation measured after at least six months. The authors calculated RRs and 95% CI for smoking cessation for each study and meta-analysis using a random-effects model.

Assume a significance level of 0.05 or 5% has been specified for the various hypothesis tests.

Table 18.3 Comparison of MI versus no treatment with an outcome of smoking cessation in four RCTs.

Study	MI		No treatment		Weight	RR	95% CI	
	n	N	n	N			Lower	Upper
1	3	28	4	31	4.2	0.83	0.2	3.39
2	48	235	49	199	67.3	0.83	0.58	1.18
3	3	27	0	28	1	7.25	0.39	134.07
4	19	77	18	59	27.5	XXXX	0.47	1.4
Total	73	367	71	317	100	0.84	0.63	1.12

Heterogeneity chi-squared = 2.16 (df = YYYY) $P = 0.54$.

I^2 (variation in RR attributable to heterogeneity) = 0%

Estimate of between-study variance tau-squared = 0.

Test for overall effect: $Z = 1.18$, $p = 0.24$.

Source: data from Lindson et al. (2019).

18.1 From the data in Table 18.3 calculate XXXX, the missing RR for Study 4.
    A 0.81
    B 0.89
    C 1.05
    D 1.78
    E 2.34

18.2 What are the degrees of freedom (labelled YYYY in Table 18.3) for the chi-squared test of heterogeneity?
    A 1
    B 2
    C 3
    D 4
    E 5

18.3 Table 18.3 reports that the *P*-value for the test for heterogeneity is $P = 0.54$.
Which, if any, of the following statements is CORRECT?
    A The result is statistically significant.
    B The probability of getting this difference or more extreme by chance if the studies are homogenous is 0.54.
    C The probability of getting this difference or one more extreme is 0.54.
    D There is sufficient evidence to reject the null hypothesis.
    E The individual trial results are consistent with the same population effect.

18.4 Table 18.3 reports that the *P*-value for the test for overall effect is $P = 0.24$.
Which, if any, of the following statements is CORRECT?
    A The result is not statistically significant.
    B The probability of getting this difference or one more extreme, when the null hypothesis (of no overall effect) is true, is 0.24.

    C The probability of getting this difference or one more extreme is 0.24.
    D There is sufficient evidence to reject the null hypothesis.
    E The individual trial results are consistent with no overall population effect.

18.5 Table 18.3 reports that the overall or pooled 95% CI for the RR across the four trials for stopping smoking in the MI group compared to the no treatment control group is 0.63 to 1.12. Which, if any, of the following statements is CORRECT?

    A The above 95% CI definitely contains the true population RR for stopping smoking in the MI group compared to the no treatment control group.
    B The 95% CI is calculated as ± 3 standard errors away from the mean difference.
    C There is a probability of 0.95 that the population RR for stopping smoking in the MI group compared to the no treatment control group lies between 0.63 and 1.12.
    D The 95% CI does not contain the true population RR for stopping smoking in the MI group compared to the no treatment control group.
    E The above 95% CI is likely to contain the true population RR for stopping smoking in the MI group compared to the no treatment control group.

19   Common Mistakes and Pitfalls

Medical Statistics: A Textbook for the Health Sciences, Fifth Edition. Stephen J. Walters, Michael J. Campbell, and David Machin.
© 2021 John Wiley & Sons Ltd. Published 2021 by John Wiley & Sons Ltd.
Companion website: www.wiley.com/go/walters/medicalstatistics

Summary

Some common errors found in the medical literature are described. They comprise: misleading graphs (such as 3D charts; lack of true zero on the vertical axis, plotting the change of a variable over time against the initial value); presentation of data in tables; analysing paired data ignoring the matching; within group versus between group analysis; unit of analysis problems; post hoc power calculations; testing for baseline imbalances in RCTs; predicting or extrapolating beyond the observed range of data; problems in using the *t*-test, repeated measurement studies, regression to the mean and confusing statistical and clinical significance.

19.1 Introduction

As Cole et al. (2004) point out many of the statistical errors that occur in the medical literature are frequently not very major and could be overcome with a little more care by the writing team and by more vigilance from any reviewers. For example, using a *t*-test when it is dubious that the data are Normally distributed, or failing to provide enough information for the reader to discover exactly how a test was carried out. There are frequent examples of poor presentation of data in figures and tables. In addition, one can find presentations in the abstract or results irrelevant to the problem being tackled by the paper. These errors do not usually destroy a paper's total credibility; they merely detract from its quality and serve to irritate the reader. However, some errors stem from a fundamental misunderstanding of the underlying reasoning in statistics, and these can produce spurious or incorrect analyses.

19.2 Misleading Graphs and Tables

Two- or Three-Dimensional Charts

Table 19.1 shows the method of delivery for new births at hospitals in England in 2016 and 2017. It is common practice to display such data as a three-dimensional (3D) bar chart or pie chart (Figure 19.1). However, this should never be done as 3D charts are especially difficult to read and interpret (as we discussed in Chapter 2). The area displayed in a pie chart or bar chart should be proportional to the relative frequencies for each group. However, when the charts are displayed as three-dimensional this relationship is lost as what is displayed becomes a volume. Only the front faces are proportional to the numbers in the categories and so only these should be displayed. In particular, categories with only a few individuals are given undue weight in 3D charts as the top face is much more prominent. Above all else, a graph should be simple and accurately reflect the data so that the reader can easily understand the information being conveyed. In the 3D chart the area of the 'Forceps low' segment looks bigger than the area of the 'Ventouse' segment but the number is larger in the latter category. It is preferable to display the data in Table 19.1 as a one-dimensional pie chart or better still as a bar chart (as in Figure 19.2). Where there is no natural ordering to the categories it can again be helpful to order them by size.

Table 19.1 Method of delivery of births at NHS hospitals in England in 2016 and 2017 (*N* = 627 362).

Method of delivery	n	%
Spontaneous vertex	368 641	58.8%
Spontaneous other	1811	0.3%
Forceps low	20 744	3.3%
Forceps other	24 575	3.9%
Ventouse	34 295	5.5%
Breech	2576	0.4%
Caesarean elective	76 163	12.1%
Caesarean emergency	98 557	15.7%
	627 362	100.0%

Source: NHS Digital.

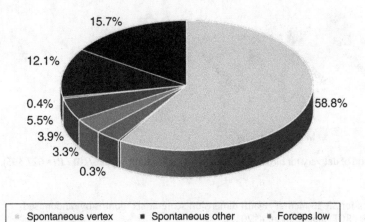

Figure 19.1 Three-dimension pie chart of method of delivery for births at NHS hospitals in England in 2016/2017 (*N* = 627 362).

Dynamite Plunger Plots

One of the easiest ways to display data badly is to display as little information as possible. This includes not labelling axes and titles adequately, and not giving units. In addition, what information that is displayed can be obscured by including unnecessary and distracting details. Consider the following table (Table 19.2) of summary statistics for SF-36 Mental Health dimension score at six months by randomised group from the Lifestyle Matters RCT (Mountain et al. 2017).

A common way to display these data badly is to present the means for each group and their associated standard errors using a bar chart with error bars, the so called 'dynamite plunger plots' as shown in Figure 19.3.

This chart violates many of the recommendations in Chapter 2 and yet is commonplace. Whilst only four pieces of information are displayed (group means and their standard errors) much ink is wasted drawing the bars. The scale begins at the origin, so that the variability of the data is compressed into a small area. There is no information about the number of observations in each group. Most importantly for these data, the raw data are hidden behind a summary statistic. It may be that the purpose of displaying these data is to compare the group means, in which case a better way

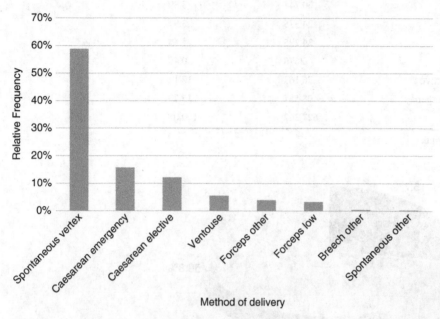

Figure 19.2   Bar chart of method of delivery for births at NHS hospitals in England in 2016/2017 (*N* = 627 363).

Table 19.2   Summary statistics for SF-36 Mental Health dimension score at six months by randomised group from the Lifestyle Matters RCT (Mountain et al. 2017).

SF-36 Mental Health dimension score at six-month post-randomisation	Randomised group	
	Lifestyle Matters Intervention	**Control**
Mean	77	76
Median	85	80
Standard error of mean	2	2
Standard deviation	18	19
Minimum	5	5
Maximum	100	100
25th percentile	70	65
75th percentile	90	90
N	136	126

would be to merely report these statistics in the text. However, if the reason for displaying data such as these is to compare the spread of values in the two groups, the standard errors for the individual means are of little use. It is better just showing the actual data, using a dot plot as described in Chapter 2 and shown in Figure 19.4 below.

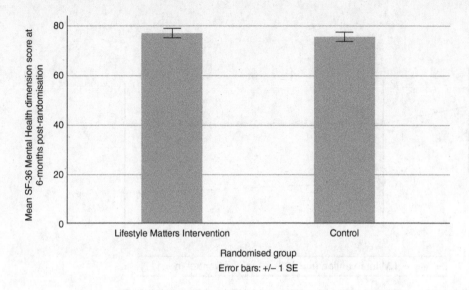

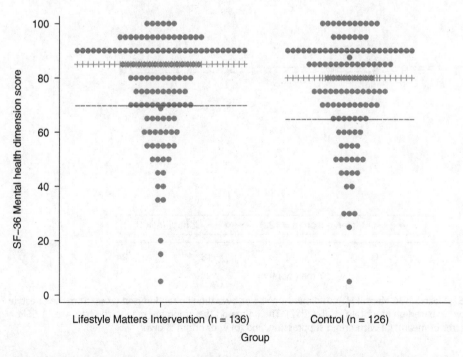

Figure 19.4   Dot plot of SF-36 Mental Health dimension score at six months by randomised group with group medians and lower quartiles. *Source:* based on Mountain et al. (2017).

Supress the Origin or Change the Baseline

A frequently used method of exaggerating trends over time is to suppress the origin. The Figure 19.5a reports the mean SF-36 Mental Health dimension scores over time by randomised group from the Lifestyle Matters RCT (Mountain et al. 2017). The treatment effect looks very

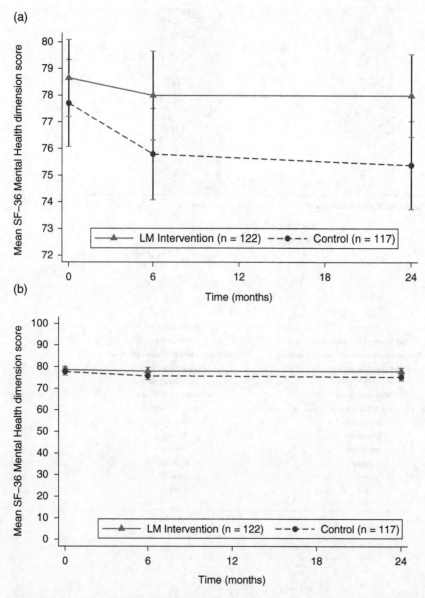

Figure 19.5 Mean SF-36 Mental Health dimension scores over time by randomised group from the Lifestyle Matters. *Source:* based on Mountain et al. (2017). The points on the graph are means, the bars are ±1 SEM (standard error of mean); (a) with origin suppression, and (b) with origin shown.

dramatic with a clear separation between the lines and groups at 6- and 24-months post-randomisation. However, the SF-36 Mental Health dimension is scored on a 0 (poor) to 100 (good) health scale. By starting the *Y*-axis at score of 72 and ending with a score of 80, a relatively small increase in scores of around 2 to 3 points looks very dramatic. This is an example of a graph that supresses the origin or lack of the true zero on the vertical axis. If the graph is redrawn with a *Y*-axis scale ranging from 0 to 100, which reflects the true range of possible scores for the outcome, then Figure 19.5b shows that the is little separation between the lines and groups at 0, 6- and 24-month post-randomisation and the lines are almost horizontal. This does not imply that displayed data should never supress the origin; meaningful change can occur even when it appears as a small percentage of the overall mean. However, it should be made clear in the figure that the origin has been supressed, which is not the case for Figure 19.5a.

Presenting Data in Tables

Table 19.3 shows the mean Shoulder Pain and Disability Index (SPADI) scores over time by treatment group from the SELF RCT (Littlewood et al. 2016) to evaluate the clinical effectiveness of a self-managed single exercise programme versus usual physiotherapy treatment for rotator cuff tendinopathy. The rotator cuff is a common name for the group of four distinct muscles and their tendons that provide strength and stability during motion of the shoulder. The primary outcome for this trial was the SPADI outcome measured at baseline (randomisation), 3-, 6- and 12-months post-randomisation. The SPADI is scored on a 0 (no pain/disability) to 100 scale with higher scores indicating higher levels of pain and disability (Roach et al. 1991).

In Table 19.3 it is hard to identify the structure of the data. The title is not very informative and for example does not include the overall sample size. It is not clear what the numbers mean: is a high SPADI score good or bad? Since the outcome is measured on a 0–100 scale there is spurious numerical precision and decimal places add to clutter. It is difficult to identify the size and direction of the effect. There is no difference in group means, between the usual physiotherapy and self-managed exercise groups, and no confidence intervals are reported for the between randomised group comparisons. It is not clear what the abbreviations such as SE and df mean. There is no sample size reported for any of the comparisons. There is repeated/multiple hypothesis/significance testing as well as testing for differences at baseline.

Table 19.3 Mean SPADI scores over time by randomised treatment group from the SELF RCT.

SPADI outcome	Treatment group					Independent samples		
	Usual physiotherapy		Self-managed exercise		*t*-test for equality of means			
Time (months)	Mean	SE	Mean	SE	*t*	df	Sig. (two-tailed)	
0	48.967	2.7726	49.121	2.8201	0.039	83	0.969	
3	30.706	3.4267	32.389	3.8849	0.326	58	0.746	
6	23.980	3.9483	16.648	3.7321	−1.344	46	0.186	
12	21.376	5.6890	14.856	4.9196	−0.852	37	0.400	

Source: data from Littlewood et al. (2016).

Table 19.4 presents the same data in the format suggested by Table 17.1. The reader should find that the results are now more clearly presented and address the issues highlighted. The number of participants with outcome data at each time point in each group is now reported. Summary statistics are presented to one decimal place and a confidence interval for the difference in group means is now reported for the two summary measures. In the footnotes to the table all abbreviations are explained; the scale of outcome and what a high or low score means as well as what the direction of the treatment effect is reported. Further examples of how to display data properly are given by Freeman et al. (2008).

19.3 Plotting Change Against Initial Value

Adjusting for Baseline

In many clinical studies, baseline characteristics of the subjects themselves may be very influential on the value of the subsequent endpoint assessed. For example, in the context of clinical trials in children with neuroblastoma it is known that prognosis in those with metastatic disease is worse than in those without. Indeed, the difference between these two groups is likely to exceed any difference observed between alternative treatments tested within a randomised trial. In other situations, the outcome measure of interest may be a repeat value of that assessed at baseline. Thus, in the example of Table 19.4 pain in the patients with rotator cuff tendinopathy was measured at the beginning of the study, and at 3, 12, and 24 month post-randomisation follow-up and a summary measure for pain for each patient was subsequently calculated in order to compare treatments. In such circumstances, investigators are often tempted to graph this change against the baseline: the logic being to correct in some way for the different (perhaps considerable) baseline levels observed.

Worked Example – Weight Change

The birthweight and weight at one month of 10 babies randomly selected from a larger group is given in Table 19.5.

The research question is: "Do the lighter babies have a different rate of growth early in life than the heavier ones?" The graph of the change in weight or growth over the one-month period against the birthweight is shown in Figure 19.6a. It would appear from this figure that the smaller babies grow fastest as the growth (the y-axis) declines as the birthweight increases (the x-axis). Indeed, the correlation between birthweight and weight gain is $r = -0.79$ which has df = 8 and $p = 0.0061$.

The negative correlation observed in Figure 19.6a appears to lead to the conclusion that weight gain is greatest in the 'smallest at birth' babies but this is a fallacious argument.

In fact, if we take any sets of paired *random* numbers (say) A and B and plotted $(A - B)$ on the y-axis against B on the x-axis a scatter plot indicating a negative association would be obtained. This is because the $-B$ is in the y-term and the $+B$ in the x-term and as a consequence we are guaranteed some degree of negative correlation between y and x. The presence of this intrinsic component in any similar correlation makes the test of significance for an association between a change and the initial value invalid. Thus, with the $r = -0.79$ of Figure 19.6a, we do not know how much of this negative value is due to the above phenomenon.

However, provided that the two sets of data have approximately the same variability, a valid test of significance can be provided by correlating $(A - B)$ with $(A + B)/2$. Somewhat surprising if we now plotted $A - B$ on the y-axis against $(A + B)/2$ on the x-axis for random numbers A and B we

Table 19.4 Mean SPADI scores over time by randomised treatment group from the SELF RCT with all valid patients at each time point.

SPADI outcome[a]	Usual physiotherapy			Self-managed exercise			Difference in means[b]	95% CI Lower	Upper	P-value[c]
Time (months)	n	Mean	SD	n	Mean	SD				
0	43	49.0	(18.0)	42	49.1	(18.3)				
3	33	30.7	(19.7)	27	32.4	(20.2)				
6	25	24.0	(19.7)	23	16.6	(17.9)				
12	21	21.4	(26.1)	18	14.9	(20.9)				
Mean follow-up SPADI score	33	27.9	(19.3)	28	25.3	(21.1)	2.6	−7.8	12.9	0.62
SPADI AUC	20	25.4	(16.7)	17	21.7	(14.9)	3.7	−7.0	14.4	0.48

[a] The Shoulder Pain and Disability Index (SPADI) is scored on a 0 (no pain/disability) to 100 scale with higher scores indicating higher levels of pain and disability.
[b] A positive difference in means indicates the self-managed exercise group has the better health.
[c] SD: standard deviation; CI: confidence interval; AUC: area under the curve. *P*-value from two independent samples *t*-test.
Source: data from Littlewood et al. (2016).

Table 19.5 Birthweight and one-month weight of 10 infants.

Birthweight (g)	One-month weight (g)	Weight gain (One month − Birth)	Mean (One month + Birth)/2
2566	3854	1288	3210.0
2653	4199	1546	3426.0
2997	5492	2495	4244.5
3292	5317	2025	4304.5
3643	4019	376	3831.0
3888	4685	787	4286.5
4065	4576	511	4320.0
4202	4293	91	4247.0
4219	4569	350	4394.0
4369	3700	−669	4035.0

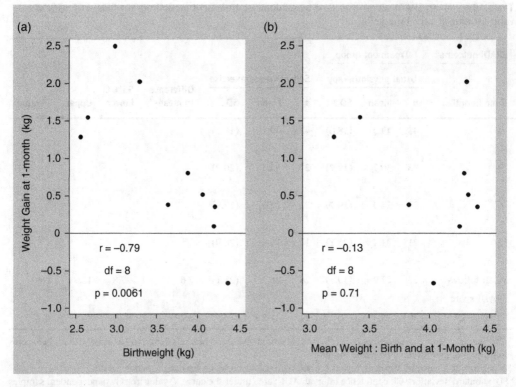

Figure 19.6 Growth of 10 babies in one month against (a) birthweight and (b) mean of birth and one-month weight.

would not get an intrinsic negative correlation but one close to zero which could be positive or negative its magnitude differing from zero only by the play of chance.

Example – Weight Change

Figure 19.6b shows weight-gain plotted against the mean of birth and one-month weights. The corresponding correlation coefficient is $r = -0.13$ and with df = 8 this yields $p = 0.71$. Although the negative relationship is still apparent, the evidence for a relationship is now much weaker.

Regression to the Mean

Figure 2.10 shows an example in which the total steps-per-day walked by one subject, assessed by a pedometer worn on the hip, was recorded every day for 100 days. Imagine an individual with a randomly varying number of steps-per-day was observed in the example of Figure 2.10, and that the number of steps walked per day has an approximately Normal distribution about the mean level for that individual with a certain SD. Suppose we wait until an observation occurs which is two SDs above the mean, perhaps the observation on day 80 in Figure 2.10, then the chance that the next value is smaller than this quite extreme observation with value close to (mean + 2SD) is about 0.975 or 97.5%. We are assuming here that the successive values are independent of each other and this may not be entirely the case. Nevertheless, the chance of the next observation being less than this quite extreme observation will be high. This phenomenon is termed *regression to the mean* but, as we have illustrated, despite its name it is not confined to regression analysis. It also occurs in intervention studies that target individuals who have a high value of a risk variable, such as cholesterol. In such a group, the values measured later will, by chance, often be lower even in the absence of any intervention effect.

In intervention studies having the same entry requirement for both groups can compensate for the regression to the mean. In this situation, if the interventions were equally effective then both groups would regress by the same amount. Thus, it would not be a problem in a comparative trial in which the interventions are randomised. However, it can appear in more insidious guises, for example by choosing a locality that for one year only has had a high cot death rate; even if nothing is done, the cot death rate for that district is likely to fall in the next year. In randomised studies, were we to have a priori evidence that the baseline results should be comparable, then the correct method to adjust for baseline is multiple regression as described in Chapter 9. The dependent variable is the outcome, and the independent variables include the baseline and a binary variable for the intervention. The same result is obtained if the dependent variable is the difference between the outcome and baseline and the intervention the single independent variable, but the former is easier to understand and more generalisable.

Example from the Literature – Change in Fasting Serum Cholesterol
The data of Figure 19.7a is taken from a study conducted by Findlay et al. (1987) and gives the change in fasting serum cholesterol (FSC) between before (T0) and after 30 (T30) weeks of physical training for a marathon.

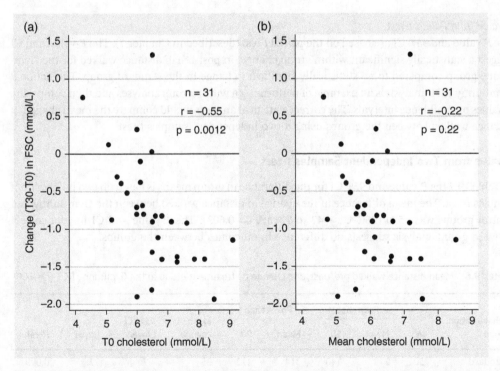

Figure 19.7 Change in fasting serum cholesterol after 30 weeks of marathon training against (a) initial and (b) mean cholesterol. (*Source:* based on data extracted from Findlay et al. 1987).

The correlation of $r = -0.55$, df $= 29$, with $p = 0.0012$, suggests strongly that those with high initial FSC levels changed the most. However, the resulting correlation of the change in FSC with the mean, (T0 + T30)/2, level of Figure 19.7b is $r = -0.22$ and $p = 0.22$. This implies that the negative association with initial levels may be less strong than that indicated by the observed correlation of -0.55.

It is interesting to note that if the individual with the greatest increase in FSC $= 1.3$ mmol l^{-1} is excluded from the calculations then the above correlations become -0.65 and -0.41 with corresponding P-values of 0.0001 and 0.026 respectively. This illustrates how sensitive these calculations can be to outlying data points.

19.4   Within Group Versus Between Group Analyses

We give a fictitious example, which is based, however, on a number of published accounts. One of the usual treatments for the lung condition chronic obstructive pulmonary disease (COPD) is a six-week course of pulmonary rehabilitation (PR) in hospital to increase the amount of exercise these patients are capable of doing. A new PR course called GymBunny has been developed which lasts six weeks. An RCT has been conducted to compare the effectiveness of the new GymBunny compared to standard PR. One-hundred COPD patients were randomised to standard PR ($n = 50$) or GymBunny PR ($n = 50$). The primary outcome was the change in distance walked (in metres) from pre- (baseline) to post-rehabilitation (six- to eight-week post-randomisation) on the endurance shuttle walk test. Table 19.6 summarises the distance walked pre, post, and change by intervention group.

P-*value from Paired* t-*test*

The P-value and 95% CI are based on the paired t-test (described in Chapter 7). The P-value and CI suggest a statistically significant within group change, in post-rehab distance walked for the GymBunny group compared to no statistically significant change in the standard group. The fictional GymBunny RCT analysis is an example of performing a within group analyses and then comparing P-values or confidence intervals. The correct statistical analysis would compare the mean change in distance walked between the groups using a two independent samples t-test.

P-value from Two Independent Samples *t*-test

In Table 19.7 the P-value and 95% CI for the difference in group means is based on two independent samples t-test. The mean difference in the change in distance walked between the GymBunny and control groups was 15 m (95% CI: -42 to 72 m; $P = 0.603$). The P-value and CI for the correct between group analysis suggests no difference in outcomes between the groups.

Table 19.6   Mean distance walked pre, post, and change by treatment group in the GymBunny RCT ($n = 100$).

| Rehabilitation Group | N | Pre-rehab | | Post-rehab | | Mean change | 95% CI | | P-value |
		Mean	SD	Mean	SD		Lower	Upper	
Standard	50	279	140	314	412	35	−7	77	0.099
GymBunny	50	280	137	330	371	50	10	90	0.015

Table 19.7 Mean change in distance walked by treatment group in the GymBunny RCT (*n* = 100).

Outcome	N	GymBunny Mean	SD	N	Standard Mean	SD	Difference in means	95% CI Lower	Upper	*P*-value
					Pulmonary rehabilitation group					
Change in distance walked (metres)	50	50	140	50	35	147	15	−42	72	0.603

The SELF RCT (Littlewood et al. 2016) reported the results of both a within group (paired *t*-test) analysis changes on the SPADI from baseline to all three follow-up points and between group analyses of mean SPADI scores at 3, 6, and 12 months using the two independent samples *t*-test. Although the within group analysis demonstrated statistically significant and clinically important within group changes on the SPADI from baseline to all three follow-up points: there were no statistically significant differences between the groups across all the outcomes at 3, 6, or 12 months.

19.5   Analysing Paired Data Ignoring the Matching

We give another fictitious example, which is based, however, on a number of published accounts. An RCT was undertaken in 50 patients undergoing bilateral (both left and right) total knee joint replacement to assess the effectiveness of a new knee joint manufactured from 'cobalt' compared to the usual stainless-steel joint. Patients were randomised to have either left or right knee joint replaced with cobalt with the other knee joint replaced with stainless steel. The primary outcome was whether or not the knee joint failed (within two years of surgery) and required replacement. The same team of surgeons performed all the operations. Table 19.8 summarises the results.

The absolute difference in joint failure rate was 16% (95% CI: 1 to 31%) in favour of the cobalt joint and the chi-squared test *P*-value of 0.037 suggests a statistically significant difference in knee joint failure rates between the cobalt and stainless steel joints with the latter group having the higher failure rate.

Table 19.8 Comparison of new joint failure rate at two years by type of joint cobalt or stainless steel.

Outcome: knee joint failure	Cobalt group	(%)	Stainless steel group	(%)	Total
Yes	5	(10%)	13	(26%)	28
No	45		37		82
Total	50		50		100

χ^2 = 4.34 on 1 df; P-value = 0.037.

Table 19.9 Paired comparison of new joint failure rate at two years by type of joint cobalt or stainless steel.

| | Outcome | Cobalt knee joint | | |
		Yes	No	Total
Control	Yes	1	12	13
stainless	No	4	33	37
steel joint	Total	5	45	50

$\chi^2_{\text{McNemar}} = 3.06$ on 1 df; $P - \text{value} = 0.080$.

However, the data in Table 19.8 are paired. Although 100 knee joints were replaced this was in 50 patients. We cannot assume the outcome, knee joint failure, is independent between the left and right knee in the same patient. The data are paired so the statistical analysis should take this into account. Chapter 8 described a test of paired proportions called McNemar's test. Table 19.9 shows the results of McNemar's test on the paired data in the 2×2 table.

The paired difference in joint failure rate is 16% (95% CI: 0 to 31%) reduction in favour of the cobalt joint. The McNemar's test from the paired analysis gives $P = 0.08$ and suggests weaker statistical evidence of a difference in knee joint failure rates between the cobalt and stainless-steel joints and is the opposite of the results of the unpaired analysis. The fictional cobalt RCT analysis is an example of analysing paired data ignoring the pairing.

19.6   Unit of Analysis

For duplicated body parts such as joints (knee, ankle, hip and elbow), eyes, ears, kidneys and teeth, the unit of analysis, that is the person or the (say) joint, must be made clear. For example, the corn plaster trial, (of Farndon et al. 2013), described in Chapter 2 aimed to investigate the effectiveness of salicylic acid plasters compared with usual scalpel debridement for the treatment of foot corns. Table 2.1 shows that participants in the trial could have multiple corns. Participants with multiple corns were asked to nominate one corn, usually the most painful or largest, which was classed as the 'index' corn and used as the primary outcome measure. The venous leg ulcer study (VenUS) series of RCTs for comparing different treatments for venous leg ulcers started off, in VenUS1, by defining the primary end-point as complete healing of *all* the ulcers on the trial leg (Iglesias et al. 2004). For the subsequent follow-on trials VenUS II, VenUS III, and VenUS IV (Dumville et al. 2009; Watson et al. 2011; Ashby et al. 2014) they refined the definition of the primary outcome as the time to complete healing of the *largest eligible ulcer* (the reference ulcer on the reference leg).

19.7   Testing for Baseline Imbalances in an RCT

Most reports of an RCT show a table with baseline demographic and clinical characteristics for each treatment group. However, testing for baseline imbalances in a properly randomised trial is futile, although the results of hypothesis test (and *P*-values) are still reported in some journal articles

(Waterlander et al. 2012a,b, 2013a, 2013b) after requests from peer reviewers and journal editors (de Boer et al. 2015). Such testing is discouraged by the CONSORT guidelines. Assuming that randomisation has been done properly, we can expect 5% of the baseline variables to differ significantly between the groups (at level 5%) just by chance. In addition, there is no a priori reason to believe the imbalance in baseline covariates are predictive of outcome.

Baseline imbalance is important, however, and could be due to chance or some subversion of the randomisation procedure. However, one should not, generally, simply include the covariates that are imbalanced in the final analysis. One issue is that other trials may not have such imbalances and so there can be problems with reproducibility. However, a sensible analyst would do several analyses to check that inclusion of covariates, not thought predictive before the trial but different in the treatment arms, does not change the treatment estimate. If it does change, then there will be uncertainty as to the true treatment effect, which should be included in the discussion of the RCT.

19.8   Repeated Measures

As discussed in Section 17.1, a common study design is one in which a subject receives a treatment and then a response to that treatment is measured on several occasions over a period of time. Thus, in the early development stage of a new drug, subjects may receive a single injection of the compound under study then blood samples are taken at intervals and tested in order to determine the pharmacokinetic (i.e. what the body does to a drug) profile. Typically, in this kind of study levels of the measure of concern initially rise, reach a peak and then gradually fall as the body excretes the compound. Other common situations are when the response post-baseline is relatively soon after an intervention with little change thereafter or one in which the profile appears to follow an approximately linear change.

Example – Postprandial Plasma Glucose Concentrations

As part of a study conducted by Drucker et al. (2008), Figure 19.8 shows the postprandial plasma glucose concentrations (mmol l^{-1}), measured at several times over 300 min in 27 patients with type 2 diabetes, following a standardised meal. Assessments were made before commencing Exanatide once a week and then again after 14 weeks of therapy.

The points on the graph are means, the bars are SEM (standard error of mean) so that if we consider the first Week-14 mean of (about) 9.5 with SEM = 0.5, then this implies that the corresponding SD = $0.5 \times \sqrt{27} = 2.6$ mmol l^{-1}. This in turn suggests that the measures at this point may range from about $9.5 - (2 \times 2.6) = 4.3$ to $9.5 + (2 \times 2.6) = 14.7$ mmol l^{-1}. This calculation suggests that for the Week-14 measures there is considerable variation about the mean profile illustrated. It also suggests that at 100 minutes many of the baseline observed values will be beyond the illustrated y-axis limit of 15 mmol l^{-1}. Although in this presentation the substantial variation is essentially disguised, it is not entirely clear how such data can be displayed without being potentially misleading. One suggestion is to present the mean profiles (omitting the SEM bars) on a background of clouds of (very small) points from the respective groups. However, individual profiles still remain obscured and these may be very different from subject to subject. Alternatively, one might select a subset of subjects and plot (in this case perhaps 5 of 27) their baseline and week 14 profiles faintly in the background.

Although not used in Figure 19.8, a common approach in these profile studies is to compare the groups concerned at each time point using an independent groups or paired test as appropriate and indicate on the graph at each observation point those differences that are 'not statistically

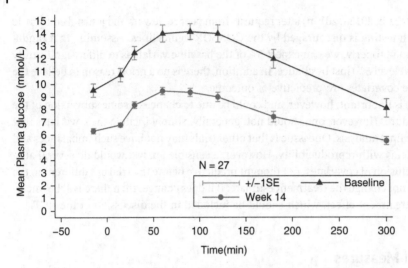

Figure 19.8 Time profiles of postprandial plasma glucose concentrations in patients with type 2 diabetes at baseline and at week 14 following once weekly Exanatide. (*Source:* based on Drucker et al. 2008, figure 5A).

significant' by NS, by a ∗ when $P < 0.05$, ∗∗ $P < 0.01$ and ∗∗∗ $P < 0.001$. Although this gives a quick impression of differences between groups, their use is not encouraged. Importantly, this format does not provide the actual magnitude of the P-values, and neither are those given that are associated with NS. As we discussed in Chapter 17, with assessments made at several time points the approach implies that many statistical significance tests have been conducted and this multiple testing makes the corresponding P-values unreliable.

Often the stated purpose of the significance test is to ask the question, 'when does the response under one treatment differ from the response under another?' Thus, suppose the baseline and Week-14 plasma glucose levels at each of the different time points in Figure 19.8 had been compared. It is a strange logic that perceives the difference between two groups of continuous variables changing from not significantly different to significantly different between two adjacent time points. Suppose the time points were only one minute (or one second) apart rather than several minutes, then it would certainly seem very strange to test for a difference between successive time points – yet in reality, if the curve is truly changing, then they will be different even if they are very close together at a particular point. Thus, it is not sensible to say they are significantly different even if two values (far apart in time) are very different. It is the whole curve that one wishes to compare between groups rather than individual points along the profiles.

Invalid Approaches

The implication of the upper error bars used in Figure 19.8 is that the true curve could be plausibly drawn through any point that did not take it outside the ranges of the lower (not shown) and upper error bars. This is not true for several separate reasons. Since the error bars are essentially 68% CIs (one standard error either side of the mean), then crudely there is a 68% chance that the true mean is within the interval. As there are eight observations then, if these are regarded as independent, the chance of the true line passing through each of intervals is $0.68^8 = 0.045$. This is small and hence the true curve is unlikely to be passing through all of them. However, the observations are certainly not independent, so this calculation gives only a guide to the true probability that the curve passes through all the intervals. Nevertheless, it does suggest that this probability is likely to be small.

Additionally, the average curve calculated from a set of individual curves may differ markedly from the shape of the individual profiles, as is indicated in Figure 19.9.

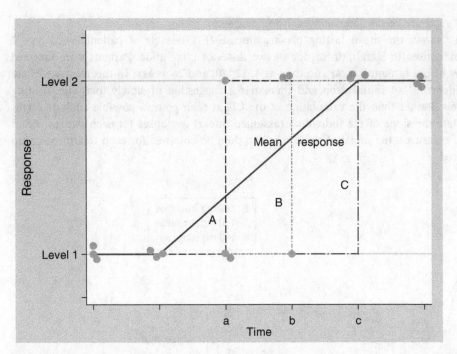

Figure 19.9   Response curves from three individuals and their mean response calculated at each time point. (*Note:* so as not to obscure the individuals of the two and three data points in each of the corresponding clusters, they are jittered about their common value.)

Example – Mean Response Over Time

In Figure 19.9 individual response curves are labelled A, B, and C, each of which simply experience a sudden change from level 1 to level 2 values but these changes occur at different times *a*, *b*, and *c* for the three subjects. However, if the mean response is calculated at each time point *a*, *b*, and *c*, these give the impression of a gradual change from level 1, through 1.33 and 1.67 to level 2.

Valid Approaches

Having plotted the individual response curves, as discussed in Chapter 17, a better approach is to try to find a small number of statistics that effectively summarise the data. For example, in Figure 19.9, each individual can be summarised by the time at which they change from level 1 to level 2. These are times *a*, *b*, and *c*. Similarly, in Figure 19.8 the area under the curve from 0 to 300 min will effectively summarise the change in plasma glucose over the period. Some possible summary statistics for repeated measures profiles are summarised in Figure 19.10, all of which can then be used in an analysis as if they were raw observations; one for each subject.

(a)   area under the curve (AUC)

(b)   maximum (or minimum) value achieved

(c)   time taken to reach the maximum (or minimum)

(d)   slope of the fitted regression line.

Once the subject summary is obtained, the mean and SD of all the subjects in a group can be determined and comparisons between groups then made by, for example, a *t*-test

---

Figure 19.10   Possible summary statistics for the profile of each subject in a repeated measures study.

Example – Liraglutide Versus Sitagliptin for Type 2 Diabetes

Figure 19.11 shows the mean fasting plasma glucose (FPG) levels of patients with type 2 diabetes randomised to Sitagliptin or one of two doses of Litaglutide. Patients were assessed immediately before randomisation and then at 4, 12, 20, and 26 weeks. In this example, there is clear evidence of an initial drop and thereafter a suggestion of slowly increasing fasting glucose levels. Rather than the calculation of the CIs at each point a possible analysis might be to calculate the slope of the individual (assumed linear) responses for each patient. From these single measures, the mean of the slopes can then be obtained for each treatment group and compared.

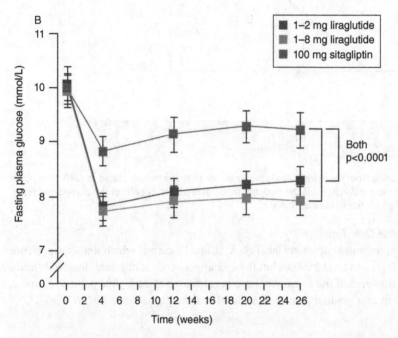

Figure 19.11 Fasting plasma glucose concentrations. (*Source:* after Pratley et al. 2010, figure 3).

In situations where the slopes of the above lines are assumed to be zero, then the summary measure for each individual is simply the mean of all the post-baseline observations for that subject.

Although not entirely correct, as the autocorrelation between successive assessments in the same subject is ignored, a linear regression could be fitted to all the post-baseline data from the individuals in (say) the 100 mg Sitagliptin group, and the corresponding straight line plotted on the graph starting at 4 and extending to 26 weeks. Clouds of individual subject values could then be added, although again these will not illustrate individual profiles, and may not be very successful in illustrating the within treatment group variability as the values from two Liraglutide groups are likely to be very overlapping.

Without formal analysis, the key points of Figure 19.11 are: (i) at four weeks FPG has fallen dramatically from a mean of 10 to a mean of 8.5 mmol l^{-1}, (ii) thereafter levels rise slowly to about 8.6 mmol l^{-1}, (iii) for the whole post-baseline period levels with Sitagliptin are about 1 mmol l^{-1} above those in patients receiving Liraglutide irrespective of dose.

19.9 Clinical and Statistical Significance

Once a study has been designed and conducted, the data collated and analysed, the conclusions have to be carefully summarised. There are two aspects to consider, depending on whether or not the result under consideration is statistically significant.

1) Given a large enough study, even small differences can become statistically significant. Thus, in a clinical trial of two hypotensive agents, with 500 subjects on each treatment, one treatment reduced blood pressure on average by 30 mmHg and the other by 32 mmHg. Suppose the pooled standard deviation was 15.5 mmHg, then the two-sample z-test, which can be used since the samples are very large, gives $z = 2.04$, $P = 0.041$. This is a statistically significant result that may be quoted in the abstract of the report as '*A* was significantly better than *B*, P-value $= 0.041$', without any mention that it was a mere 2 mmHg better. Such a small difference is unlikely to be of any practical importance to individual patients. Thus, the result is *statistically significant* but not *clinically important*.

2) On the other hand, given a small study, quite large differences can fail to be statistically significant. For example, in a clinical trial of a placebo versus a hypotensive agent, each group with only 10 patients, the change in blood pressure for the placebo was 17 mmHg and for the hypotensive drug it was 30 mmHg. If the pooled standard deviation was 15.5 mmHg, by the two-sample t-test: $t = 1.88$, df $= 18$ and $P = 0.06$. This fails to reach the conventional 5% significance level and may be declared *not statistically significant*. However, the potential benefit from a reduction in blood pressure of 13 mmHg is substantial and so the result should not be ignored. In this case, it would be misleading to state in the abstract: 'There was no significant difference between the drugs *A* and *B*'. It would be better to quote the extra gain achieved of 13 mmHg, together with a 95% CI of -2 to 28 mmHg. Further studies can be conducted and the results from this study included in a meta-analysis (Chapter 18).

19.10 Post Hoc Power Calculations

Sample size estimation and power calculation are essentially a priori, i.e. before the data is collected. After we have carried out the study it is the observed data that will determine the size and direction of the treatment effect and the width of any confidence interval estimates for this treatment effect. The a priori power is immaterial to this. Power is the probability of rejecting the null hypothesis in a (future) study. In other words, power is the probability of obtaining a statistically significant P-value if the null hypothesis is truly false (and the pre-specified alternative hypothesis is true). Once the study has been conducted, this probability is either 1 (if the null hypothesis was rejected) or else 0. Thus, post hoc power is fundamentally flawed. After the study, meaningful quantifications of uncertainty are CIs and P-values. It is the size of the treatment effect and the width of the confidence intervals and their interpretation that are important. The width of the confidence interval depends on the precision or standard error of the estimated treatment effect, which is itself dependent on the variability of the outcome and the study sample size. The only parameter we need to consider from the initial power calculation is the size of the anticipated or target effect we considered to be clinically meaningful, the minimum clinically important difference (MCID) and how our observed treatment effect and associated confidence intervals appear in relation to this MCID (Walters 2009b).

19.11 Predicting or Extrapolating Beyond the Observed Range of Data

Figure 19.12 shows a scatterplot of the relationship between obesity (defined as a body mass index of greater than or equal to 30 kg m^{-2}) in adults aged 16 and over from the Health Survey for England (2017, https://digital.nhs.uk/data-and-information/publications/statistical/health-survey-for-england/2017) over time from 1993 to 2017, separately for males and females. The raw data is shown in Table 19.10. Over the 25-year period there appears to be a positive linear relationship between calendar year and the increasing prevalence of obesity for both males and females. The corresponding observed Pearson correlation coefficients (see Chapter 9) were 0.94 for males and 0.95 for females respectively; suggesting a 'very strong relationship' using the interpretation guidelines in Table 9.2.

Figure 19.13 shows the same plot as the Figure 19.12 but this time with the individual linear regression lines for males and females imposed on the plot and the horizontal time axis extended to 2070.

The statistical models described by the extended regression lines would predict that by 2065 over 50% of the England's male and female population would be obese. If the relationship between obesity prevalence and time in future years continues to be linear, as observed between 1993 and 2017, this may well turn out to be the case. However, at this point in time, we have no idea of the relationship between obesity prevalence and time in future years. In may be that the relationship between the two variables is curved or non-linear. Consequently, in general, it is not advisable to use the graph or such models to make predictions outside the range of values in the observed data. If extrapolation is used to make predictions beyond the range of the observed data then the assumptions you are making about the future unobserved relationship between the variables should be made very clear. A fitted statistical model is only a guide to a relationship so, for example, one rarely believes that the pattern of the true relationship is exactly linear, in the way described by the model.

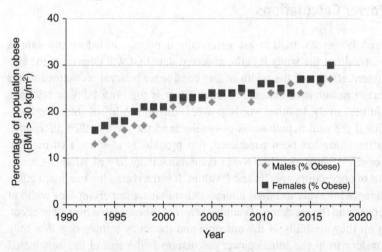

Figure 19.12 Scatterplot of obesity prevalence amongst male and female adults, aged 16 or more, in England (1993–2017).

Table 19.10 Prevalence of obesity in adults aged 16 and over, with a valid height and weight measurement, by survey year and sex from Health Survey for England 1993–2017.

Survey year	Males % obese	Females % obese	Survey sample size
1993	13	16	15 284
1994	14	17	14 679
1995	15	18	14 436
1996	16	18	15 061
1997	17	20	7939
1998	17	21	14 330
1999	19	21	6903
2000	21	21	6963
2001	21	23	13 681
2002	22	23	6478
2003	22	23	13 056
2004	23	23	5579
2005	22	24	6339
2006	24	24	12 027
2007	24	24	5929
2008	24	25	12 836
2009	22	24	3961
2010	26	26	6987
2011	24	26	7038
2012	24	25	6878
2013	26	24	7347
2014	24	27	6943
2015	27	27	6793
2016	26	27	6499
2017	27	30	6530

Obese = BMI 30 kg m^{-2} or more.
Source: Health Survey for England, NHS Digital.

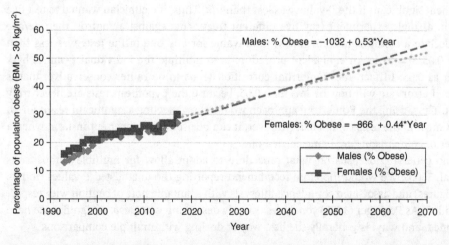

Males: % Obese = −1032 + 0.53*Year

Females: % Obese = −866 + 0.44*Year

Figure 19.13 Obesity prevalence amongst male and females adults in England 1993–2017.

19.12 Exploratory Data Analysis

'Fishing Expeditions'

There is an important distinction to be made between studies that test well-defined hypotheses and studies where the investigator does not specify the hypotheses in advance. It is human nature to wish to collect as much data as possible on subjects entered in a study and, having once collected the data, it is incumbent on the investigator to analyse it all to see if new and unsuspected relationships are revealed.

In these circumstances it is important, *a priori*, to separate out the main hypothesis (to be tested) and subsidiary hypotheses (to be explored). Within the 'to be explored' category of so-called 'fishing expeditions' or 'data-dredging exercises' the notion of statistical significance, as discussed in Chapter 7, plays no part at all. If used, it can only be as a guide to the relative importance of different results. As one statistician has remarked: 'If you torture the data long enough it will eventually confess!' Subsidiary hypotheses that are statistically significant should be presented in an exploratory manner as results needing further testing with other studies. For clinical trials, this is particularly the case for any subgroup analysis. Doctors are always interested to see whether a particular treatment works only for a particular category of patient. The difficulty is that the subgroup is not usually specified in advance. Results of subgroup analysis, where the subgroups are discovered during the data processing, should always be treated with caution until confirmed by other studies.

If the data set is large, a different approach to 'fishing' is to divide it into two, usually equal and randomly chosen, sets. One set is used for the exploratory analysis. This then generates the hypotheses that can be tested in the second set of data.

Multiple Comparisons

In some cases, it may be sensible to carry out a number of hypothesis tests on a single data set. Clearly if one carried out a large number of such tests, each with significance level set at 5%, then, even in the absence of any real effects, some of the tests would be significant by chance alone.

There are a number of solutions to controlling the consequentially inflated (above 5%) Type I error rate. A simple ad hoc method is to use a Bonferroni correction. The idea is that if one were conducting k significance tests, then to get an overall type I error rate of α, one would only declare any one of them significant if the P-value was less than α/k. Thus, if a clinician wanted to test five hypotheses in a single experiment (say five different treatments against a control) then he/she would not declare a result significant unless the P-value for any one of the tests was less than $\alpha_{Bonferroni} = 0.05/5 = 0.01$. An equivalent procedure is to multiple the individual P-values by k and retain α as 0.05. In fact, the Bonferroni correction tends to be rather conservative; that is the true Type I error rate will now be less than 0.05, because the hypothesis tests are never truly independent. Thus, using the Bonferroni approach would miss detecting a significant result for an uncertain number of the tests conducted. However, it can be useful to temper enthusiasm when a large number of comparisons are being carried out!

There is no general consensus on what procedure to adopt allow for multiple comparisons (Altman et al. 2000). We would therefore recommend reporting the unadjusted P-values (to two significant figures) and associated confidence intervals with a suitable note of caution with respect to interpretation. As Perneger (1998) concludes: 'simply describing what tests of significance have been performed, and why, is generally the best way of dealing with multiple comparisons'.

19.13   Misuse of *P*-values

Some of the above examples describe misuse of *P*-values, but the practice is so prevalent that it had led a number of journals to ban their use altogether. As is clear from our previous discussions we think this is a step too far, but it is worth summarising the issues here.

1) A non-significant *P*-value for a comparison of two groups does not mean the groups are similar; simply we have not enough evidence to claim they are different (absence of evidence is not evidence of absence).
2) *P*-values critically depend on the sample size, which is not part of the original hypothesis.
3) *P*-values test a specific hypothesis. Ideally, hypotheses should be few. Sometimes authors will use *P*-values as a signal detector, e.g. comparing baseline variables at the start of a study to suggest imbalances. Firstly, as we stated earlier if the study is truly randomised, then any differences in baseline will be due to chance. Secondly, the interpretation of a *P*-value as a probability is lost.
4) The use of an arbitrary cut off to determine 'significant' is a lazy convention. The actual *P*-value should be quoted, and all the evidence concerning whether there is a true difference taken into account.

19.14   Points When Reading the Literature

1) Are the distributional assumptions underlying parametric tests such as the *t*-test satisfied? Is there any way of finding out?
2) If a correlation coefficient is tested for significance is the null hypothesis of zero correlation a sensible one?
3) Is the study a repeated measures type? If so, beware! Read the paper by Matthews et al. (1990) for advice on handling these types of data.
4) Are the results clinically important as well as statistically significant? If the results are statistically *not* significant, is equivalence between groups being claimed? If the result is statistically significant, what is the size of the effect? Is there a confidence interval quoted?
5) Have a large number of tests been carried out that have not been reported? Were the hypotheses generated by an exploration of the data set, and then confirmed using the same data set?
6) Be aware of graphs that have truncated the scales and suppressed the origin or changed the baseline.
7) Do not use the graph or regression model to predict outside of the range of observations. Do not assume just because you have an equation that shows you can predict *y* from *x* that this implies that *x* causes *y*.

Appendix

Statistical Tables

Table T1   The Standard Normal distribution. The value tabulated is the probability, α, that a random variable, Normally distributed with mean zero and standard deviation one, will be greater than z_α or less than $-z_\alpha$.

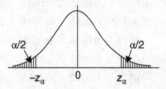

Z	0.00	0.01	0.02	0.03	0.04	0.05	0.06	0.07	0.08	0.09
0.00	1.0000	0.9920	0.9840	0.9761	0.9681	0.9601	0.9522	0.9442	0.9362	0.9283
0.10	0.9203	0.9124	0.9045	0.8966	0.8887	0.8808	0.8729	0.8650	0.8572	0.8493
0.20	0.8415	0.8337	0.8259	0.8181	0.8103	0.8026	0.7949	0.7872	0.7795	0.7718
0.30	0.7642	0.7566	0.7490	0.7414	0.7339	0.7263	0.7188	0.7114	0.7039	0.6965
0.40	0.6892	0.6818	0.6745	0.6672	0.6599	0.6527	0.6455	0.6384	0.6312	0.6241
0.50	0.6171	0.6101	0.6031	0.5961	0.5892	0.5823	0.5755	0.5687	0.5619	0.5552
0.60	0.5485	0.5419	0.5353	0.5287	0.5222	0.5157	0.5093	0.5029	0.4965	0.4902
0.70	0.4839	0.4777	0.4715	0.4654	0.4593	0.4533	0.4473	0.4413	0.4354	0.4295
0.80	0.4237	0.4179	0.4122	0.4065	0.4009	0.3953	0.3898	0.3843	0.3789	0.3735
0.90	0.3681	0.3628	0.3576	0.3524	0.3472	0.3421	0.3371	0.3320	0.3271	0.3222
1.00	0.3173	0.3125	0.3077	0.3030	0.2983	0.2937	0.2891	0.2846	0.2801	0.2757
1.10	0.2713	0.2670	0.2627	0.2585	0.2543	0.2501	0.2460	0.2420	0.2380	0.2340
1.20	0.2301	0.2263	0.2225	0.2187	0.2150	0.2113	0.2077	0.2041	0.2005	0.1971
1.30	0.1936	0.1902	0.1868	0.1835	0.1802	0.1770	0.1738	0.1707	0.1676	0.1645
1.40	0.1615	0.1585	0.1556	0.1527	0.1499	0.1471	0.1443	0.1416	0.1389	0.1362
1.50	0.1336	0.1310	0.1285	0.1260	0.1236	0.1211	0.1188	0.1164	0.1141	0.1118
1.60	0.1096	0.1074	0.1052	0.1031	0.1010	0.0989	0.0969	0.0949	0.0930	0.0910
1.70	0.0891	0.0873	0.0854	0.0836	0.0819	0.0801	0.0784	0.0767	0.0751	0.0735

(Continued)

Medical Statistics: A Textbook for the Health Sciences, Fifth Edition. Stephen J. Walters, Michael J. Campbell, and David Machin.
© 2021 John Wiley & Sons Ltd. Published 2021 by John Wiley & Sons Ltd.
Companion website: www.wiley.com/go/walters/medicalstatistics

Table T1   (Continued)

Z	0.00	0.01	0.02	0.03	0.04	0.05	0.06	0.07	0.08	0.09
1.80	0.0719	0.0703	0.0688	0.0672	0.0658	0.0643	0.0629	0.0615	0.0601	0.0588
1.90	0.0574	0.0561	0.0549	0.0536	0.0524	0.0512	0.0500	0.0488	0.0477	0.0466
2.00	0.0455	0.0444	0.0434	0.0424	0.0414	0.0404	0.0394	0.0385	0.0375	0.0366
2.10	0.0357	0.0349	0.0340	0.0332	0.0324	0.0316	0.0308	0.0300	0.0293	0.0285
2.20	0.0278	0.0271	0.0264	0.0257	0.0251	0.0244	0.0238	0.0232	0.0226	0.0220
2.30	0.0214	0.0209	0.0203	0.0198	0.0193	0.0188	0.0183	0.0178	0.0173	0.0168
2.40	0.0164	0.0160	0.0155	0.0151	0.0147	0.0143	0.0139	0.0135	0.0131	0.0128
2.50	0.0124	0.0121	0.0117	0.0114	0.0111	0.0108	0.0105	0.0102	0.0099	0.0096
2.60	0.0093	0.0091	0.0088	0.0085	0.0083	0.0080	0.0078	0.0076	0.0074	0.0071
2.70	0.0069	0.0067	0.0065	0.0063	0.0061	0.0060	0.0058	0.0056	0.0054	0.0053
2.80	0.0051	0.0050	0.0048	0.0047	0.0045	0.0044	0.0042	0.0041	0.0040	0.0039
2.90	0.0037	0.0036	0.0035	0.0034	0.0033	0.0032	0.0031	0.0030	0.0029	0.0028
3.00	0.0027	0.0026	0.0025	0.0024	0.0024	0.0023	0.0022	0.0021	0.0021	0.0020
3.10	0.0019	0.0019	0.0018	0.0017	0.0017	0.0016	0.0016	0.0015	0.0015	0.0014
3.20	0.0014	0.0013	0.0013	0.0012	0.0012	0.0012	0.0011	0.0011	0.0010	0.0010
3.30	0.0010	0.0009	0.0009	0.0009	0.0008	0.0008	0.0008	0.0008	0.0007	0.0007
3.40	0.0007	0.0006	0.0006	0.0006	0.0006	0.0006	0.0005	0.0005	0.0005	0.0005
3.50	0.0005	0.0004	0.0004	0.0004	0.0004	0.0004	0.0004	0.0004	0.0003	0.0003

Table T2   Student t-distribution. The value tabulated is t_α such that if X is distributed as Student's t-distribution with df degrees of freedom, then α is the probability that $X \le -t_\alpha$ or $X \ge t_\alpha$.

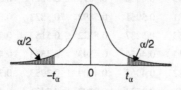

	α							
df	0.20	0.10	0.05	0.04	0.03	0.02	0.01	0.001
1	3.078	6.314	12.706	15.895	21.205	31.821	63.657	636.619
2	1.886	2.920	4.303	4.849	5.643	6.965	9.925	31.599
3	1.638	2.353	3.182	3.482	3.896	4.541	5.841	12.924
4	1.533	2.132	2.776	2.999	3.298	3.747	4.604	8.610
5	1.476	2.015	2.571	2.757	3.003	3.365	4.032	6.869
6	1.440	1.943	2.447	2.612	2.829	3.143	3.707	5.959
7	1.415	1.895	2.365	2.517	2.715	2.998	3.499	5.408
8	1.397	1.860	2.306	2.449	2.634	2.896	3.355	5.041

Table T2 (Continued)

df	α							
	0.20	**0.10**	**0.05**	**0.04**	**0.03**	**0.02**	**0.01**	**0.001**
9	1.383	1.833	2.262	2.398	2.574	2.821	3.250	4.781
10	1.372	1.812	2.228	2.359	2.527	2.764	3.169	4.587
11	1.363	1.796	2.201	2.328	2.491	2.718	3.106	4.437
12	1.356	1.782	2.179	2.303	2.461	2.681	3.055	4.318
13	1.350	1.771	2.160	2.282	2.436	2.650	3.012	4.221
14	1.345	1.761	2.145	2.264	2.415	2.624	2.977	4.140
15	1.341	1.753	2.131	2.249	2.397	2.602	2.947	4.073
16	1.337	1.746	2.120	2.235	2.382	2.583	2.921	4.015
17	1.333	1.740	2.110	2.224	2.368	2.567	2.898	3.965
18	1.330	1.734	2.101	2.214	2.356	2.552	2.878	3.922
19	1.328	1.729	2.093	2.205	2.346	2.539	2.861	3.883
20	1.325	1.725	2.086	2.197	2.336	2.528	2.845	3.850
21	1.323	1.721	2.080	2.189	2.328	2.518	2.831	3.819
22	1.321	1.717	2.074	2.183	2.320	2.508	2.819	3.792
23	1.319	1.714	2.069	2.177	2.313	2.500	2.807	3.768
24	1.318	1.711	2.064	2.172	2.307	2.492	2.797	3.745
25	1.316	1.708	2.060	2.167	2.301	2.485	2.787	3.725
26	1.315	1.706	2.056	2.162	2.296	2.479	2.779	3.707
27	1.314	1.703	2.052	2.158	2.291	2.473	2.771	3.690
28	1.313	1.701	2.048	2.154	2.286	2.467	2.763	3.674
29	1.311	1.699	2.045	2.150	2.282	2.462	2.756	3.659
30	1.310	1.697	2.042	2.147	2.278	2.457	2.750	3.646
31	1.309	1.696	2.040	2.144	2.275	2.453	2.744	3.633
32	1.309	1.694	2.037	2.141	2.271	2.449	2.738	3.622
33	1.308	1.692	2.035	2.138	2.268	2.445	2.733	3.611
34	1.307	1.691	2.032	2.136	2.265	2.441	2.728	3.601
35	1.306	1.690	2.030	2.133	2.262	2.438	2.724	3.591
36	1.306	1.688	2.028	2.131	2.260	2.434	2.719	3.582
37	1.305	1.687	2.026	2.129	2.257	2.431	2.715	3.574
38	1.304	1.686	2.024	2.127	2.255	2.429	2.712	3.566
39	1.304	1.685	2.023	2.125	2.252	2.426	2.708	3.558
40	1.303	1.684	2.021	2.123	2.250	2.423	2.704	3.551
41	1.303	1.683	2.020	2.121	2.248	2.421	2.701	3.544
42	1.302	1.682	2.018	2.120	2.246	2.418	2.698	3.538
43	1.302	1.681	2.017	2.118	2.244	2.416	2.695	3.532
44	1.301	1.680	2.015	2.116	2.243	2.414	2.692	3.526

(Continued)

Table T2 (Continued)

df	α 0.20	0.10	0.05	0.04	0.03	0.02	0.01	0.001
45	1.301	1.679	2.014	2.115	2.241	2.412	2.690	3.520
46	1.300	1.679	2.013	2.114	2.239	2.410	2.687	3.515
47	1.300	1.678	2.012	2.112	2.238	2.408	2.685	3.510
48	1.299	1.677	2.011	2.111	2.237	2.407	2.682	3.505
49	1.299	1.677	2.010	2.110	2.235	2.405	2.680	3.500
50	1.299	1.676	2.009	2.109	2.234	2.403	2.678	3.496
51	1.298	1.675	2.008	2.108	2.233	2.402	2.676	3.492
52	1.298	1.675	2.007	2.107	2.231	2.400	2.674	3.488
53	1.298	1.674	2.006	2.106	2.230	2.399	2.672	3.484
54	1.297	1.674	2.005	2.105	2.229	2.397	2.670	3.480
55	1.297	1.673	2.004	2.104	2.228	2.396	2.668	3.476
56	1.297	1.673	2.003	2.103	2.227	2.395	2.667	3.473
57	1.297	1.672	2.002	2.102	2.226	2.394	2.665	3.470
58	1.296	1.672	2.002	2.101	2.225	2.392	2.663	3.466
59	1.296	1.671	2.001	2.100	2.224	2.391	2.662	3.463
60	1.296	1.671	2.000	2.099	2.223	2.390	2.660	3.460
61	1.296	1.670	2.000	2.099	2.222	2.389	2.659	3.457
62	1.295	1.670	1.999	2.098	2.221	2.388	2.657	3.454
63	1.295	1.669	1.998	2.097	2.220	2.387	2.656	3.452
64	1.295	1.669	1.998	2.096	2.220	2.386	2.655	3.449
65	1.295	1.669	1.997	2.096	2.219	2.385	2.654	3.447
66	1.295	1.668	1.997	2.095	2.218	2.384	2.652	3.444
67	1.294	1.668	1.996	2.095	2.217	2.383	2.651	3.442
68	1.294	1.668	1.995	2.094	2.217	2.382	2.650	3.439
69	1.294	1.667	1.995	2.093	2.216	2.382	2.649	3.437
70	1.294	1.667	1.994	2.093	2.215	2.381	2.648	3.435
71	1.294	1.667	1.994	2.092	2.215	2.380	2.647	3.433
72	1.293	1.666	1.993	2.092	2.214	2.379	2.646	3.431
73	1.293	1.666	1.993	2.091	2.213	2.379	2.645	3.429
74	1.293	1.666	1.993	2.091	2.213	2.378	2.644	3.427
75	1.293	1.665	1.992	2.090	2.212	2.377	2.643	3.425
76	1.293	1.665	1.992	2.090	2.212	2.376	2.642	3.423
77	1.293	1.665	1.991	2.089	2.211	2.376	2.641	3.421
78	1.292	1.665	1.991	2.089	2.211	2.375	2.640	3.420
79	1.292	1.664	1.990	2.088	2.210	2.374	2.640	3.418
80	1.292	1.664	1.990	2.088	2.209	2.374	2.639	3.416
81	1.292	1.664	1.990	2.087	2.209	2.373	2.638	3.415
82	1.292	1.664	1.989	2.087	2.209	2.373	2.637	3.413

Table T2 (Continued)

df	α 0.20	0.10	0.05	0.04	0.03	0.02	0.01	0.001
83	1.292	1.663	1.989	2.087	2.208	2.372	2.636	3.412
84	1.292	1.663	1.989	2.086	2.208	2.372	2.636	3.410
85	1.292	1.663	1.988	2.086	2.207	2.371	2.635	3.409
86	1.291	1.663	1.988	2.085	2.207	2.370	2.634	3.407
87	1.291	1.663	1.988	2.085	2.206	2.370	2.634	3.406
88	1.291	1.662	1.987	2.085	2.206	2.369	2.633	3.405
89	1.291	1.662	1.987	2.084	2.205	2.369	2.632	3.403
90	1.291	1.662	1.987	2.084	2.205	2.368	2.632	3.402
91	1.291	1.662	1.986	2.084	2.205	2.368	2.631	3.401
92	1.291	1.662	1.986	2.083	2.204	2.368	2.630	3.399
93	1.291	1.661	1.986	2.083	2.204	2.367	2.630	3.398
94	1.291	1.661	1.986	2.083	2.204	2.367	2.629	3.397
95	1.291	1.661	1.985	2.082	2.203	2.366	2.629	3.396
96	1.290	1.661	1.985	2.082	2.203	2.366	2.628	3.395
97	1.290	1.661	1.985	2.082	2.202	2.365	2.627	3.394
98	1.290	1.661	1.984	2.081	2.202	2.365	2.627	3.393
99	1.290	1.660	1.984	2.081	2.202	2.365	2.626	3.392
100	1.290	1.660	1.984	2.081	2.201	2.364	2.626	3.390
110	1.289	1.659	1.982	2.078	2.199	2.361	2.621	3.381
120	1.289	1.658	1.980	2.076	2.196	2.358	2.617	3.373
130	1.288	1.657	1.978	2.075	2.194	2.355	2.614	3.367
140	1.288	1.656	1.977	2.073	2.192	2.353	2.611	3.361
150	1.287	1.655	1.976	2.072	2.191	2.351	2.609	3.357
160	1.287	1.654	1.975	2.071	2.190	2.350	2.607	3.352
170	1.287	1.654	1.974	2.070	2.188	2.348	2.605	3.349
180	1.286	1.653	1.973	2.069	2.187	2.347	2.603	3.345
190	1.286	1.653	1.973	2.068	2.187	2.346	2.602	3.342
200	1.286	1.653	1.972	2.067	2.186	2.345	2.601	3.340
210	1.286	1.652	1.971	2.067	2.185	2.344	2.599	3.337
220	1.285	1.652	1.971	2.066	2.184	2.343	2.598	3.335
230	1.285	1.652	1.970	2.065	2.184	2.343	2.597	3.333
240	1.285	1.651	1.970	2.065	2.183	2.342	2.596	3.332
250	1.285	1.651	1.969	2.065	2.183	2.341	2.596	3.330
300	1.284	1.650	1.968	2.063	2.180	2.339	2.592	3.323
400	1.284	1.649	1.966	2.060	2.178	2.336	2.588	3.315
500	1.283	1.648	1.965	2.059	2.176	2.334	2.586	3.310
∞	1.282	1.645	1.9602	2.054	2.1704	2.327	2.5763	3.2915

Table T3 The χ^2 distribution. The value tabulated is $\chi^2(\alpha)$, such that if X is distributed as χ^2 with df degrees of freedom, then α is the probability that $X \geq \chi^2$.

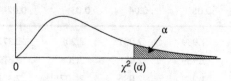

df					α				
	0.20	0.10	0.05	0.04	0.03	0.02	0.01	0.001
1	1.64	2.71	3.84	4.22	4.71	5.41	6.63	10.83
2	3.22	4.61	5.99	6.44	7.01	7.82	9.21	13.82
3	4.64	6.25	7.81	8.31	8.95	9.84	11.34	16.27
4	5.99	7.78	9.49	10.03	10.71	11.67	13.28	18.47
5	7.29	9.24	11.07	11.64	12.37	13.39	15.09	20.52
6	8.56	10.64	12.59	13.20	13.97	15.03	16.81	22.46
7	9.80	12.02	14.07	14.70	15.51	16.62	18.48	24.32
8	11.03	13.36	15.51	16.17	17.01	18.17	20.09	26.12
9	12.24	14.68	16.92	17.61	18.48	19.68	21.67	27.88
10	13.44	15.99	18.31	19.02	19.92	21.16	23.21	29.59
11	14.63	17.28	19.68	20.41	21.34	22.62	24.72	31.26
12	15.81	18.55	21.03	21.79	22.74	24.05	26.22	32.91
13	16.98	19.81	22.36	23.14	24.12	25.47	27.69	34.53
14	18.15	21.06	23.68	24.49	25.49	26.87	29.14	36.12
15	19.31	22.31	25.00	25.82	26.85	28.26	30.58	37.70
16	20.47	23.54	26.30	27.14	28.19	29.63	32.00	39.25
17	21.61	24.77	27.59	28.44	29.52	31.00	33.41	40.79
18	22.76	25.99	28.87	29.75	30.84	32.35	34.81	42.31
19	23.90	27.20	30.14	31.04	32.16	33.69	36.19	43.82
20	25.04	28.41	31.41	32.32	33.46	35.02	37.57	45.31
21	26.17	29.62	32.67	33.60	34.76	36.34	38.93	46.80
22	27.30	30.81	33.92	34.87	36.05	37.66	40.29	48.27
23	28.43	32.01	35.17	36.13	37.33	38.97	41.64	49.73
24	29.55	33.20	36.42	37.39	38.61	40.27	42.98	51.18
25	30.68	34.38	37.65	38.64	39.88	41.57	44.31	52.62
26	31.79	35.56	38.89	39.89	41.15	42.86	45.64	54.05
27	32.91	36.74	40.11	41.13	42.41	44.14	46.96	55.48
28	34.03	37.92	41.34	42.37	43.66	45.42	48.28	56.89
29	35.14	39.09	42.56	43.60	44.91	46.69	49.59	58.30
30	36.25	40.26	43.77	44.83	46.16	47.96	50.89	59.70
50	58.16	63.17	67.50	68.80	70.42	72.61	76.15	86.66
200	216.61	226.02	233.99	236.35	239.27	243.19	249.45	267.54
500	526.40	540.93	553.13	556.71	561.14	567.07	576.49	603.45

Table T4 *F*-distribution. The value tabulated is $F(\alpha, \nu_1, \nu_2)$ such that if X has distributed an *F*-distribution with ν_1 and ν_2 degrees of freedom, then α is the probability that $X \geq F(\alpha, \nu_1, \nu_2)$.

ν_2	α	ν_1 1	2	3	4	5	6	7	8	9	10	20	∞
1	0.10	39.86	49.50	53.59	55.83	57.24	58.20	58.91	59.44	59.86	60.19	61.74	63.33
1	0.05	161.45	199.50	215.71	224.58	230.16	233.99	236.77	238.88	240.54	241.88	248.01	254.31
1	0.01	4052.18	4999.50	5403.35	5624.58	5763.65	5858.99	5928.36	5981.07	6022.47	6055.85	6208.73	6365.68
2	0.10	8.53	9.00	9.16	9.24	9.29	9.33	9.35	9.37	9.38	9.39	9.44	9.49
2	0.05	18.51	19.00	19.16	19.25	19.30	19.33	19.35	19.37	19.38	19.40	19.45	19.50
2	0.01	98.50	99.00	99.17	99.25	99.30	99.33	99.36	99.37	99.39	99.40	99.45	99.50
3	0.10	5.54	5.46	5.39	5.34	5.31	5.28	5.27	5.25	5.24	5.23	5.18	5.13
3	0.05	10.13	9.55	9.28	9.12	9.01	8.94	8.89	8.85	8.81	8.79	8.66	8.53
3	0.01	34.12	30.82	29.46	28.71	28.24	27.91	27.67	27.49	27.35	27.23	26.69	26.13
4	0.10	4.54	4.32	4.19	4.11	4.05	4.01	3.98	3.95	3.94	3.92	3.84	3.76
4	0.05	7.71	6.94	6.59	6.39	6.26	6.16	6.09	6.04	6.00	5.96	5.80	5.63
4	0.01	21.20	18.00	16.69	15.98	15.52	15.21	14.98	14.80	14.66	14.55	14.02	13.46
5	0.10	4.06	3.78	3.62	3.52	3.45	3.40	3.37	3.34	3.32	3.30	3.21	3.10
5	0.05	6.61	5.79	5.41	5.19	5.05	4.95	4.88	4.82	4.77	4.74	4.56	4.36
5	0.01	16.26	13.27	12.06	11.39	10.97	10.67	10.46	10.29	10.16	10.05	9.55	9.02
6	0.10	3.78	3.46	3.29	3.18	3.11	3.05	3.01	2.98	2.96	2.94	2.84	2.72
6	0.05	5.99	5.14	4.76	4.53	4.39	4.28	4.21	4.15	4.10	4.06	3.87	3.67
6	0.01	13.75	10.92	9.78	9.15	8.75	8.47	8.26	8.10	7.98	7.87	7.40	6.88
7	0.10	3.59	3.26	3.07	2.96	2.88	2.83	2.78	2.75	2.72	2.70	2.59	2.47
7	0.05	5.59	4.74	4.35	4.12	3.97	3.87	3.79	3.73	3.68	3.64	3.44	3.23
7	0.01	12.25	9.55	8.45	7.85	7.46	7.19	6.99	6.84	6.72	6.62	6.16	5.65
8	0.10	3.46	3.11	2.92	2.81	2.73	2.67	2.62	2.59	2.56	2.54	2.42	2.29
8	0.05	5.32	4.46	4.07	3.84	3.69	3.58	3.50	3.44	3.39	3.35	3.15	2.93
8	0.01	11.26	8.65	7.59	7.01	6.63	6.37	6.18	6.03	5.91	5.81	5.36	4.86
9	0.10	3.36	3.01	2.81	2.69	2.61	2.55	2.51	2.47	2.44	2.42	2.30	2.16

(Continued)

Table T4 (Continued)

v_2	α	v_1											
		1	2	3	4	5	6	7	8	9	10	20	∞
9	0.05	5.12	4.26	3.86	3.63	3.48	3.37	3.29	3.23	3.18	3.14	2.94	2.71
9	0.01	10.56	8.02	6.99	6.42	6.06	5.80	5.61	5.47	5.35	5.26	4.81	4.31
10	0.10	3.29	2.92	2.73	2.61	2.52	2.46	2.41	2.38	2.35	2.32	2.20	2.06
10	0.05	4.96	4.10	3.71	3.48	3.33	3.22	3.14	3.07	3.02	2.98	2.77	2.54
10	0.01	10.04	7.56	6.55	5.99	5.64	5.39	5.20	5.06	4.94	4.85	4.41	3.91
20	0.10	2.97	2.59	2.38	2.25	2.16	2.09	2.04	2.00	1.96	1.94	1.79	1.61
20	0.05	4.35	3.49	3.10	2.87	2.71	2.60	2.51	2.45	2.39	2.35	2.12	1.84
20	0.01	8.10	5.85	4.94	4.43	4.10	3.87	3.70	3.56	3.46	3.37	2.94	2.42
30	0.10	2.88	2.49	2.28	2.14	2.05	1.98	1.93	1.88	1.85	1.82	1.67	1.46
30	0.05	4.17	3.32	2.92	2.69	2.53	2.42	2.33	2.27	2.21	2.16	1.93	1.62
30	0.01	7.56	5.39	4.51	4.02	3.70	3.47	3.30	3.17	3.07	2.98	2.55	2.01
40	0.10	2.84	2.44	2.23	2.09	2.00	1.93	1.87	1.83	1.79	1.76	1.61	1.38
40	0.05	4.08	3.23	2.84	2.61	2.45	2.34	2.25	2.18	2.12	2.08	1.84	1.51
40	0.01	7.31	5.18	4.31	3.83	3.51	3.29	3.12	2.99	2.89	2.80	2.37	1.80
50	0.10	2.81	2.41	2.20	2.06	1.97	1.90	1.84	1.80	1.76	1.73	1.57	1.33
50	0.05	4.03	3.18	2.79	2.56	2.40	2.29	2.20	2.13	2.07	2.03	1.78	1.44
50	0.01	7.17	5.06	4.20	3.72	3.41	3.19	3.02	2.89	2.78	2.70	2.27	1.68
100	0.10	2.76	2.36	2.14	2.00	1.91	1.83	1.78	1.73	1.69	1.66	1.49	1.21
100	0.05	3.94	3.09	2.70	2.46	2.31	2.19	2.10	2.03	1.97	1.93	1.68	1.28
100	0.01	6.90	4.82	3.98	3.51	3.21	2.99	2.82	2.69	2.59	2.50	2.07	1.43
∞	0.10	2.71	2.30	2.08	1.94	1.85	1.77	1.72	1.67	1.63	1.60	1.42	1.01
∞	0.05	3.84	3.00	2.60	2.37	2.21	2.10	2.01	1.94	1.88	1.83	1.57	1.01
∞	0.01	6.64	4.61	3.78	3.32	3.02	2.80	2.64	2.51	2.41	2.32	1.88	1.01

Table T5 Random numbers table.

94071	63090	23901	93268	53316	87773
67970	29162	60224	61042	98324	30425
91577	43019	67511	28527	61750	55267
84334	54827	51955	47256	21387	28456
03778	05031	90146	59031	96758	57420
58563	84810	22446	80149	99676	83102
29068	74625	90665	52747	09364	57491
90047	44763	44534	55425	67170	67937
54870	35009	84524	32309	88815	86792
23327	78957	50987	77876	63960	53986
03876	89100	66895	89468	96684	95491
14846	86619	04238	36182	05294	43791
94731	63786	88290	60990	98407	43473
96046	51589	84509	98162	39162	59469
95188	25011	29947	48896	83408	79684

Each digit 0 to 9 is independent of every other digit and is equally likely to occur.

Solutions to Multiple-Choice Exercises

Chapter 2

2.1 A. Figure 2.11 is a bar chart – it is displaying categorical data and there are some gaps between the bars.

2.2 B. The data are categorical with more than two categories which are not ordered so they are nominal categorical data.

2.3 E

2.4 C

2.5 D

2.6 E. The sum of the 10 corn sizes is 44 mm so the mean is 44/10 = 4.4 mm.

2.7 D. The number of patients in the sample is even (10); so the median is the average of the fifth and sixth ordered values of 4 and 4. So the median is $(4 + 4)/2 = 4$ mm.

2.8 B. The modal corn size is 2 mm and three patients have this corn size.

2.9 C. The smallest corn size is 2 mm and the largest is 10 mm so the range is 2 to 10 mm.

2.10 C. We have 10 observations, the bottom or lower half of the data has 5 observations; so the cut-point for the first or lower quartile is the observation that splits the five lowest ranked observations into two halves again. Thus, the lower quartile is the third ordered observation or 2 mm.

    Similarly, the upper quartile is calculated from the top half of the data (i.e. the observations with the largest values). The top or upper half of the data has five observations; so again the cut-point for the upper quartile is the observation that splits the five highest ranked observations, ordered observations 6 to 10, into two halves again. Thus, the upper quartile is the eighth ordered observation or 5 mm. So the interquartile range (IQR), for the corn size data, is from 2.0 to 5.0 mm.

2.11 E. The sum of the squared deviations from the mean is 58.4 mm^2. The number in the sample minus 1 or $(n - 1)$ is $10 - 1 = 9$. The variance is 58.4/9 = 6.49 or 6.5 mm^2 rounded to 1 decimal place.

2.12 B. The standard deviation is the square root of the variance $\sqrt{6.49} = 2.5$ mm.

Chapter 3

3.1 E. 147 out of 210 or 0.70 in the Band-aid group had a healed ulcer at 12 months.

3.2 C. 123/205 or 0.60 in the control group had a healed ulcer at 12 months.

3.3 E. The difference in healing rates is $0.70 - 0.60 = 0.10$.

Medical Statistics: A Textbook for the Health Sciences, Fifth Edition. Stephen J. Walters, Michael J. Campbell, and David Machin.
© 2021 John Wiley & Sons Ltd. Published 2021 by John Wiley & Sons Ltd.
Companion website: www.wiley.com/go/walters/medicalstatistics

3.4 E. NNT = 1/0.1 = 10.

3.5 C. Relative $\text{risk}_{\text{Band-aid/Control}} = 0.70/0.60 = 1.17$.

3.6 B. Relative $\text{risk}_{\text{Control/Band-aid}} = 0.60/0.70 = 0.86$.

3.7 E. Odds for healing at 12 months in Band-aid group = $0.7/(1 - 0.7) = 2.33$.

3.8 C. Odds for healing at 12 months in control group = $0.6/(1 - 0.6) = 1.50$.

3.9 D. Odds ratio for healing at 12 months in the Band-aid compared to control group = 2.33/1.50 = 1.56.

3.10 A. Odds ratio for healing at 12 months in the control group compared to Band-aid = 1.50/2.33 = 0.64.

Chapter 4

4.1 D is incorrect, when the outcome can never happen the probability is 0 (not 1).

4.2 D. The probability of three heads is $0.5 \times 0.5 \times 0.5 = 0.125$.

4.3 B. With a 10-sided die 5 faces have a label of 6 or more so the probability is 5/10 or 0.5.

4.4 E is incorrect. As the variance gets larger the curve gets flatter, since the area should be unity.

4.5 D is correct. Approximately 5% of the observation from a Normal distribution lies outside the mean ± 2 SD. The more precise value is 4.6%.

4.6 D is correct. Approximately 32% of the observation from a Normal distribution lies outside the mean ± 1 SD. The more precise value is 31.7%.

4.7 (i) A. The blood pressure of 120 mmHg is 20 mmHg below the mean (of 140 mmHg) or 2 SD below, i.e. $z = \dfrac{120 - 140}{10} = -2$. Since the blood pressure data is assumed to be Normally distributed then approximately 5% or 0.05 of the data is above or below ± 2SD from the mean. Since the areas in the tails of the Normal distribution are symmetric then approximately half the area or probability is above +2SD or 0.025, and half the area or probability is below -2 SD. So the probability of having a BP of 120 mmHg or less (2 SD below the mean) is approximately 0.025.

(ii) B. The BPs of 130 and 150 mmHg are 10 mmHg above and below the mean (of 140 mmHg) or 1 SD (since the SD is assumed to be 10 mmHg). Since the blood pressure data is assumed to be Normally distributed then approximately 32% or 0.32 of the data is above or below ± 1SD from the mean; conversely $1 - 0.32$ or 0.68 or the area or probability is within ± 1SD from the mean.

4.8 (i) C. Since the birthweight data is Normally distributed with a mean of 3.5 kg then half of the data or area will be above the mean and half below the mean. Therefore, the probability of giving birth to a baby weighting more than 3.5 kg (the mean) is 0.5.

(ii) C. The birthweight of 4 kg is 0.5 kg above the mean birthweight (of 3.5 kg) or 1 SD above, i.e. $z = \dfrac{4.0 - 3.5}{0.5} = 1$. Since the birthweight data is assumed to be Normally distributed then approximately 16% or 0.16 of the data is above 1 SD from the mean.

(iii) A. The birthweight of 4.5 kg is 1.0 kg above the mean birthweight (of 3.5 kg) or 2 SD above, i.e. $z = \dfrac{4.5 - 3.5}{0.5} = 2$. Since the birthweight data is assumed to be Normally distributed then approximately 2.5% or 0.025 of the data is above 2 SD from the mean.

Chapter 5

5.1 Options A, B, C, and D are correct statements about the standard error. Option E is incorrect. The standard error of the mean is $\dfrac{\text{sd}}{\sqrt{n}}$.

5.2 B. The standard error of the mean birthweight is $\text{SE} = \dfrac{\text{sd}}{\sqrt{n}} = \dfrac{500}{\sqrt{100}} = 50 \text{ g}$.

5.3 C. The standard error of the mean birthweight is $\text{SE} = \dfrac{\text{sd}}{\sqrt{n}} = \dfrac{500}{\sqrt{25}} = 100 \text{ g}$.

5.4 Options B and C are correct. Option B is correct because the calculation of a confidence interval is based around the observed sample mean. Option C is the definition of a 95% confidence interval. Option A is incorrect since the CI does not always include the true mean. D is incorrect because the population mean is not a random variable and has no probability attached to it. E is incorrect because it should be '95% of possible samples.'

5.5 D. The SE is 50 g so an approximate 95% confidence interval is mean $-$ 2SE to mean $+$ 2SE or $\{3500 + (2 \times 50)\}$ to $\{3500 - (2 \times 50)\}$ or 3400 g to 3600 g.

5.6 C. The SE is 100 g so an approximate 95% confidence interval is mean $-$ 2SE to mean $+$ 2SE or $\{3500 + (2 \times 100)\}$ to $\{3500 - (2 \times 100)\}$ or 3300 g to 3700 g.

5.7 E. A is incorrect because the result is not 'definitely'. The CI may contain the true value but we cannot say that it definitely will. B is incorrect because it should be $+/-$ 2 standard errors. C is incorrect because population parameters do not have probabilities attached to them.
D is incorrect D is incorrect because the CI probably does contain the true population mean. E is correct because the CI may or is likely to contain the true value but we cannot say that it definitely will.

5.8 E. This is the definition of a 95% confidence interval.

5.9 A. The standard error of the recruitment rate per month (r) is $\text{SE}(r) = \sqrt{\dfrac{r}{n}} = \sqrt{\dfrac{1.8}{13}} = 0.37$.

5.10 D. The 95% CI for the recruitment rate is $r - \{1.96 \times \text{SE}(r)\}$ to $r + \{1.96 \times \text{SE}(r)\}$
or $1.8 - \{1.96 \times 0.37\}$ to $1.8 + \{1.96 \times 0.37\} = 1.1$ to 2.5.

5.11 B. When there are no observed events, $r = 0$ and hence $p = 0/n = 0$ (0%), the recommended confidence interval simplifies to 0 to $\dfrac{z^2}{(n + z^2)}$ or 0 to $\dfrac{1.96^2}{(23 + 1.96^2)} = 0.143$ or 0 to 14.3%. Note that the '3 over n' rule gives $3/23 = 0.13$ or 13.

Chapter 6

6.1 B, C, D, E are all correct. A is incorrect because it does not mention the null hypothesis.

6.2 A, B, and C are correct. D is incorrect because A is true. E is incorrect because we increase the risk of a Type I error by going from a 1% to 5% level of statistical significance.

6.3 B is the only correct statement.

6.4 A, B, D, E are correct. C is incorrect because it does not mention the null hypothesis.

6.5 D is correct – the 95% confidence interval includes zero (no effect or no statistically significant difference) and includes -1 mm and is potentially a clinically important reduction in corn size favouring the corn plaster group. A,B,C are incorrect because the confidence interval includes 0. E is incorrect because the confidence interval includes an important result.

6.6 A is correct – the confidence interval excludes zero (so is compatible with a non-zero effect or statistically significant difference) and includes −1mm and is potentially a clinically important reduction in corn size favouring the corn plaster group. B is incorrect because CI includes an important result. C is incorrect because the CI includes results less than an important result. D and E are incorrect because the result is statistically significant

6.7 A is correct – the confidence interval excludes zero (so is compatible with a non-zero effect or statistically significant difference) and includes −0.5mm and is potentially a clinically important reduction in corn size favouring the corn plaster group. B is incorrect because CI includes an important result. C is incorrect because the CI includes results less than an important result. D and E are incorrect because the result is statistically significant

Chapter 7

7.1 B. The data are paired with the subjects measured before and after exercise so the paired t-test is appropriate. The other tests do not account for pairing.

7.2 C

7.3 A. The standard deviation (sd) of the differences is 10.894 and the sample size is $n = 8$. The $\text{SE} = \dfrac{\text{sd}}{\sqrt{n}} = \dfrac{10.894}{\sqrt{8}} = 3.852$ or 3.9 rounded to 1 decimal place. However, for subsequent calculations will use the SE to three decimal places.

7.4 D. Using the paired t-test and Table T2 with $8 - 1 = 7$ degrees of freedom, $t_{8,\,0.05} = 2.365$ giving the 95% CI for the mean paired difference as $16.300 - [2.365 \times 3.852]$ to $16.300 + [2.365 \times 3.852] = 7.191$ to 25.409 or rounding to one decimal place: 7.2 to 25.4.

7.5 B. The degrees of freedom are $n - 1 = 8 - 1 = 7$.

7.6 D. The paired t-test statistic is $t = \dfrac{\bar{d}}{\text{SE}(\bar{d})} = \dfrac{16.300}{3.852} = 4.232$ or 4.2 rounded to one decimal place.

7.7 A. From Table T2 the probability or areas in the tails of the t-distribution with 7 degrees of freedom and a t-value of 4.2 is a P-value between 0.01 and 0.001. Using a computer the more precise probability is $P = 0.0039$.

7.8 E is not an assumption of the two independent samples t-test. A, B, C, D are assumptions.

7.9 D The difference in means is $55.67 - 49.43 = 6.24$ or 6.2 rounded to one decimal place.

7.10 C The degrees of freedom are $n_1 + n_2 - 2$ or $18 + 21 - 2 = 37$.

7.11 C. The pooled SD is $\text{SD}_{\text{pooled}} = \sqrt{\dfrac{(n_1-1)s_1^2 + (n_2-1)s_2^2}{n_1 + n_2 - 2}} = \sqrt{\dfrac{(18-1)20.26^2 + (21-1)16.24^2}{18 + 21 - 2}} = 18.20$.

The $\text{SE}(\bar{x}_1 - \bar{x}_2) = \text{SD}_{\text{pooled}} \times \sqrt{\dfrac{1}{n_1} + \dfrac{1}{n_2}} = 18.20 \times \sqrt{\dfrac{1}{18} + \dfrac{1}{21}} = 5.82 = 5.8$ rounded to one decimal place.

7.12 C. The test statistic is $t = \dfrac{\bar{x}_1 - \bar{x}_2}{\text{SE}(\bar{x}_1 - \bar{x}_2)} = \dfrac{55.67 - 49.43}{5.82} = 1.07$ or 1.1 rounded to one decimal place.

7.13 E. From Table T2 the probability or areas in the tails of the t-distribution with 37 degrees of freedom and a t-value of 1.1 is a P-value >0.20. A more precise probability is $P = 0.29$.

7.14 A. Using the t-test and Table T2 with $18 + 21 - 2 = 37$ degrees of freedom, $t_{37,\,0.05} = 2.026$ giving the 95% CI for the mean paired difference as $6.24 - [2.026 \times 5.82]$ to $6.24 + [2.026 \times 5.82] = -5.55$ to 18.03 or rounding to one decimal place: −5.6 to 18.0.

Chapter 8

8.1 B. The proportion of corns healed at six months in the corn plaster group is $27/74 = 0.3649$ or 0.36 rounded to two decimal places.

8.2 A. The proportion of corns healed at six months in the scalpel group is $24/80 = 0.3000$ or 0.30 rounded to two decimal places.

8.3 D. The difference in response or proportions is $0.365 - 0.300 = 0.065$.

8.4 C. Using the method of Table 5.4, with $p_1 = 0.3649$, $n_1 = 74$ and $p_2 = 0.3000$, $n_2 = 80$; the SE (of the difference in proportions) is $\sqrt{\dfrac{p_1(1-p_1)}{n_1} + \dfrac{p_2(1-p_2)}{n_2}} = \sqrt{\dfrac{0.3649 \times 0.6351}{74} + \dfrac{0.3000 \times 0.7000}{80}} = 0.076$. So, the 95% CI is $0.065 - [1.96 \times 0.076]$ to $0.065 + [1.96 \times 0.076] = -0.084$ to 0.214 or after rounding to 2 decimal places -0.08 to 0.21.

8.5 D is not an assumption of the chi-squared test. The assumptions for the validity of the chi-squared test about the cell counts are based on the expected cell counts: not the observed cell counts.

8.6 B. The chi-squared test statistic is
$$\frac{(27 - 24.506)^2}{24.506} + \frac{(24 - 26.494)^2}{26.494} + \frac{(47 - 49.494)^2}{49.494} + \frac{(56 - 53.506)^2}{53.506} = 0.730.$$

8.7 A. The degrees of freedom for the chi-squared test with contingency table with r rows and c columns are $(r - 1) \times (c - 1)$. So for a 2×2 contingency table the degrees of freedom are $(2 - 1) \times (2 - 1) = 1$.

8.8 E. The P-value from a chi-squared value 0.730 of with one degree freedom is 0.393. So it is greater than 0.20.

8.9 A is incorrect. Any CI 'may' contain the true population value, but we cannot say for certain that the CI will actually contain the true population value.

Chapter 9

9.1 B is false. Regression (not correlation) can be used to predict one variable from another. The others are false

9.2 B. It is clearly a negative correlation and not perfect correction which would imply $r = -1$

9.3 D. It is clearly a positive correlation and neither 0 or 1

9.4 D It is a positive correlation but not strong enough for $r = 0.8$

9.5 C. e-rehab distance is 0.

9.6 D When x increases from 0 to 500, y increases from 200 to 800 so slope $=(800-200)/500 = 1.2$

9.7 D

9.8 B. The confidence intervals for the regression coefficients all include zero except for pre-rehabilitation distance walked.

9.9 D. The predicted post-rehabilitation distance walked is $589.5 + (-4.5 \times 60) + (-92.3 \times 0) + (1.1 \times 100) = 429.5$ m.

9.10 E. The R^2 value is 0.20 so $1 - R^2 = 1 - 0.20 = 0.80$ is the proportion of variability not explained by the covariates.

Chapter 10

10.1 B and C. Previous treatment is nominal since it is categorical. It is also a binary variable since it can only take two values.

10.2 E. The Wald z statistic for the group coefficient is $-0.798/0.231 = -3.455$.

10.3 E. From Table T1 the P-value for a Z-value of 3.46 is 0.0005.

10.4 D

10.5 OR = $\exp(-0.798) = 0.45$.

10.6 C. The 95% CI is $\exp[-0.788 - (1.96 \times 0.231)]$ to $\exp[-0.788 + (1.96 \times 0.231)] = 0.286$ to 0.708 or 0.29 to 0.71 rounded to two decimal places.

10.7 E A is incorrect because there is a possibility the CI does not include the true value. B is incorrect because it should be 2SEs away from the log odds. C is incorrect because it treats the population odds ratio as a random variable. D is incorrect because the CI includes 1 and so the result is not statistically significant and we do not know if it is clinically important.

10.8 E. The predicted probability is

$$\frac{\exp\left[(-0.003 \times 50) + (-0.798 \times 0) + (0.189 \times 0) + (0.425 \times 0) - 0.128\right]}{1 + \exp\left[[(-0.003 \times 50) + (-0.798 \times 0) + (0.189 \times 0) + (0.425 \times 0) - 0.128]\right]}$$

$= 0.431$ rounded to 0.43.

10.9 A. The predicted probability is

$$\frac{\exp\left[(-0.003 \times 50) + (-0.798 \times 1) + (0.189 \times 0) + (0.425 \times 0) - 0.128\right]}{1 + \exp\left[[(-0.003 \times 50) + (-0.798 \times 1) + (0.189 \times 0) + (0.425 \times 0) - 0.128]\right]}$$

$= 0.254$ rounded to 0.25.

10.10 B. The odds ratio is $\dfrac{0.15/(1-0.15)}{0.30/(1-0.30)} = 0.41$.

10.11 A. B is incorrect because the CI includes a clinically important result, C is incorrect because the CI includes clinically unimportant results and D and E are incorrect because the result is statistically significant.

Chapter 11

11.1 B

11.2 D

11.3 D. The number at risk at 300 days is $64 + 53 + 8 = 125$.

11.4 B. We are comparing $g = 3$ groups so the degrees of freedom for the logrank test is $= g - 1 = 2$.

11.5 B, D and E are true.

11.6 C

11.7 A. The Wald z statistic for the PIG (versus PEG) group coefficient is $0.343/0.329 = 1.043$.

11.8 B. From Table T1 the P-value for a Z-value of 1.04 is 0.2983 so $P > 0.20$.

11.9 E. Only the variables age and weight loss have confidence intervals for the hazard ratio which do not include one.

11.10 D. The hazard ratio = $\exp(0.343) = 1.41$.

11.11 B. The 95% CI for the HR is $\exp[0.343 - (1.96 \times 0.329)]$ to $\exp[0.343 + (1.96 \times 0.329)] = 0.739$ to 2.685 or 0.74 to 2.69 rounded to two decimal places.

Chapter 12

12.1 E. $P_{\text{Agree}} = \dfrac{x_{00} + x_{11}}{N_{\text{Repeat}}} = \dfrac{23 + 20}{50} = 0.86.$

12.2 D. $P_{\text{Chance}} = \dfrac{(x_{00} + x_{01})(x_{00} + x_{10})}{N_{\text{Repeat}}^2} + \dfrac{(x_{10} + x_{11})(x_{01} + x_{11})}{N_{\text{Repeat}}^2} = \dfrac{(23 + 6)(23 + 1)}{50^2}$

$$+ \dfrac{(1 + 20)(6 + 20)}{50^2} = 0.497$$

and $\kappa = \dfrac{P_{\text{Agree}} - P_{\text{Chance}}}{1 - P_{\text{Chance}}} = \dfrac{0.860 - 0.497}{1 - 0.497} = 0.72.$

12.3 D

12.4 E. $\alpha_{\text{Cronbach}} = \dfrac{k}{k-1}\left(1 - \dfrac{\sum s_i^2}{s_T^2}\right)$

$$= \dfrac{6}{6-1}\left(1 - \dfrac{(0.85^2 + 1.48^2 + 1.49^2 + 1.32^2 + 1.25^2 + 1.66^2)}{6.33^2}\right)$$

$$= 0.864 \text{ or } 0.86 \text{ rounded to two decimal places.}$$

12.5 A, C, and D are true.

12.6 C is true.

12.7 C. $s_{\text{Within}}^2 = \{(-3)^2 + (-1)^2 + (-8)^2 (-2)^2 + (-2)^2 + 0^2 + (-2)^2 + (-1)^2 + 0^2 + 4^2\}/(2 \times 10)$

$$= 103/20 = 5.15.$$

and $\text{Var}(\bar{x}_i) = 5.636.$ Hence, $s_{\text{Between}}^2 = 5.636 - 5.15/2 = 3.061$

$$\text{ICC} = \dfrac{s_{\text{Between}}^2}{s_{\text{Within}}^2 + s_{\text{Between}}^2} = \dfrac{3.061}{5.15 + 3.061} = 0.373 \text{ or } 0.37 \text{ rounded to two decimal places.}$$

Chapter 13

13.1 D. The prevalence is $50/250 = 0.20$ or 20%

13.2 A. The sensitivity is $40/50 = 0.80$ or 80%

13.3 E. The specificity is $195/200 = 0.975$ or 98%

13.4 B. The PPV is $40/45 = 0.889 = 89\%$

13.5 C. The NPV is $195/205 = 0.951 = 95\%$

13.6 C. The overall proportion correctly diagnosed is $(40 + 195)/250 = 0.94$ or 94%

13.7 E. The rest are correct.

13.8 E. The rest are correct.

13.9 E. The rest are correct.

13.10 A. E is only correct if the false positives and false negatives are weighted equally.

Chapter 14

14.1 C. The proportion of smokers who died is 9132/28627 = 0.319.

14.2 A. The risk of dying or the proportion of non-smokers who died is 940/5813 = 0.162.

14.3 D. The absolute risk difference is 0.319 − 0.162 = 0.157.

14.4 C. The relative risk for dying for smokers versus non-smokers is 0.319/0.162 = 1.969 or 1.97 rounded to 2 decimal places.

14.5 D. The natural logarithm of the RR, log(RR) = log(1.97) = 0.678 and the SE(logRR) =

$$\sqrt{\left(\frac{1}{a} - \frac{1}{a+c} + \frac{1}{b} - \frac{1}{b+d}\right)} = \sqrt{\left(\frac{1}{9132} - \frac{1}{9132+19495} + \frac{1}{940} - \frac{1}{940+4873}\right)} = 0.031.$$

The 95% CI for the RR is exp[0.678 − (1.96 × 0.031)] to exp[0.678 + (1.96 × 0.031)] or 1.854 to 2.093 or 1.85 to 2.09 rounded to two decimal places.

14.6 C. The odds ratio is OR = $\dfrac{ad}{bc} = \dfrac{688 \times 59}{650 \times 21}$ = 2.973 or 2.97 rounded to two decimal places.

14.7 C. The natural logarithm of the OR, log(OR) = log(2.973) = 1.090 and the

$$SE(logOR) = \sqrt{\left(\frac{1}{a} + \frac{1}{b} + \frac{1}{c} + \frac{1}{d}\right)} = \sqrt{\left(\frac{1}{688} + \frac{1}{650} + \frac{1}{21} + \frac{1}{59}\right)} = 0.260.$$

The 95% CI for the OR is exp[1.090 − (1.96 × 0.260)] to exp[1.090 + (1.96 × 0.260)] or 1.786 to 4.948 or 1.79 to 4.95 rounded to two decimal places.

14.8 E. The odds ratio for a matched case-control study is OR = $\dfrac{f}{g} = \dfrac{42}{19}$ = 2.211 or 2.21 rounded to two decimal places.

14.9 E. McNemar's test statistic $\chi^2_{McN} = \dfrac{(f-g)^2}{f+g} = \dfrac{(42-19)^2}{42+19}$ = 8.672 or 8.67 rounded to two decimal places.

14.10 B. The lower and upper 95% CI limits for the odds ratio are:

$$OR_{Lower} = 2.211^{(1-1.96/\sqrt{8.672})} = 1.30 \text{ to } OR_{Upper} = 2.211^{(1+1.96/\sqrt{8.672})} = 3.75.$$

Chapter 15

15.1 (A) F. The main comparison is between arms, and since these contain different subjects it is not a paired design.

(B) T. The trial is double blind by design, but it is possible that subjects may guess if they are on the intervention.

(C) T. The previous study had shown a bigger effect, so the power of the trial would be higher to detect this effect.

(D) T. The investigators wish to show that they can reduce cotinine in the intervention.

(E) F. The authors do not say how randomisation was to be carried out and so one cannot verify if the method is correct.

15.2 (A) T. Subjects are compared with each other.

(B) F. Selection bias is not ruled out by within subject comparisons.

(C) T. The trial by Berkowitz is highly susceptible to carryover bias, in that subjects given the home delivery in the first period might be persuaded to buy healthy food in the second period.

(D) T. A cross-over trial has to give enough time for the treatment to take effect, and so with two periods that is twice the total time of a parallel trial.

(E) T. One needs fewer subjects in a cross-over trial than a parallel group trial since much of the variability in the outcome measure is eliminated by comparing pairs.

15.3 (A) T. Subjects were not blind to treatment, since they knew they were using a pump or an MDI. The HbA1c% could be measured blind to treatment.

(B) F. The courses were randomised, not the subjects within courses.

(C) F. One of the difficulties of this sort of trial is the decision about withdrawing treatment if it is funded by a research grant, especially if the treatment is shown to be successful.

(D) F. The confidence interval included zero.

(E) T. $248/26 \approx 5$.

Chapter 16

16.1 D is not required – we are calculating a sample size for a continuous outcome so the proportion is not required.

16.2 D is incorrect – the sample size goes up (not down) with increasing power.

16.3 D is incorrect – the Type I error is the probability of rejecting the null hypothesis when it is true.

16.4 A is incorrect – the Type II error is the probability of not rejecting the null hypothesis when it is really false.

16.5 C is not required – we are calculating a sample size for a binary outcome so the standard deviation is not required.

16.6 C is incorrect – the standardised effect size Δ goes down with a larger SD.

16.7 E. The standardised effect size $\Delta_{Plan} = \delta_{Plan}/\sigma_{Plan}$ is $8/20 = 0.40$.

16.8 D. For 80% power using the simple formula $= 16\left(\dfrac{\sigma_{Plan}}{\delta_{Plan}}\right)^2 = \dfrac{16}{\Delta_{Plan}^2} = \dfrac{16}{0.40^2} = 100$ per group. So $2 \times 100 = 200$ in total.

16.9 E. For 90% power using the simple formula $= 21\left(\dfrac{\sigma_{Plan}}{\delta_{Plan}}\right)^2 = \dfrac{21}{\Delta_{Plan}^2} = \dfrac{21}{0.40^2} = 131.25$ per group or 132 rounded up. So $2 \times 132 = 264$ in total.

16.10 E. The standardised effect size $\Delta_{Plan} = \delta_{Plan}/\sigma_{Plan}$ is $10/20 = 0.50$.

16.11 C. Using Table 16.1 or the formula (16.5) in the technical details section the sample size per group is 291 per group or 2×291 or 582 in total.

16.12 D. Using formula (16.5) in the technical details section with 90% power

$$n_{Binary} = \frac{(1.96 + 1.2816)^2[0.30(1-0.30) + 0.20(1-0.20)]}{(0.30 - 0.20)^2} = \frac{10.51 \times 0.37}{0.01} = 388.8 \text{ per group}$$

the sample size per group is 389 per group or 2×389 or 778 in total.

Chapter 17

17.1 A, B, C are correct. D is monotone missingness. E is Intermittent missingness

17.2 A, D, E are correct. B Complete case analysis assume MCAR. C Multiple imputation assumes MAR

17.3 B is not a method of imputing missing data. The others are correct.

17.4 A is incorrect – the correct definition of the bootstrap is that it involves repeatedly drawing random samples from the original data *with replacement*. The others are correct.

17.5 E. The jackknife is not a method of estimating a bootstrap confidence interval. The others are correct

Chapter 18

18.1 A. The risk ratio for study 4 is $\dfrac{19/77}{18/59} = 0.81$.

18.2 C. The degrees of freedom are the number of studies, k, minus one, i.e. df $= k - 1 = 4 - 1 = 3$.

18.3 B and E are correct. A is incorrect because P>0.05. C is incorrect because there is no mention of the null hypothesis D is incorrect because A is incorrect

18.4 A, B, E are correct. C is incorrect because there is no mention of the null hypothesis. D is incorrect because P>0.05

18.5 E is correct. A is incorrect because the 95% CI does not definitely contain the true population RR, B is incorrect because the CI is based on the log RR and is +/− 2 standard errors. C is informally correct, but the strict definition is that the probability refers to 95% of CIs taken from samples of the population include the true value, D Is incorrect because the CI by definition includes the observed estimate.

References (Chapter numbers in square brackets)

Ahmed, H.U., El-Shater Bosaily, A., Brown, L.C. et al. (2017). Diagnostic accuracy of multi-parametric MRI and TRUS biopsy in prostate cancer (PROMIS): a paired validating confirmatory study. *Lancet* 389 (10071): 815–822. [13].

Allen, S.I., Foulds, J., Pachas, G.N. et al. (2017). A two-site, two-arm, 34-week, double-blind, parallel-group, randomized controlled trial of reduced nicotine cigarettes in smokers with mood and/or anxiety disorders: trial design and protocol. *BMC Public Health* 17 (1): 100. [15].

Al-Shahi, R., Pal, N., Lewis, S.C. et al. (2014). Observer agreement in the angiographic assessment of arteriovenous malformations of the brain. *Stroke* 33: 1501–1509. [12].

Altman, D.G. (1991). *Practical Statistics for Medical Research*. London: Chapman & Hall.

Altman, D.G., Machin, D., Gardner, M.J., and Bryant, T. (eds.) (2000). *Statistics with Confidence: Confidence Intervals and Statistical Guidelines*, 2e. London: BMJ Books [7, 19].

Amrhein, V., Greenland, S., and McShane, B. (2019). Scientists rise up against statistical significance. *Natu* 567: 305–307. [5].

Armitage, P., Berry, G., and Matthews, J.N.S. (2002). *Statistical Methods in Medical Research*, 4e. Oxford: Blackwell Science [7].

Ashby, R., Gabe, R., Ali, S. et al. (2014). VenUS IV (Venous leg Ulcer Study IV): compression hosiery versus compression bandaging in the treatment of venous leg ulcers: a randomised controlled trial, mixed treatment comparison and decision analytic model. *Health Technology Assessment* 18 (57): 1–293. [19].

ATAC Triallists (2002). Anastrozole alone or in combination with tamoxifen versus tamoxifen alone for adjuvant treatment of postmenopausal women with early breast cancer: first results of the ATAC randomised trial. *The Lancet* 359 (9324): 2131–2139. [15].

Avery, K.N.L., Williamson, P.R., Gamble, C. et al. (2017). Informing efficient randomised controlled trials: exploration of challenges in developing progression criteria for internal pilot studies. *BMJ Open* 7: e013537. [16].

Begley, C.G. and Ioannidis, J.P. (2015). Reproducibility in science: improving the standard for basic and preclinical research. *Circulation Research* 116: 116–126. [18].

Bell, M.L. and Fairclough, D.L. (2014). Practical and statistical issues in missing data for longitudinal patient reported outcomes. *Statistical Methods in Medical Research* 23 (5): 440–459. [17].

Bentur, L., Lapidot, M., Livnat, G. et al. (2009). Airway reactivity in children before and after stem cell transplantation. *Pediatric Pulmonology* 44: 845–850. https://doi.org/10.1002/ppul.20964. [8].

Berkowitz, S.A., Delahanty, L.M., Terranova, J. et al. (2019). Medically tailored meal delivery for diabetes patients with food insecurity: A randomized cross-over trial. *J Gen Intern Med* 34: 396–404. [15].

Bland, M. (2000). *An Introduction to Medical Statistics*, 3e. Oxford: Oxford University Press.

Medical Statistics: A Textbook for the Health Sciences, Fifth Edition. Stephen J. Walters, Michael J. Campbell, and David Machin.
© 2021 John Wiley & Sons Ltd. Published 2021 by John Wiley & Sons Ltd.
Companion website: www.wiley.com/go/walters/medicalstatistics

Bland, M. (2015). *An Introduction to Medical Statistics*, 4e. Oxford: Oxford University Press [6].

Bland, J.M. and Altman, D.G. (1986). Statistical methods for assessing agreement between two methods of clinical measurement. *Lancet* 1: 307–310. [12].

Bland, J.M. and Altman, D.G. (1997). Statistics notes: Cronbach's alpha. *BMJ* 314: 572. [12].

de Boer, M.R., Waterlander, W.E., Kuijper, L.D.J. et al. (2015). Testing for baseline differences in randomized controlled trials: an unhealthy research behavior that is hard to eradicate. *International Journal of Behavioral Nutrition and Physical Activity* 12: 4. [19].

Brown, S.R., Tiernan, J.P., Watson, A.J.M. et al. (2016). Haemorrhoidal artery ligation versus rubber band ligation for the management of symptomatic second-degree and third-degree haemorrhoids (HubBLe): a multicentre, open-label, randomised controlled trial. *The Lancet* 388 (10042): 356–364. [5,8].

Browne, R.H. (1995). On the use of a pilot sample for sample size determination. *Statistics in Medicine* 14 (17): 1933–1940. [16].

Calman, K.C. (1996). Cancer: science and society and the communication of risk. *BMJ* 13 (7060): 799–802. [3].

Campbell, M.J. (2006). *Statistics at Square Two*, 2e. Oxford: BMJ Books Blackwell [17].

Campbell, M.J. and Walters, S.J. (2014). *How to Design, Analyse and Report Cluster Randomised Trials in Medicine and Health Related Research*. Chichester: Wiley Blackwell [15].

Campbell, M.J., Hodges, N.G., Thomas, H.F. et al. (2005). A 24 year cohort study of mortality in slate workers in North Wales. *Journal of Occupational Medicine* 55: 448–453. [14].

Campbell, M.J., Hemming, K., and Taljaard, M. (2019). The stepped wedge cluster randomised trial: what it is and when it should be used. *The Medical Journal of Australia* 210 (6): 253–254. [15].

Cancer Research UK (2019) Phases of clinical trials Cancer Research UK Available from: https://www.cancerresearchuk.org/about-cancer/find-a-clinical-trial/what-clinical-trials-are/phases-of-clinical-trials (accessed 19/11/19) [15].

Cao, S., Yang, C., Gan, Y., and Lu, Z. (2015). The health effects of passive smoking: an overview of systematic reviews based on observational epidemiological evidence. *PLoS ONE* 10: e0139907. https://doi.org/10.1371/journal.pone.0139907 [1].

Carpenter, J. and Bithell, J. (2000). Bootstrap confidence intervals: when, which, what? A practical guide for medical statisticians. *Statistics in Medicine* 19: 1141–1164. [17].

Christie, D. (1979). Before and after comparisons: a cautionary tale. *BMJ* 279: 1629–1630. [14].

Cleophas, T.J. and Zwinderman, A.H. (2017). *Modern Meta-Analysis*. Switzerland: Springer [18].

Cohen, J. (1988). *Statistical Power Analysis*, 2. NJ Lawrence Erlbaum Associates: Hillsdale [16].

Cole, T.J., Altman, D.G., Ashby, D. et al. (2004). BMJ statistical errors. *BMJ* 58: 211–212. [19].

Collett D, (2015). Modelling Survival Data in Medical Research. (3). London Chapman and Hall/CRC [11].

Cook, J., Hislop, J., Adewuyi, T.E. et al. (2014). Assessing methods to specify the targeted difference for a randomised controlled trial – DELTA (Difference ELicitation in TriAls) review. *Health Technology Assessment* 18: 28. [16].

Cook, J.A., Julious, S.A., Sones, W. et al. (2018). DELTA 2 guidance on choosing the target difference and undertaking and reporting the sample size calculation for a randomised controlled trial. *Trials* 19 (1): 606. [16].

Cox, M., O'Connor, C., Biggs, K. et al. (2018). The feasibility of early pulmonary rehabilitation and activity after COPD exacerbations: external pilot randomised controlled trial, qualitative case study and exploratory economic evaluation. *Health Technology Assessment* 22 (11): 1–204. [15].

Davison, A.C. and Hinkley, D.V. (1997). *Bootstrap Methods and their Applications*. Cambridge: Cambridge University Press [17].

DerSimonian, R. and Laird, N. (1986). Meta-analysis in clinical trials. *Controlled Clin Trials* 7: 177–188. [14].

Diggle, P.J., Heagerty, P., Liang, K.-Y., and Zeger, S. (2002). *Analysis of Longitudinal Data*, 2e. Oxford: Oxford University Press [17].

Doll, R. and Hill, A.B. (1950). Smoking and carcinoma of the lung. Preliminary report. *BMJ* 2: 739–748. [14].

Doll, R. and Peto, R. (1976). Mortality in relation to smoking: 20 years' observations on male British doctors. *BMJ* 273 (ii): 1525–1536. [14].

Doll, R., Peto, R., Boreham, J., and Sutherland, I. (2004). Mortality in relation to smoking: 50 years' observations on male British doctors. *BMJ* 328 (7455): 1519. [1].

Drucker, D.J., Buse, J.N., Taylor, K. et al. (2008). Exenatide once weekly versus twice daily for the treatment of type 2 diabetes: a randomised, open-label, non-inferiority study. *Lancet* 372: 1240–1249. [19].

Dumville, J.C., Worthy, G., Soares, M.O. et al. (2009). VenUS II: a randomised controlled trial of larval therapy in the management of leg ulcers. *Health Technology Assessment* 13 (55): 1–182. [19].

Efron, B. and Tibshirani, R.J. (1993). *An Introduction to the Bootstrap*. New York: Chapman & Hall [17].

Egger, M., Davey-Smith, G., and Altman, D. (eds.) (2001). *Systematic Reviews in Health Care: Meta-Analysis in Context*, 2e. BMJ Books: London [18].

Eldridge, S.M., Chan, C.L., Campbell, M.J. et al. (2016). CONSORT 2010 statement: extension to randomised pilot and feasibility trials. *BMJ* 355: i5239. [15].

Elmore, J.G., Barnhill, R.L., Elder, D.E. et al. (2017). Pathologists' diagnosis of invasive melanoma and melanocytic proliferations: observer accuracy and reproducibility study. *BMJ* 357: j2813. [1].

Enstrom, J.E., Kabat, G.C., and Smith, D. (2003). Environmental tobacco smoke and tobacco related mortality in a prospective study of Californians, 1960-98. *BMJ* 326 (7398): 1057. [1].

Everitt, B.S. (2001). *Statistics for Psychologists*. Mahwah, New Jersey: Lawrence Erlbaum Associates [17].

Everitt, B.S. (2002). *A Handbook of Statistical Analyses Using S-Plus*, 2e. Boca Raton, Florida: Chapman & Hall/CRC [17].

Eypasch, E., Leferinga, R., Kuma, C.K., and Troidl, H. (1995). Education and debate. Probability of adverse events that have not yet occurred: a statistical reminder. *BMJ* 311: 619. [5].

Fagerland, M.W., Lydersen, S., and Laake, P. (2017). *The Statistical Analysis of Contingency Tables*. Boca Raton: CRC Press [8, 14].

Fairclough, D.L. (2010). *Design and Analysis of Quality of Life Studies in Clinical Trials*, 2e. New York: Chapman & Hall [17].

Farndon, L.J., Vernon, W., Walters, S.J. et al. (2013). The effectiveness of salicylic acid plasters compared with 'usual' scalpel debridement of corns: a randomised controlled trial. *Journal of Foot and Ankle Research* 6 (1): 40. [2,3,4 5,6,7,8,10, 16,19].

Fayers, P.M. and Machin, D. (2016). *Quality of Life: The Assessment, Analysis & Interpretation of Patient-Reported Outcomes*, 3e. Chichester: Wiley [12, 17].

Findlay, I.N., Taylor, R.S., Dargie, H.J. et al. (1987). Cardiovascular effects of training for a marathon run in unfit middle-aged men. *British Medical Journal* 295: 521–524. [19].

Foley, K.G., Morgan, C., Roberts, S.A., and Crosby, T. (2017). Impact of positron emission tomography and endoscopic ultrasound length of disease difference on treatment planning in patients with oesophageal cancer. *Clinical Oncology* 29: 760–766. [12].

Fotheringham, J., Barnes, T., Dunn, L. et al. (2017). Rationale and design for SHAREHD: a quality improvement collaborative to scale up shared haemodialysis care for patients on centre based haemodialysis. *BMC Nephrology* 18 (1): 335. [15].

Freeman, J.V., Walters, S.J., and Campbell, M.J. (2008). *How to Display Data*. Oxford: BMJ Books, Blackwell [19].

Frison, L. and Pocock, S.J. (1992). Repeated measures in clinical trials: analysis using mean summary statistics and its implications for design. *Statistics in Medicine* 11: 1685–1704. [17].

Furness, S., Connor, J., Robinson, E. et al. (2003). Car colour and risk of car crash injury: population based case control study. *BMJ* 327 (7429): 1455–1456. [3].

Gangadi, M., Margetaki, A., Gavana, M. et al. (2016). Prevalence of asthma and asthma-like symptoms in Greece: early results of the E.ME.NO study. *European Respiratory Journal* 48: PA4237. [14].

Gazzuola Rocca, L., Smith, C.Y., Grossardt, B.R. et al. (2017). Adverse childhood or adult experiences and risk of bilateral oophorectomy: a population-based case–control study. *BMJ Open* 7: e016045. [14].

GBD 2016 Alcohol Collaborators (2018). The burden of disease in Russia from 1980 to 2016: a systematic analysis for the global burden of disease study 2016. *The Lancet* 392 (10152): 1015–1035. [6].

Gorecki, C., Brown, J.M., Cano, S. et al. (2013). Development and validation of a new patient-reported outcome measure for patients with pressure ulcers: the PU-QOL instrument. *Health and Quality of Life Outcomes* 11: 95. [12].

Greenfield, D.M., Walters, S.J., Coleman, R.E. et al. (2007). Prevalence and consequences of androgen deficiency in young male cancer survivors in a controlled cross-sectional study. *Journal of Clinical Endocrinology & Metabolism* 92 (9): 3476–3482. [7].

Hancock, B.W., Wheatley, K., Harris, S. et al. (2004). Adjuvant interferon in high-risk melanoma: the AIM-HIGH study – United Kingdom coordinating committee on cancer research randomized study of adjuvant low-dose extended-duration interferon alfa-2a in high-risk resected malignant melanoma. *Journal of Clinical Oncology* 22: 53–61. [11].

Hansen, T.W., Thijs, L., Li, Y. et al. (2010). International database on ambulatory blood pressure in relation to cardiovascular outcomes investigators. Prognostic value of reading-to-reading blood pressure variability over 24 hours in 8938 subjects from 11 populations. *Hypertension* 55: 1049–1057. Epub 2010 Mar 8. [1].

Heeren, T. and D'Agostino, R. (1987). Robustness of the two independent samples t-test when applied to ordinal scaled data. *Statistics in Medicine* 6: 79–90. [7].

Hemming, K., Taljaard, M., McKenzie, J.E. et al. (2018). Reporting of stepped wedge cluster randomised trials: extension of the CONSORT 2010 statement with explanation and elaboration. *BMJ* 363: k1614. [15].

Hepworth, S.J., Schoemaker, M.J., Muir, K.R. et al. (2006). Mobile phone use and risk of glioma in adults: case-control study. *BMJ* 332 (7546): 883–887. [14].

Hernán, M.A. and Robins, J.M. (2017). *Causal Inference*. Chapman & Hall/CRC [14].

Hill CL (2015). Development of an Osteogenesis Imperfecta (OI) specific Quality of Life measure. PhD Thesis, University of Sheffield. [12].

Hill, C.L., Baird, W.O., and Walters, S.J. (2014). Quality of life in children and adolescents with Osteogenesis Imperfecta: a qualitative interview based study. *Health Qual Life Outcomes* 12: 54. [12].

Hind, D., Drabble, S., Arden, M. et al. (2019). Supporting medication adherence for adults with cystic fibrosis: a randomised feasibility study. *BMC Pulmonary Medicine* 19 (1): 77. [4,5].

Hislop, J. et al. (2014). Methods for specifying the target difference in a randomised controlled trial: the Difference ELicitation in TriAls (DELTA) syematic review. *PLoS Med* 11 (5): e1001645. [16].

Hollis, S. and Campbell, F. (1999). What is meant by intention to treat analysis? Survey of published randomised controlled trials. *BMJ* 319 (7211): 670–674. [15].

IARC (International Agency for Research on Cancer) (2012) Personal Habits and Indoor Combustions, Volume 100 E. A Review of Human Carcinogens.; IARC Monogr Eval Carcinog Risks Hum 100 1–53 [1].

IARC (International Agency for Research on Cancer) (2018). Drinking coffee, mate and very hot beverages. IARC Working Group. Lyon, France IARC Monogr Eval Carcinog Risks Hum 116. [1].

Iglesias, C., Nelson, A., Cullum, N., and Torgerson, D. (2004). VenUS1: a randomised controlled trial of two types of bandage for treating venous leg ulcers. *Health Technology Assessment* 8 (29): 1–105. [19].

Information Services Division (ISD) (2017) Cancer Mortality in Scotland (2016). Edinburgh: Information Services Division. Accessed 1 April 2020]. Available from: https://www.isdscotland.org/Health-Topics/Cancer/Publications/2017-10-31/2017-10-31-Cancer-Mortality-Report.pdf [14]

Jankowski, J.A., de Caestecker, J., Love, S.B. et al. (2018). Esomeprazole and aspirin in Barrett's oesophagus (AspECT): a randomised factorial trial. *The Lancet* 392 (10145): 400–408. [15].

Jha, S., Moran, P., Greenham, H., and Ford, C. (2007). Sexual function following surgery for urodynamic stress incontinence. *Int Urogynecol J Pelvic Floor Dysfunt* 18 (8): 845–850. [16].

Jha, S., Walters, S.J., Bortolami, O. et al. (2018). Impact of pelvic floor muscle training on sexual function of women with urinary incontinence and a comparison of electrical stimulation versus standard treatment (IPSU trial): a randomised controlled trial. *Physiotherapy* 104 (1): 91–97. [16].

Julious, S.A. (2005). Sample size of 12 per group rule of thumb for a pilot study. *Pharmaceutical Statistics: Journal of Applied Statistics in the Pharmaceutical Industry* 4 (4): 287–291. [15, 16].

Julious, S.A. and Mullee, M.A. (1994). Confounding and Simpson's paradox. *BMJ* 309 (6967): 1480–1481. [14].

Juniper, E.F., Guyatt, G.H., Feeny, D.H. et al. (1996). Measuring quality of life in children with asthma. *Quality of Life Research* 5: 35–46. [12].

Keen, C., Skilbeck, J., Ross, H. et al. (2018). Is it feasible to conduct a randomised controlled trial of pretransplant exercise (prehabilitation) for patients with multiple myeloma awaiting autologous haematopoietic stem cell transplantation? Protocol for the PREeMPT study. *BMJ Open* 8: e021333. [5,7,8].

Koletsi, D. and Pandis, N. (2016). The chi-square test for trend. *American Journal of Orthodontics and Dentofacial Orthopedics* 150 (6): 1066–1067. [8].

Koo, T.K. and Li, M.Y. (2016). A guideline of selecting and reporting intraclass correlation coefficients for reliability research. *Journal of Chiropractic Medicine* 15 (2): 155–163. [12].

Kourlaba, G., Relakis, J., Kontodimas, S. et al. (2016). A systematic review and meta-analysis of the epidemiology and burden of venous thromboembolism among pregnant women. *International Journal of Gynecology & Obstetrics* 132 (1): 4–10. [3].

Leeflang, M.M., Rutjes, A.W., Reitsma, J.B. et al. (2013). Variation of a test's sensitivity and specificity with disease prevalence. *CMAJ: Canadian Medical Association Journal* 185 (11): E537–E544. [13].

Li, H. and Johnson, T. (2014). Wilcoxon's signed-rank statistic: what null hypothesis and why it matters. *Pharmaceutical Statistics* 13 (5): 281–285. [7].

Lindson, N., Thompson, T.P., Ferrey, A. et al. (2019). Motivational interviewing for smoking cessation. *Cochrane Database of Systematic Reviews* 7: CD06936. [18].

Littlewood, C., Bateman, M., Brown, K. et al. (2016). A self-managed single exercise programme versus usual physiotherapy treatment for rotator cuff tendinopathy: a randomised controlled trial (the SELF study). *Clinical Rehabilitation* 30 (7): 686–696. [19].

Loomis, D., Guyton, K.Z., Grosse, Y. et al. (2016). Carcinogenicity of drinking coffee, matmaté, and very hot beverages. *The Lancet Oncology*, Published online 15 June 2016; doi:https://doi.org/10.1016/S1470-2045(16)30239-X [1].

Macfarlane, G.J., Biggs, A.M., Maconochie, N. et al. (2003). Incidence of cancer among UK Gulf war veterans: cohort study. *BMJ* 327 (7428): 1373. [14].

Machin, D. and Campbell, M.J. (2005). *Design of Studies for Medical Research*. Chichester: Wiley [14].

Machin, D. and Fayers, P.M. (2010). *Randomized Clinical Trials: Design, Practice and Reporting*. Chichester: Wiley [15].

Machin, D., Campbell, M.J., Tan, S.B., and Tan, S.H. (2018). *Sample Sizes for Clinical, Laboratory and Epidemiological Studies*. 4th edition. Chichester: Wiley Blackwell [16].

Matthews, J.N.S., Altman, D.G., Campbell, M.J., and Royston, P. (1990). Analysis of serial measurements in medical research. *British Medical Journal* 300: 230–235. [17].

Merza, Z., Edwards, N., Walters, S.J. et al. (2003). Patients with chronic pain and abnormal pituitary function require investigation. *Lancet* 361: 2203–2204. [4].

Moher, D., Liberati, A., Tetzlaff, J. et al. (2009). Preferred reporting items for systematic reviews and meta-analyses: the PRISMA statement. *PLoS Medicine* 6 (6): e1000097. [18].

Morrell, C.J., Walters, S.J., Dixon, S. et al. (1998). Cost-effectiveness of community leg ulcer clinics: randomised controlled trial. *BMJ* 316: 1487–1491. [11].

Morrell, C.J., Spiby, H., Stewart, P. et al. (2000). Costs and effectiveness of community postnatal support workers: randomised controlled trial. *BMJ* 321 (7261): 593–598. [17].

Morrell, C.J., Slade, P., Warner, R. et al. (2009). Clinical effectiveness of health visitor training in psychologically informed approaches for depression in postnatal women: pragmatic cluster randomised trial in primary care. *BMJ* 338: 1–12. [13].

Mountain, G., Windle, G., Hind, D. et al. (2017). A preventative lifestyle intervention for older adults (lifestyle matters): a randomised controlled trial. *Age and Ageing* 46: 627–634. [19].

Nicholl, J. (2007). Case-mix adjustment in non-randomised observational evaluations: the constant risk fallacy. *Journal of Epidemiology and Community Health* 61: 1010–1013. [14].

van Nood, E., Vrieze, A., Nieuwdorp, M. et al. (2013). Duodenal infusion of donor faces for recurrent Clostridium difficile. *New England Journal of Medicine* 368: 407–415. [8].

O'Cathain, A., Walters, S.J., Nicholl, J.P. et al. (2002). Use of evidence based leaflets to promote informed choice in maternity care: randomised controlled trial in everyday practice. *BMJ* 324: 643–646. [4, 5].

O'Sullivan, J.J., Derrick, G., Griggs, P. et al. (1999). Ambulatory blood pressure in schoolchildren. *Archives of Disease in Childhood* 80 (6): 529–532. [1].

Pearson, A.D., Pinkerton, C.R., Lewis, I.J. et al. (2008). High-dose rapid and standard induction chemotherapy for patients aged over 1 year with stage 4 neuroblastoma: a randomised trial. *The Lancet Oncology* 9 (3): 247–256. [11].

Pearson, T., Campbell, M.J., and Maheswaran, R. (2016). Acute effects of aircraft noise on cardiovascular admissions – an interrupted time-series analysis of a six-day closure of London Heathrow Airport caused by volcanic ash. *Spatial and Spatio-temporal Epidemiology* 18: 38–43. [14].

Pedersen, S.A., Gaist, D., Schmidt, S.A. et al. (2018). Hydrochlorothiazide use and risk of nonmelanoma skin cancer: a nationwide case-control study from Denmark. *Journal of the American Academy of Dermatology* 78 (4): 673–681. [10].

Perneger, T.V. (1998). What's wrong with Bonferroni adjustments? *British Medical Journal* 316: 1236–1238. [19].

Pettiti, D. (1994). Meta-analysis, decision analysis and cost-effectiveness analysis. In: *Methods for Quantitative Synthesis in Medicine*, 2e. New York, NY: Oxford University Press [18].

Piaggio, G., Elbourne, D.R., Pocock, S.J. et al. (2012). Reporting of noninferiority and equivalence randomized trials: extension of the CONSORT 2010 statement. *Journal of the American Medical Association* 308 (24): 2594–2604. [15].

Pratley, R.E., Nauck, M., Bailey, T. et al. (2010). Liraglifide versus sitagliptin for patients with type 2 diabetes who do not have adequate glycaemic control with metformin: a 26-week, randomised, parallel-group, open-label trial. *Lancet* 375: 1447–1456. [19].

Preston, N.J., Fayers, P., Walters, S.J. et al. (2013). Recommendations for managing missing data, attrition and response shift in palliative and end-of-life care research: part of the MORECare research method guidance on statistical issues. *Palliative Medicine* 27 (10): 899–907. [17].

ProGas Study Group (2015). Gastrostomy in patients with amyotrophic lateral sclerosis (ProGas): a prospective cohort study. *The Lancet Neurology* 14 (7): 702–709. [11].

Pye, C., Chatters, R., Cohen, J. et al. (2018). Induced endometrial trauma (endometrial scratch) in the mid-luteal menstrual cycle phase preceding first cycle IVF/ICSI versus usual IVF/ICSI therapy: study protocol for a randomised controlled trial. *BMJ Open* 8 (5): e020755. [15].

Reddington, M., Walters, S.J., Cohen, J. et al. (2017). Does early intervention improve outcomes in physiotherapy management of lumbar radicular syndrome? A mixed-methods study protocol. *BMJ Open* 7: e014422. [16].

Reddington, M., Walters, S.J., Cohen, J. et al. (2018). Does early intervention improve outcomes in the physiotherapy management of lumbar radicular syndrome? Results of the POLAR pilot randomised controlled trial. *BMJ Open* 8 (7): e021631. [15,16,17].

REPOSE Study Group (2017). Relative effectiveness of insulin pump treatment over multiple daily injections and structured education during flexible intensive insulin treatment for type 1 diabetes: cluster randomised trial (REPOSE). *BMJ* 356: j1285. [15].

Rigby, A.S., Armstrong, G.K., Campbell, M.J., and Summerton, N. (2004). A survey of statistics in three UK general practice journals. *BMC Medical Research Methodology* 13: 28. [1].

Roach, K.E., Budiman-Mak, E., Songsiridej, N., and Lertratanakul, Y. (1991). Development of a shoulder pain and disability index. *Arthritis Care and Research* (4): 143–149. [19].

Rothwell, J.C., Julious, S.A., and Cooper, C.L. (2018). A study of target effect sizes in randomised controlled trials published in the Health Technology Assessment Journal. *Trials* 19 (1): 544. [16].

Sargent, R.P., Shepard, R.M., and Glantz, S.A. (2004). Reduced incidence of admissions for myocardial infarction associated with public smoking ban: before and after study. *BMJ* 328 (7446): 977–980. [14].

Schulz, K.F., Altman, D.G., and Moher, D. (2010). CONSORT 2010 statement: updated guidelines for reporting parallel group randomized trials. *Annals of Internal Medicine* 152 (11): 726–732. [15].

Sharwood, L.N., Elkington, J., Meuleners, L. et al. (2013). Use of caffeinated substances and risk of crashes in long distance drivers of commercial vehicles: case-control study. *BMJ* 346: f1140. [10].

Sim, J. and Lewis, M. (2012). The size of a pilot study for a clinical trial should be calculated in relation to considerations of precision and efficiency. *Journal of Clinical Epidemiology* 65 (3): 301–308. [16].

Simpson AG (2004). *A comparison of the ability of cranial ultrasound, neonatal neurological assessment and observation of spontaneous general movements to predict outcome in preterm infants.* PhD Thesis, University of Sheffield. [4,5,8].

Sivaguru A., Gaines P.A., Walters S., Beard J., Venables G.S.(1998) Neuropsychological outcome after carotid angioplasty: randomised controlled trial. *The Challenge of Stroke. The Lancet Conference, Montreal, Canada,* Lancet 352(S4) 44. [9].

Stegeman, B.H., de Bastos, M., Rosendaal, F.R. et al. (2013). Different combined oral contraceptives and the risk of venous thrombosis: systematic review and network meta-analysis. *BMJ* 347: f5298. [3].

Sterne, J.A.C. and Egger, M. (2001). Funnel plots for detecting bias in meta-analysis: guidelines on choice of axis. *Journal of Clinical Epidemiology* 54: 1046–1055. [18].

Strasak, A.M., Zaman, Q., Marinell, G. et al. (2007). The use of statistics in medical research. *The American Statistician* 61: 47–55. https://doi.org/10.1198/000313007X170242 [1].

Streiner, D.L., Norman, G.R., and Cairney, J. (2015). *Health Measurement Scales: A Practical Guide to their Development and Use.* Oxford: Oxford University Press [14].

Sullivan, l.M. and D'Agostino, R.B. (2003). Robustness and power of analysis of covariance applied to ordinal scaled data as arising in randomized controlled trials. *Statistics in Medicine* 22: 1317–1334. [7].

Sutton, A.J., Abrams, K.R., Jones, D.R. et al. (2000). *Methods for Meta-Analysis in Medical Research*, vol. 348. Chichester: Wiley [18].

Tai, B.C. and Machin, D. (2014). *Regression Methods for Medical Research*. Chichester: Wiley Blackwell [11].

Teare, M., Dimairo, M., Shephard, N. et al. (2014). Sample size requirements to estimate key design parameters from external pilot randomised controlled trials: a simulation study. *Trials* 15 (1): 264–264. [15,16].

Thomas, K.J., MacPherson, H., Thorpe, L. et al. (2006). Randomised controlled trial of a short course of traditional acupuncture compared with usual care for persistent non-specific low back pain. *BMJ* 333 (7569): 623. [17].

Thomas, S.A., Coates, E., das Nair, R. et al. (2016). Behavioural Activation Therapy for Depression after Stroke (BEADS): a study protocol for a feasibility randomised controlled pilot trial of a psychological intervention for post-stroke depression. *Pilot and Feasibility Studies* 2 (1) [7].

Thomas, S.A., Drummond, A.E.R., Lincoln, N.B. et al. (2019). Behavioural activation therapy for post-stroke depression: the BEADS feasibility RCT. *Health Technology Assessment* 23 (47): 1–176. [16].

Viechtbauer, W. (2010). Conducting meta-analyses in R with the metafor package. *Journal of Statistical Software* 36 (3): 1–48. [18].

Walters SJ (2004). *The use of bootstrap methods for estimating sample size and analysing health-related quality of life outcomes (particularly the SF-36)*. PhD thesis, University of Sheffield [10]

Walters, S.J. (2009a). *Quality of Life Outcomes in Clinical Trials and Health Care Evaluation: A Practical Guide to Analysis and Interpretation*. Chichester: Wiley [17].

Walters, S.J. (2009b). Consultants' forum: should post hoc sample size calculations be done? *Pharmaceutical Statistics* 8 (2): 163–169. [19].

Walters, S.J. (2012). Analyzing time to event outcomes with a Cox regression model. *WIREs Computational Statistics* 4: 310–315. https://doi.org/10.1002/wics.1197 [11].

Walters, S.J. (2014). *What is a Cox Model?* 3e. Harvard Medical Communications [11].

Walters, S.J., dos Anjos Henriques-Cadby, I.B., Bortolami, O. et al. (2017). Recruitment and retention of participants in randomised controlled trials: a review of trials funded and published by the United Kingdom Health Technology Assessment Programme. *BMJ Open* 7 (3): e015276. [16].

Wasserstein, R.L. and Lazar, N.A. (2016). The ASA's statement on p-values: context, process, and purpose. *The American Statistician* https://doi.org/10.1080/00031305.2016.1154108 [6].

Waterhouse, J.C., Walters, S.J., Oluboyede, Y., and Lawson, R.A. (2010). A randomised 2 × 2 trial of community versus hospital pulmonary rehabilitation for chronic obstructive pulmonary disease followed by telephone or conventional follow-up. *Health Technology Assessment* 14 (6): 1–164. [6].

Waterlander, W.E., Steenhuis, I.H.M., de Boer, M.R. et al. (2012a). The effects of a 25% discount on fruits and vegetables: results of a randomized trial in a three-dimensional web-based supermarket. *International Journal of Behavioral Nutrition and Physical Activity* 9: 11. [19].

Waterlander, W.E., Steenhuis, I.H.M., de Boer, M.R. et al. (2012b). Introducing taxes, subsidies or both: the effects of various food pricing strategies in a web-based supermarket randomized trial. *Preventive Medicine* 54: 323–330. [19].

Waterlander, W.E., de Boer, M.R., Schuit, A.J. et al. (2013a). Price discounts significantly enhance fruit and vegetable purchases when combined with nutrition education: a randomized controlled supermarket trial. *The Journal of Clinical Nutrition* 97 (4): 886–895. [19].

Waterlander, W.E., Steenhuis, I.H.M., de Boer, M.R. et al. (2013b). Effects of different discount levels on healthy products coupled with a healthy choice label, special offer label or both: results from a web-based supermarket experiment. *International Journal of Behavioral Nutrition and Physical Activity* 10: 59. [19].

Watson, J., Kang'ombe, A., Soares, M. et al. (2011). VenUS III: a randomised controlled trial of therapeutic ultrasound in the management of venous leg ulcers. *Health Technology Assessment* 15 (13) [19].

Whitehead, A. (2002). *Meta-Analysis of Controlled Clinical Trials*, vol. 7. Wiley [18].

Whitehead, A., Sully, B., and Campbell, M.J. (2014). Pilot and feasibility studies: is there a difference from each other and from a randomised controlled trial? *Contemporary Clinical Trials* 38 (1): 130–133. [15].

Whitehead, A.L., Julious, S.A., Cooper, C.L., and Campbell, M.J. (2016). Estimating the sample size for a pilot randomised trial to minimise the overall trial sample size for the external pilot and main trial for a continuous outcome variable. *Statistical Methods in Medical Research* 25 (3): 1057–1073. [16].

Whittaker, R., McRobbie, H., Bullen, C. et al. (2016). Mobile phone-based interventions for smoking cessation. *Cochrane Database of Systematic Reviews* 4 [18].

Writing Group for the Women's Health Initiative Investigators (2002). Risks and benefits of estrogen plus progestin in healthy postmenopausal women: principal results from the Women's Health Initiative randomized controlled trial. *Journal of the American Medical Association* 288: 321–333. [1].

Index

Medical Statistics: A Textbook for the Health Sciences, Fifth Edition. Stephen J. Walters, Michael J. Campbell, and David Machin.
© 2021 John Wiley & Sons Ltd. Published 2021 by John Wiley & Sons Ltd.
Companion website: www.wiley.com/go/walters/medicalstatistics